THE PRESERVATION OF MEMORY

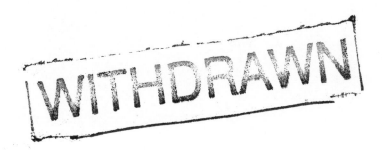

An increase in average life expectancy has given rise to a number of pressing health challenges for the 21st century. Age-related memory loss, whether due to a neuro-degenerative condition such as Alzheimer's disease, or as a product of the normal process of ageing, is perhaps the most significant of the health problems of old age presently confronting our society. *The Preservation of Memory* explores non-invasive, empirically sound strategies that can be implemented to ensure long-lasting and effective retention of information.

The chapters in this volume describe and evaluate both well-established and novel methods for improving and strengthening memory for people with and with-out dementia. They also look at ways in which effective detection and care can be implemented and describe empirical findings that can be translated into every-day practice. The contributors take a multidisciplinary approach, motivated by the desire to look beyond and across boundaries to find new areas of knowledge and opportunities for future research.

The Preservation of Memory will be useful reading for students and researchers focusing upon memory, ageing and dementia, and also for mental health practitio-ners, social workers and carers of persons living with dementia or other memory impairments.

Davide Bruno is Senior Lecturer in Psychology at Liverpool Hope University, UK.

THE PRESERVATION
OF MEMORY

Edited by Davide Bruno

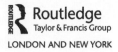

Routledge
Taylor & Francis Group

LONDON AND NEW YORK

First published 2016
by Routledge
2 Park Square, Milton Park, Abingdon, Oxon OX14 4RN

and by Routledge
711 Third Avenue, New York, NY 10017

Routledge is an imprint of the Taylor & Francis Group, an informa business

British Library Cataloguing in Publication Data
A catalogue record for this book is available from the British Library

Library of Congress Cataloging-in-Publication Data
The preservation of memory / edited by Davide Bruno. — 1 Edition.
     pages cm
  Includes bibliographical references and index.
  1. Memory.   I. Bruno, Davide, editor.
  BF390.P74 2016
  153.1'2—dc23
  2015024407

ISBN: 978-1-138-84018-8 (hbk)
ISBN: 978-1-138-84019-5 (pbk)
ISBN: 978-1-315-73292-3 (ebk)

Typeset in Bembo
by Apex CoVantage, LLC
Printed in Great Britain by Ashford Colour Press Ltd

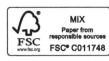

To Ingrid

CONTENTS

CONTRIBUTORS

Harriet A. Allen, University of Nottingham, UK
Mark Barrett-Baxendale, Liverpool Hope University, UK
Holly Blake, University of Nottingham, UK
Charlotte Bonardi, University of Nottingham, UK
Noeleen M. Brady, University College Cork, Ireland
Davide Bruno, Liverpool Hope University, UK
Tina Chen, University of Massachusetts Amherst, USA
Daniel P. A. Clark, Liverpool Hope University, UK
Stephanie Leal, University of California Irvine and Johns Hopkins
    University, USA
Iracema Leroi, Manchester Academic Health Sciences Centre,
    University of Manchester, UK
Niamh Malone, Liverpool Hope University, UK
Gerasimos Markopoulos, Bath Spa University, UK
Jan R. Oyebode, University of Bradford, UK
Nunzio Pomara, Nathan S. Kline Institute for Psychiatric Research and
    New York University-Langone School of Medicine, USA
Donna Redgrave, RMD Memory Matters Theatre Company, UK
Chelsea Reichert, Nathan S. Kline Institute for Psychiatric Research, USA
David Reid, Liverpool Hope University, UK
Damien Renner, Liverpool Hope University, UK
Richard A. P. Roche, Maynooth University, Ireland
Caren M. Rotello, University of Massachusetts Amherst, USA
Andrew Rutherford, Keele University, UK
Peter Sawyer, Lancaster University, UK
John J. Sidtis, Nathan S. Kline Institute for Psychiatric Research and
    New York University-Langone School of Medicine, USA

Grahame Smith, Liverpool John Moores University, UK
Sarah Jane Smith, University of Bradford, UK
Carla M. Strickland-Hughes, University of Florida, USA
Gemma Stringer, Manchester Academic Health Sciences Centre,
    University of Manchester, UK
Alistair Sutcliffe, Lancaster University, UK
Hissam Tawfik, Liverpool Hope University, UK
Richard J. Tunney, University of Nottingham, UK
Paul Verhaeghen, Georgia Institute of Technology, USA
Robin L. West, University of Florida, USA
Michael Yassa, University of California Irvine, USA

PREFACE

Dementia has entered our collective awareness in recent years, with books and movies dedicated to describing its effects, and daily news items chronicling the search for a cure, inevitably leading to new questions. Among these, for example, are how to differentiate between the pathology of dementia and the non-pathological progression of normal ageing; how to reduce the risk of becoming affected by dementia in later life; and how to treat and live with the disease once it has developed. This book deals with these questions and aims to provide a snapshot of the field of study of the ageing memory, and its preservation.

This edited book is a collaborative effort and sees the contribution of academics working on both sides of the Atlantic. The chapters embrace a range of disciplines that touch upon issues to do with ageing and dementia, including cognitive psychology, neuroscience, e-health, psychiatry and the social sciences. The multidisciplinary approach is motivated by a desire to look beyond and across boundaries in an attempt to find new areas of knowledge, new approaches and new opportunities.

The book is structured in four parts. Part I, *Introduction to remembering: the basics of memory,* is dedicated to covering the main concepts and theories behind memory, ageing and pathological ageing. We begin with an overview of the main effects of age and dementia on short- and long-term memory, and a bit of history (Chapter 1); and then move on to explore the age-related changes that happen in the hippocampus, a brain region that is severely affected in Alzheimer's disease, in humans and non-humans (Chapter 2). In Chapter 3, the effects of age on recognition memory are examined with the help of state-trace analysis; and, finally, Chapter 4 focuses on age-related changes in how we remember the origin of what we remember.

Part II, titled *Assessment and prediction,* is dedicated to the attempts to determine who is more at risk of developing dementia, among normal elderly. First, a computerized system designed to detect subtle hints of cognitive decline via everyday computer use is described (Chapter 5); to follow, Chapter 6 looks at a community-based project dedicated to memory screening, and its results.

Part III, *From the laboratory to the home: practical applications for ageing populations,* includes chapters reflecting on possible uses of existing knowledge in cognitive psychology and neuroscience for the purposes of helping older individuals achieve better memory results. Chapter 7 explores the impact of context on age-related memory changes; Chapter 8 provides an account of the survival processing strategy to learning, which could find applications to aid memory in ageing populations and in people with memory impairment; finally, the last two chapters in Part III are dedicated to how physical (Chapter 9) and mental (Chapter 10) exercise can positively impact memory ability and preservation.

In Part IV, *Facing the memory challenge in dementia,* the focus shifts more specifically to dementia, and the final four chapters present different, non-pharmacological approaches to countering its effects. Chapter 11 shows how theatre can be integrated within care to improve support of people with dementia; Chapter 12 describes a living lab approach to the development of assistive technologies for dementia, where all parties are equally involved in the decision process; Chapter 13 is dedicated to discussing person-centred interventions to enhance the well-being of people with dementia; and, finally, the last chapter of the book describes a concrete example of how assistive technologies can be created to help people with dementia perform simple, everyday tasks while protecting their independence and individuality.

PART I

Introduction to remembering

The basics of memory

1

THE EFFECTS OF NORMAL AND PATHOLOGICAL AGEING ON MEMORY

Andrew Rutherford and Davide Bruno

1.1 Introduction

Memory has been suggested as the central aspect of human thought, so answers to key questions about human nature will depend on an understanding of memory (Radvansky, 2005). Memory occupies this role not only because it contains all we know, but also because it provides us with all the ways we have learned to think and act, ranging from how to address scientific, mechanical or social problems to how to walk in a straight line. Memory is not only the basis or a crucial influence on everything we do, it is also the source of our sense of self. Given these roles, it is unsurprising memory impairment and loss can be devastating, both practically and emotionally, not only for the person suffering the memory problem(s), but for all involved (e.g., Corkin, 2013; Wearing, 2005).

This chapter considers how the normal ageing process affects human memory, and how memory is affected by the neurodegenerative pathologies thought to cause dementia. However, to facilitate understanding, some pertinent aspects of the psychology of memory, such as the ways in which memory is examined and explained, and the contemporary theoretical account of normal memory are reviewed briefly, prior to describing how normal ageing and abnormal neurodegeneration influences memory.

1.2 Memory research perspectives and approaches

Although memory has been a matter of interest, if not fascination, throughout most of recorded history (e.g., Turkington & Harris, 2001), the *scientific* investigation of memory began with the demonstration by German psychologist Herman Ebbinghaus (1885) that scientific methods could be applied as successfully to study mental phenomena, such as memory, as they were applied to study physical phenomena.

Memory continues to be a major area of research in psychology generally and for cognitive psychology in particular, but contemporary memory research also receives input from neuroscience.

Cognitive psychology aims to give account of the information processing operations underlying cognition – including memory. In terms of Marr's (1982; Poggio, 2012) three information processing abstractions, cognitive psychology is concerned with computational theory, and representational and algorithmic forms of process account. In contrast, the focus of neuroscience is the (neural) hardware and its implementation of these processes. These two perspectives overlap at the interface between the representational and algorithmic, and the neural implementation abstractions of psychological processes, with interdisciplinary research conducted at the intersection of these two perspectives labelled as cognitive neuroscience. Nevertheless, in terms of the history of memory research, it is only recently cognitive psychology and neuroscience theories have had anything to say to each other. Previously, neither cognitive psychology theory nor neuroscience theory exerted any significant constraints on the other, and for some time, this provided cognitive psychology-free neuroscience, and neuroscience-free cognitive psychology.

Psychologists examine memory by presenting material and then observing what can be remembered. Logic dictates at least three stages or operations must underlie memory to enable such remembering: the encoding of material into memory, the storage of the encoded material over a period of time, and then the successful retrieval of the required material from the memory store. Depending on the study purpose, psychologists apply different manipulations at one or more of these stages, but it is useful to bear in mind that irrespective of the stage of interest, all memory stages will have been involved when material is remembered. Encoding can be manipulated in numerous ways, such as by varying the nature of the stimuli, the stimulus presentation times, the number of stimulus presentations and the task instructions. Storage manipulation usually is in terms of how long an item is held in store before it is retrieved, while retrieval can be manipulated by varying factors such as the type and number of the cues available to be used at retrieval, and the time available to use these cues. Therefore, retrieval is manipulated by varying the nature of the task used to test memory, the majority of which provide accuracy or latency or both measures of the remembering observed. As accuracy and latency measures usually rely on overt behaviours such as speaking, writing, pointing and button pressing, they are labelled behavioural measures.

Beyond the frequently sophisticated and sometimes complex research and data analytic methods applied to study memory, two theoretical approaches are apparent across contemporary cognitive psychology and so contemporary memory research. The processing approach emphasizes the nature and role of psychological processing, while the systems approach emphasizes the structures or systems and usually the brain region(s) where processing occurs. The key term here is 'emphasizes'. Processes must operate within systems and given the evolutionary history and neurological organization of the brain, it is reasonable to assume some systematic organization of psychological processing. Therefore, the two approaches are entirely compatible, but dispute concerns the utility of emphasizing one approach over the other (e.g., Foster & Jelic, 1999; Surprenant & Neath, 2009).

The major impetus for the current neuroscience contribution to understanding cognition generally, and memory in particular, comes from technological advances in the study of neural activity around the late 1970s and early 1980s. New techniques, such as magneto-encephalography (MEG), functional magnetic resonance imaging (fMRI), positron emission tomography (PET) and transcranial magnetic stimulation (TMS) were added to the more established techniques of single cell recording (SCR) and event-related potentials (ERPs). A useful way to summarize the data obtained from MEG, fMRI and PET techniques is to generate a brain image upon which the different levels of neural activity recorded are depicted using different colours to reflect the activity levels measured, hence the label *neuroimaging techniques*. However, the contribution of neuroimaging to an understanding of cognition also has been the focus of serious criticism (Coltheart, 2004; Hartley, 2004; Henson, 2005; Uttal, 2001; 2011; 2013).

Typically, the cognitive neuroscience approach to memory involves conducting a cognitive psychology memory experiment while employing one of the neural activity measuring techniques mentioned. However, difficulties can arise satisfying the requirements for both cognitive psychology experiments and brain activity measurement. For example, there is very little room inside an MRI scanner and even specially designed equipment for the cognitive psychology experiment stimulus presentation, and behavioural response recording can be difficult to accommodate without affecting the way the person in the scanner carries out the memory task. As neuroimaging seeks to identify brain regions associated with particular tasks, with these regions very often conceived as the location of the systems responsible for executing these tasks, it is unsurprising the systems approach dominates cognitive neuroscience and is a major source of systems influence on psychological theorizing. Of course, cognitive neuroscience also applies other methods, such as studying the effect on memory and other processing of specific brain lesions in animals, and the effect of drug administration on memory storage mechanisms in animals and humans (e.g., Pomara et al., 2006). The examination of human memory and other processing after brain lesions caused by injury or disease has a long and important history in the development of cognitive psychology theory. This research area is known as neuropsychology or cognitive neuropsychology, but whether it should be re-labelled as cognitive neuroscience remains moot (e.g., Coltheart, 2004; Hartley, 2004; Salthouse, 2010).

Generally, the same research methods applied to examine normal memory are applied to examine the effect of ageing on normal memory. Cross-sectional methods, where subject groups are distinguished on the basis of age, predominate; but longitudinal methods, where subjects are studied over a period of time to investigate age-related changes in memory operation, also have been employed, sometimes in combination with cross-sectional designs (Hertzog, 1996; Salthouse, 2000).

1.3 A basic history of memory research

While a logical analysis of memory providing encoding, storage and retrieval stages is useful, it provides only an elementary outline, and far greater theoretical development is required to provide a good account of memory operation. Around the time Ebbinghaus (1885) was publishing his work in Germany, a number of other psychologists were beginning to develop theoretical ideas about the nature of memory (e.g., James, 1890), but further development of these 'cognitive' ideas dropped off the agenda as behaviourism began to dominate experimental psychology (Watson, 1913). Ebbinghaus' work was not published in English until 1913, and after eradication of mentalistic ideas, it was merged with the dominant behaviourist approach to learning, where all memory phenomena were explained in terms of stimulus/response associations. Although some important exceptions to this approach developed over this period (e.g., Tolman's cognitive maps, the Gestalt approach and Bartlett's approach to memory), it was not until the cognitive revolution in the 1950s that memory, as part of mind, became a legitimate topic for psychological theory.

One aspect omitted by the elementary outline of memory involving encoding, storage and retrieval stages is mention of the transition from an active and so temporary form of memory representation to a more permanent memory representation. This transition is labelled consolidation and, historically, it has been investigated by neuroscientists rather than psychologists (Wixted, 2004). *Synaptic consolidation* and *systems consolidation* have been described. Synaptic consolidation involves strengthening pertinent synaptic connections between neurons via a process of protein synthesis in the first hours after encoding. It generally is agreed episodic memory components are stored in the cortex, but the hippocampus is required at retrieval to provide an integrated episodic memory. Systems consolidation involves re-writing these memories in an integrated fashion to the cortex over weeks to years to provide memory retrieval independent of the hippocampus (e.g., Dudai, 2004; McClelland, McNaughton, & O'Reilly, 1995; Wixted & Cai, 2013).

1.3.1 Atkinson and Shiffrin's multi-store model of memory

If memory phenomena are explained exclusively by different stimulus/response associations, then only a relatively simple unitary memory store is required. The notion of a unitary memory or memory system was one of the theoretical positions challenged by one of the first cognitive psychological accounts of memory – Atkinson and Shiffrin's (1968) multi-store model of memory. This also is known as the modal memory model because it presented an account consistent with what most opponents of unitary memory advocated. Following James' (1890) early distinction between primary and secondary memory, Atkinson and Shiffrin postulated separate short-term (STM) and long-term memory (LTM) stores, as well as modality specific sensory stores (e.g., iconic and echoic memory).

Previously, Scoville and Milner (1957) had reported findings supporting a distinction between STM and LTM. Twenty-seven-year-old Henry Molaison (known as HM to protect his privacy until his death in 2008 at the age of 82) had brain surgery to remove bilaterally sections of his medial temporal lobe thought to be the origin of his severe epileptic seizures. The operation successfully improved Henry's epilepsy, but it left him with a severe global amnesia. Henry retained his amiable personality, intelligence and awareness, and was able to interact normally with others, but unfortunately, he could not remember anything once it had departed his immediate conscious awareness. Scoville and Milner (1957) proposed Henry's memory problems were due to a failure to transfer or consolidate STM information into LTM, lending strong support to the STM-LTM distinction formalized in Atkinson and Shiffrin's (1968) multi-store memory model.

However, difficulties with Atkinson and Shiffrin's model were appreciated at the time and soon after (e.g., Baddeley, 1976). In particular, the notion of a single STM store that was also the main location for mental processing was challenged by a number of findings. For example, patient KF suffered a left hemisphere lesion adjacent to the Sylvian fissure and exhibited severely impaired auditory STM, but KF also demonstrated normal LTM (Shallice & Warrington, 1970). The observation of impaired STM with normal LTM (e.g., KF), and normal STM with impaired LTM (e.g., Henry Molaison), is known as a double disassociation of STM and LTM and lends greater support to the STM-LTM distinction, but finding impaired STM and normal LTM presents a stiff challenge to Atkinson and Shiffrin's account of STM. According to the multi-store memory model, KF's poor auditory STM deficit was due to damage to the unitary STM system, but the very fact a modality specific STM deficit is observed suggests the notion of a unitary and so multi-modal STM is incorrect – there may be a set of modality specific STMs receiving input from the set of modality specific sensory registers. Nevertheless, if KF's short-term auditory processing system was damaged, then KF still should have shown serious impairment on all auditory tasks, but particularly on tasks involving spoken language, where understanding can require subtle and speedy auditory and verbal processing discrimination. However, KF's auditory STM deficit had little consequence for his language abilities and other life activities generally. This presented a substantial problem for the STM conception in the multi-store memory model.

Baddeley also conducted a number of experiments that presented further problems for the multi-store memory model. For example, using a dual task paradigm, Baddeley (1986) demonstrated simultaneous performance of a verbal task and a visuo-spatial task was on a par with single task performance. This conflicts with expectations based on STM in the multi-store memory model, as performing the two tasks simultaneously should place substantial processing demands on the STM system to the extent that performance of one or both of these tasks should decline in comparison with single task performance. Evidence contradicting the STM conception in Atkinson and Shiffrin's (1968) multi-store memory model was accumulating and a new theoretical account able to accommodate the new evidence was required.

1.3.2 Baddeley's multicomponent working memory (M-WM) model

Baddeley's multicomponent working memory model (M-WM; e.g., Baddeley, 1986; 2000; 2007; 2012; Baddeley & Hitch,1974), illustrated schematically in Figure 1.1, presented a new conception of STM activity to accommodate data consistent and inconsistent with Atkinson and Shiffrin's (1968) account. The M-WM replaced the unitary short-term memory store in Atkinson and Shiffrin's (1968) systems-based multi-store memory model with a multicomponent system for the temporary storage and manipulation of information, and like the multi-store memory model, the M-WM exemplifies the systems approach in psychology (e.g., Surprenant & Neath, 2009). The current version of the M-WM model comprises four components.

The *central executive* (CE) is the most complex and important component. Later versions of the M-WM (e.g., Baddeley, 1996; Baddeley & Logie, 1999) presented a CE without information storage capacity, leaving a system focused exclusively on the supervisory control of attention. Attention is focused, divided and switched by allocating processing resources to relevant M-WM components to enable the required implementations.

The *episodic buffer* (EB) is the most recent addition to the M-WM (Baddeley, 2000). Although the EB can contribute to most memory tasks and provides a more direct link between the CE and LTM, its main role is providing an integrated representation of an event or entity (episode) based on information employing different representational formats. These different formats/codes arise not only from other M-WM model components, but also from LTM and perception, suggesting the EB links depicted in Figure 1.1 should be more extensive. Baddeley (2007; 2012) also claims retrieval from the EB is based on conscious awareness, which places the EB at the heart of any account of consciousness. Binding and other operations are required to integrate different representational formats, but research on the visual and verbal binding required in M-WM tasks (Baddeley, Allen, & Hitch, 2011; Baddeley, Hitch, & Allen, 2009) indicates they occur without attentional demands. This suggests M-WM has no active role in binding, with the EB only displaying the representational outcome of the binding process, which may occur quite automatically in LTM (Baddeley, 2007; 2012).

The *phonological loop* (PL) is the most theoretically developed M-WM component. It comprises a phonological store and an articulatory control process and is able to provide an account of most verbal short-term memory phenomena. Research suggests the PL's main role is to enable new vocabulary learning, but it also can be used to record short instructions (to self) to assist performance, particularly when repetitive shifts in attention from one task to another are required (cf. Luria, 1959; Vygotsky, 1962).

The *visuo-spatial sketch pad* (VSSP) processes and stores visual and spatial information. It comprises a visual cache, which stores visual form and colour information, and an inner scribe, which implements spatial processing, stores information in the visual cache and moves information between the visual cache and the CE. The visual cache and inner scribe are VSSP counterparts to the phonological store and articulatory control process in the PL (Logie, 1995; 2011).

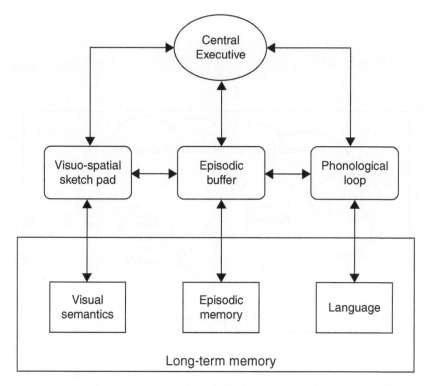

FIGURE 1.1 Baddeley's multicomponent working memory model (based on Baddeley, 2007; 2012).

Each M-WM component can operate relatively independently of the others, but all have capacity limitations. Baddeley (2007) suggested direct links between the EB and the VSSP and the PL, and all but the CE also link directly to pertinent parts of long-term memory. While the CE has processing capability only, all of the other M-WM components have both storage and processing capability. System theorists frequently assume a system has a particular location in the brain, but while Baddeley accepts the CE, VSSP and PL processing may be based primarily in the pre-frontal, parietal and occipital lobes, respectively, he considers it most likely that working memory will depend upon processes running and data stored in a variety of interconnected brain regions – especially when the EB is involved.

1.3.3 Cowan's embedded processes working memory (E-WM) model

Cowan's model of working memory (e.g., Cowan, 1988; 1995; 1999; 2001; 2005) is illustrated schematically in Figure 1.2. The E-WM comprises two levels of activated representations and processes in LTM, a central executive, and a set of activated LTM features associated with brief sensory afterimages. (Although labelled 'images', these representations will not be limited to vision.) At the first level, the set of

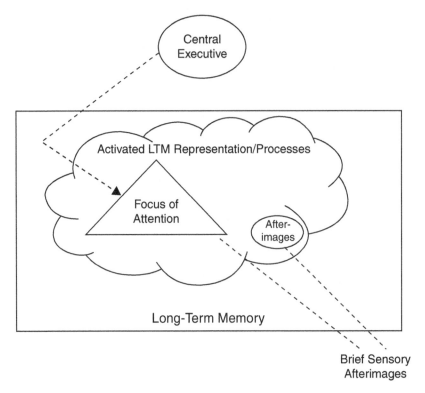

FIGURE 1.2 Cowan's embedded processes working memory model (based on Cowan, 2005).

activated LTM representations and processes (also labelled slots or chunks) involved in working memory is unlimited. However, among these is a limited set of LTM representations and processes operating at a second (higher) level of activation that constitute the focus of attention. Cowan proposes a maximum of four active LTM representations and processes (slots or chunks) can occupy the focus of attention. A central executive also is included, but this CE has a more limited role than the M-WM model CE, as it is responsible only for the conscious control of the focus of attention. Unconscious control of the focus of attention also is possible via the operation of automatic orientating in response to environmental changes. Cowan (2005) also suggests information in the sensory store (e.g., iconic memory) may need to activate LTM representations to enable inclusion within the attentional focus.

1.3.4 Overview

Cowan considers the E-WM model as providing a more general level of analysis than Baddeley's M-WM model. For example, large differences between verbal and visuo-spatial processing are acknowledged, but rather than committing to separate buffers like Baddeley, Cowan makes the more general assumption that phonological and visuo-spatial operations occur within temporarily activated areas of LTM. Cowan also raises a key issue: is storage and processing capacity limited by a single resource or do separate resources determine storage and processing capacity? Both Baddeley and Cowan consider their accounts of WM to be mutually consistent (e.g., Baddeley, 2007; 2010; 2012; Cowan, 2005), with any apparent differences due to the level of analysis applied, emphases or terminology. Cowan's focus has been explaining capacity limitations in terms of the E-WM model, with Baddeley suggesting Cowan's E-WM model may be seen as specifying the interaction between the M-WM attention-limited CE and storage-limited EB. Baddeley and Cowan also agree on the important role of interaction between WM and LTM, with the M-WM assuming such links operate at a number of different levels in ways Cowan's notion of activated LTM does not encompass (e.g., Baddeley, 2007, pp. 155–156; Baddeley, 2010, p. 140). However, both M-WM and E-WM models can be criticised for postulating the operation of relatively unspecified working memory representations and processes. Moreover, while the E-WM seems to have been applied more frequently than the M-WM in studies of normal ageing, the M-WM seems to have been applied more frequently than the E-WM in studies of pathological ageing.

1.4   Effects of normal and pathological ageing on memory

It is important to emphasize not all cognitive functions decline with age and there is also considerable individual variation in the extent to which affected functions decline (e.g., Salthouse, 2015). Nevertheless, anecdotal evidence and casual observation, as well as empirical evidence (see later), indicate thinking speed diminishes with age, as does the ability to divide attention effectively, while the ability to remember old memories with ease contrasts with the more difficult and less successful recall of more recent memories. Thinking (i.e., cognitive processing) speed and the division of attention are topics addressed by models of WM, while the difference between the ability to remember remote and recent memories is addressed by theories of LTM. Other aspects of memory, such as prospective memory, also are affected, but here the focus is age effects on WM and LTM, specifically episodic memory (cf. semantic memory).

1.4.1   Normal ageing and working memory

Studies applying Cowan's E-WM model or Baddeley's M-WM model usually examine whether the effects of ageing can be localized to a limited set of WM component processes. However, another possibility of the effect of ageing is to impair the operation of WM operations in a much more general fashion.

One general influence on WM is an increase in response time with age. Response time (RT) begins to decline around the time people reach their 20th year (e.g., Fozard, Vercruyssen, Reynolds, Hancock, & Quilter, 1994; Rabbitt, 1979).

Verhaeghen and colleagues (Verhaeghen & Carella, 2002; 2008; Verhaeghen & De Meersman, 1998a; 1998b; also see Verhaeghen, 2012) presented meta-analyses of response time data obtained from a number of studies where specific WM task conditions had been manipulated. They found older adults take just a 'little' longer to complete negative priming tasks, but take 'much' longer to complete Stroop tasks, global and local switching tasks and dual tasks. Nevertheless, separate analyses by task revealed a general slowing of processing associated with age explained the RT differences between young and old adults across Stroop task interference and no-interference conditions, across local task switch and no-switch conditions, and across the negative priming and baseline task conditions. Similar analyses of the young and old adults' RT data from dual task (single and dual) conditions and global switch (and no-switch) tasks revealed the same general slowing of processing associated with age, but additional specific age-related deficits were detected with dual and global switch tasks.

Verhaeghen and colleagues' analyses suggest the speed of cognitive processes underlying WM tasks slows with age. As this relationship appears to be linear, the reduction in cognitive processing speed between 20 and 25 years will be the same as the reduction in cognitive processing speed between 70 and 75 years, but as older adults, by definition, are further along the age scale, their RTs will be slower than younger adults. However, some tasks are even slower to complete than would be expected on the basis of this slowing of general processing speed. Presumably, tasks such as the dual and global switch tasks tax specific and impaired WM operations causing further slowing of processing beyond that attributable to general processing slowing. These findings suggest there are no specific age-related problems with older adults' resistance to interference beyond the general processing slowing with age. Salthouse (1996) presented an account of age differences in cognition based on the processing consequences of the general slowing of processing speed with age (which may be related to white matter integrity, see Kerchner et al., 2012). However, the specific age-related effects identified by Verhaeghen and colleagues' meta-analyses indicate general processing slowing with age cannot give a full account of all age-related WM problems.

As resistance to interference (inhibitory control) is examined most frequently using Stroop and negative priming tasks, and a specific failure to control interference has been suggested as a key WM component process impaired by age, the lack of age-related differences in resistance to interference is of particular interest. These data challenge this theoretical perspective, although further support in the form of accuracy data would be extremely useful. These data also identify dual tasks and global switch tasks as tapping into specific age-related impairments in WM operation and requiring further theoretical account.

Verhaeghen summarizes these data as revealing no age-related deficits in the Stroop, negative priming and local task switch tasks, all of which require WM to select relevant information by releasing attention from one stimulus aspect and connecting it to another stimulus aspect. However, age-related deficits arise with dual and global switch tasks that require the maintenance in WM of two plans, task or goal sets. This assessment has some similarity to Braver and West's (2008) goal maintenance account of age-related changes in cognition, but while maintaining more than one goal would place additional demands on the processing system and might be predicted to exert greater effect, handling more than one goal is not a key feature of the goal maintenance account.

Braver and West (2008) also note the minimal effect of age when simple/ passive span tasks are employed to occupy M-WM model storage capacity (e.g., Bopp & Verhaeghen, 2005; Zacks, Hasher, & Li, 2000). When storage capacity in the M-WM model is occupied, older adult performance should be diminished more due to their already diminished storage capacity. However, to observe age-related differences seems to require the use of complex span tasks (e.g., reading span), which tax both storage and processing (e.g., Bopp & Verhaeghen, 2005). Although the PL, VSSP and EB in the M-WM model incorporate processing capability, this draws attention to the issue raised by Cowan concerning a single resource limiting storage and processing capacity, or a separate resource limiting storage capacity and a separate resource limiting processing capacity. The RT data above suggests age exerts influence on WM processing, rather than storage, resources.

Consistent with the idea that only WM processing resources are affected by age, a substantial amount of work based on the E-WM model has suggested a reduction in older adults' ability to refresh or update the focus of attention (Johnson, Mitchell, Raye, & Greene, 2004; Johnson, Reeder, Raye, & Mitchell, 2002; Verhaeghen & Basak, 2005). Older adults also require more time to access information in activated LTM and are likely to be less successful switching information into the focus of attention (Oberauer, Demmrich, Mayr, & Kliegl, 2001; Verhaeghen, Cerella, Bopp, & Basak, 2005). Although older adults appear to have access to as many slots in activated LTM and employ the same retrieval processes as younger adults (Basak & Verhaeghen, 2011; Lange & Verhaeghen, 2009; Vaughan, Basak, Hartmann, & Verhaeghen, 2008), Verhaeghen (2012) suggests the problem may be due to the resolution of the slot contents in older adults' WM.

Several studies have suggested older adults are less able to bind the various features of a representation in WM, so the fully bound representation can be stored in and retrieved from LTM. Chalfonte and Johnson (1996) reported age-related differences for the recognition of stimulus features and stimulus feature configurations. In comparison with younger adults, older adults exhibited poorer memory for stimulus item locations, while their memory for the stimulus items and, separately, the stimulus item colours was on a par with younger adults. However, older adults' memory was poor for bound item and location, and bound item and colour information. This was particularly apparent for bound item and colour, given older adults' memory performance when these features were assessed separately. Mitchell, Johnson, Raye, Mather and D'Esposito (2000) replicated these findings when they observed equal performance by younger and older adults when individual stimulus features (stimulus items or stimulus locations) were tested, but older adults' memory performance was significantly poorer when stimulus feature combinations (stimulus items and stimulus locations) were tested.

Logie and Maylor (2009; also see Brockmole & Logie, 2013; Johnson, Logie, & Brockmole, 2010; Maylor & Logie, 2010) conducted an Internet based study in collaboration with the BBC. Five WM tasks were presented: Digit Span for immediate typed serial recall of visually presented digits; Working Memory Span for semantic processing of sentence sequences and ordered recall of the final word of each sentence; immediate recall of Feature Binding in arrays of colour, shape and location combinations; immediate recall of visually presented square matrix patterns in the Visual Patterns Task; and identifying which hand on a human figure holds a ball in different spatial orientations in the Man and Ball Task. Performance on all tasks declined with age, but considerable variation in decline was apparent across tasks. The two tasks worst affected by increasing age were the Visual Patterns Task and Feature Binding.

Studies such as those just outlined present convincing evidence for an age-related deficit in binding. However, they do not present evidence of binding occurring in WM – it simply is assumed this binding occurs in WM. In contrast to these assumptions, Baddeley's specific examination of visual and verbal binding in M-WM concluded M-WM had no active role in feature binding, which may occur automatically in LTM. Therefore, further discussion of this issue is postponed until section 1.4.3, Normal ageing and LTM.

1.4.2 Pathological ageing effects and working memory

Pathological ageing refers to all age-related changes in functional ability caused by an underlying pathology – usually these changes are more severe than typically expected given a person's age and level of education, and do not tend to follow the normal progression of non-pathological decline. In this section and in section 1.4.4, the focus will be on the effects of pathological ageing on WM and LTM, respectively, with a specific focus on the effects of the most common form of dementing illness – Alzheimer's disease (AD). The German psychiatrist Alois Alzheimer was the first to identify and describe AD in 1906, which is an acquired, progressive and persistent neurodegenerative brain disorder characterised by deterioration of cognitive function in multiple domains (Budson & Kowall, 2011), with episodic memory loss featuring early and prominently in its development. Neuropathologically, the disease begins in the hippocampus and medial-temporal lobe (MTL), and then spreads to other surrounding cortical areas (Raj et al., 2015), although some degree of diversity in the type of impairment beyond simply severity also has been observed (Stopford, Snowden, Thompson, & Neary, 2007; 2008). Given the involvement of the hippocampus (see Chapter 2), it is not surprising to find individuals with AD showing loss of memory ability early in the disease (e.g., McKhann et al., 2011; Sperling et al., 2011), starting with an inability to form new memories (anterograde amnesia), later followed by loss of information acquired earlier in life (retrograde amnesia). For these reasons, research has focused mainly on the loss of LTM (see 1.4.4) in the early stages of AD, and particularly of episodic memory, which is memory for contextualised episodes belonging to one's own experience that can be retrieved consciously (Tulving, 1983), although some studies have also shown WM dysfunction can emerge quite early in the disease progression (e.g., Belleville, Chertkow, & Gauthier, 2007; and Perry & Hodges, 1999, for review).

The classic view on the WM problems experienced by individuals with AD was formulated by Baddeley and colleagues (Baddeley, Bressi, Della Sala, Logie, & Spinnler, 1991; Baddeley, Logie, Bressi, Sala, & Spinnler, 1986; Morris & Baddeley, 1988; see also Becker, 1988). This account suggests that WM deficits depend upon CE dysfunction. Baddeley et al. (1986; 1991) compared performance across groups of participants with mild-to-moderate AD, healthy age-matched controls and young controls, and showed that AD participants presented impaired performance, compared to controls, when asked to coordinate two separate tasks at the same time. Analogously, Calderon et al. (2001) have reported AD patients performing normally on tests of visual object and space perception, perhaps indicating relatively intact VSP ability, but showing deficits in selective attention. These findings generally would highlight a CE failure, as this component (see 1.3.2) is involved in the supervisory control of attention. Following on from this pattern of findings, it typically is assumed WM failures in AD are associated with impairment of frontal lobe structures in the brain (Baddeley & Della Sala, 1996). Similarly, compared to individuals with mild cognitive impairment (MCI), which is considered a stepping stone in the development of full-blown AD, subjects with mild AD present more severe and consistent impairments in tasks requiring attention (Belleville et al., 2007). Moreover, failures in attentional tasks are thought to be predictive of whether a person with MCI will convert to AD over time (Gagnon & Belleville, 2011).

When examining early-onset AD (EOAD), a rarer form of AD beginning before the age of 65, Stopford and colleagues (e.g., Stopford et al., 2008; Stopford, Thompson, Neary, Richardson, & Snowden, 2012) have suggested mechanisms other than frontal dysfunction may be implicated in the AD-related WM impairment. These mechanisms would involve a reduction of activity in temporoparietal regions. Some support for this claim derives from the assessment of psychiatric symptoms in EOAD subjects: unlike individuals with frontotemporal dementia (FTD), a form of degeneration that typically, and specifically, affects the frontal lobes, subjects with EOAD do not usually show inappropriate social behaviours or a lack of interest in the outcome of their performance. Empirical support also comes from studies comparing WM performance between these two groups. For instance, Stopford et al. (2012), revealed EOAD subjects presented a different pattern of WM dysfunction compared to FTD subjects, often with more severe impairment in the former. Individuals with FTD generally showed attentional and executive deficits, normally linked to frontal impairment, whereas EOAD participants also presented impairments in the PL, suggesting a problem in maintaining information available for processing.

1.4.3 Normal ageing and long-term memory

A distinction frequently drawn is between semantic and episodic LTM (e.g., Rutherford, Markopoulos, Bruno, & Brady-van den Bos, 2012). Of these two sorts of memory, episodic memory declines most with increasing age (e.g., Craik & Jennings, 1992; Naveh-Benjamin & Old, 2008), but a definitive explanation of age effects in LTM generally and episodic memory specifically still is lacking, despite a number of theoretical proposals and many empirical studies (e.g., Hoyer & Verhaeghen, 2006). Here, the focus is on the reduced processing resources account (Craik, 1982; 1983) and the associative deficit hypothesis (Naveh-Benjamin, 2000; Naveh-Benjamin, Hussein, Guez, & Bar-On, 2003).

Craik (1982; 1983) suggested older adults have diminished processing resources in comparison with younger adults, so their memory encoding and retrieval processing will be less effective, resulting in poorer memory performance. To test these ideas, several experiments have employed a dual task paradigm, where a secondary, non-memory task is carried out at the same time as the memory task encoding, or retrieval operations by younger adults to determine if their memory performance diminishes in the same way as older adults' memory performance without (and sometimes with) a secondary, non-memory task. Dividing the attention of younger adults at encoding does seem to reproduce older adults' memory performance in some situations (e.g., Anderson et al., 2000). However, older adults do not always show poorer memory performance (cf. younger adults) when attention is divided at encoding, but this may be due to older adults prioritizing the encoding task, as differences between older and younger adults manifest in secondary task performance, with older adults usually exhibiting poorer performance at encoding and always exhibiting poorer performance at retrieval (Naveh-Benjamin, Craik, Guez, & Kreuger, 2005; also see Kilb & Naveh-Benjamin, 2015, for review).

The associative deficit hypothesis (ADH) proposed by Naveh-Benjamin and colleagues (Naveh-Benjamin, 2000; Naveh-Benjamin et al., 2003) assumes each episode in episodic memory is comprised of stimulus and contextual features connected in a coherent fashion to provide a distinctive representation, and older adults impaired episodic memory is due to a failure to construct and retrieve the links, bindings or associations between individual stimulus feature and context feature information units. Simons, Dodson, Bell and Schacter (2004) demonstrated older adults' poorer memory for episodic source information, and many experimental studies have demonstrated older adults age memory for associated or bound items across a variety of types of stimulus pairs is substantially worse than that of younger adults, despite older adults remembering the individual items as well as younger adults, and when memory performance levels for associated and individual items were controlled (see Naveh-Benjamin, 2012, for review).

It might be thought the attentional resources described by Craik would be used to bind feature information into episodic representations. However, consistent with Baddeley and colleagues' (Baddeley, Allen, & Hitch, 2011; Baddeley, Hitch, & Allen, 2009) findings regarding binding in WM, Craik and Kester (2000) found the effect of dividing attention and the effect of associative elaboration (i.e., amount of binding) was additive, and not interactive as would be predicted if the attention available was directed to binding operations. Where and how binding occurs is an issue requiring further research.

If diminished ability to encode or bind such information into episodic memories underlies older adults' poorer performance on episodic memory tasks, then both Craik and Naveh-Benjamin provide compatible accounts explaining why older adults have difficulty binding contextual/source information into episodic memory representations. More detailed description of how this affects memory is given by dual process accounts of memory retrieval. According to these models, recollection is the form of memory retrieval underlying what most people would regard as normal memory. It retrieves the episodic representation into which the contextual/source information is bound and provides conscious awareness of the episode. In contrast, familiarity based retrieval simply outputs a memory strength signal, which gives rise to a feeling of knowing, but without any episodic (i.e., context/source) information (e.g., Yonelinas, 2002). Therefore, dual process accounts predict recollection will exhibit age effects, with older adults' recollection being inferior to that of younger adults, with studies examining the effect of age on recollection supporting these predictions (for review, see Light, 2012).

1.4.4 Pathological ageing and long-term memory

The most prominent effect of AD on LTM is the loss of episodic memory (Grady, 2005), although semantic memory loss also has been reported (e.g., Mårdh, Nägga, & Samuelsson, 2013). Individuals with AD tend to show consistent episodic memory impairment in tests of free recall. In addition, unlike older adults with no AD, recognition memory also declines (e.g., Clark et al., 2012). The loss of episodic memory is largely consistent with the nature of AD-related neurodegeneration, which, as noted (see 1.4.2), begins in the MTL, including the hippocampus (see Chapter 2), and then spreads to other regions. Critically, MTL atrophy is thought to emerge early in the disease, and has been consistently reported by volumetric MRI studies (Jack & Petersen, 2000). Indeed, MTL structural data may predict conversion to AD up to ten years prior to the disease onset (e.g., Tondelli et al., 2012).

Focusing on free recall, it is fairly common to observe delayed performance being affected more dramatically by AD than immediate performance, and usually this is attributed to a failure to consolidate information (Bruno, Reiss, Petkova, Sidtis, & Pomara, 2013; Gomar, Bobes-Bascaran, Conejero-Goldberg, Davies, & Goldberg, 2011). For example, Lyness, Lee, Zarow, Teng and Chui (2014) showed delayed recall performance, up to five years prior to death, was sensitive to the presence of AD pathology, as determined by *post-mortem* examination. Importantly, this index was shown to be a better predictor of consensus clinical diagnosis, whereas immediate recall performance was not significantly sensitive. In particular, AD pathology is thought to prevent the process of synaptic consolidation (see 1.3) by reducing neuronal plasticity that is necessary for the formation of new synaptic connections (Borlikova et al., 2013).

1.5 Conclusions

This chapter has reviewed the essential literature pertaining to the changes in cognition, behaviour and, to a lesser extent, brain structure and function, occurring as part of the ageing process, when normal and abnormal trajectories are followed. Our focus here has been primarily on the cognitive psychology approach to the study of memory, although we have also touched upon the contributions of neuroscience. Chapter 2 provides a more thorough neuroscientific discussion of relevant age-related memory changes, focusing especially on the impact of age on the hippocampus.

In general, age-related declines in both short- and long-term memory functions have been reported for cognitively healthy older individuals when compared to younger controls, although the nature of these changes is complex and their origins remain a matter for theoretical and empirical research. Future chapters, and particularly Chapter 10, will discuss activities healthy older adults can engage in to train their memory and preserve function as much as possible. With regards to pathological ageing, the focus has been on Alzheimer's disease, and the way this form of pathological brain degeneration affects multiple memory domains, beginning with episodic memory, but also semantic and working memory.

References

Anderson, N. D., Iidaka, T., Cabeza, R., Kapur, S., McIntosh, A. R., & Craik, F. I. M. (2000). The effects of divided attention on encoding- and retrieval-related related brain activity: A PET study of younger and older adults. *Journal of Cognitive Neuroscience, 12*(5), 775–792.

Atkinson, R. C., & Shiffrin, R. (1968). Human memory: A proposed system and its control processes. In K. Spence & J. Spence (Eds.), *The psychology of learning and motivation, volume 2*. New York: Academic Press.

Baddeley, A. D. (1976). *The psychology of memory*. New York: Harper & Row.

Baddeley, A. D. (1986). *Working memory*. Oxford: Oxford University Press.

Baddeley, A. D. (1996). Exploring the central executive. *Quarterly Journal of Experimental Psychology, A 49*, 5–28.

Baddeley, A. D. (2000). The episodic buffer: A new component of working memory? *Trends in Cognitive Science, 4*, 417–423.

Baddeley, A. D. (2007). *Working memory, thought and action*. Oxford: Oxford University Press.

Baddeley, A. D. (2010). Working memory. *Current Biology, 20*(4), 136–140.

Baddeley, A. D. (2012). Working memory: Theories, models, and controversies. *Annual Review of Psychology, 63*, 1–29. doi: 10.1146/annurev-psych-120710-100422

Baddeley, A. D., Allen, R. J., & Hitch, G. J. (2011). Binding in visual working memory: The role of the episodic buffer. *Neuropsychologia, 49*(6), 1393–1400.

Baddeley, A. D., Bressi, S., Della Sala, S., Logie, R., & Spinnler, H. (1991). The decline of working memory in Alzheimer's disease. *Brain, 114*(6), 2521–2542.

Baddeley, A. D., & Della Sala, S. (1996). Working memory and executive control. *Philosophical Transactions of the Royal Society of London, 351*, 1397–1404.

Baddeley, A. D., & Hitch, G. (1974). Working memory. In G. H. Bower (Ed.), *The psychology of learning and motivation 2* (pp. 47–89). London: Academic Press.

Baddeley, A. D., Hitch, G. J., & Allen, R. J. (2009). Working memory and binding in sentence recall. *Journal of Memory & Language, 61*(3), 438–456.

Baddeley, A. D., & Logie, R. H. (1999). Working memory: The multiple-component model. In A. Miyake & P. Shah (Eds.), *Models of working memory* (pp. 28–61). Cambridge: Cambridge University Press.

Baddeley, A., Logie, R., Bressi, S., Sala, S. D., & Spinnler, H. (1986). Dementia and working memory. *The Quarterly Journal of Experimental Psychology, 38*(4), 603–618.

Bartlett, F. C. (1932). *Remembering*. Cambridge University Press: Cambridge.

Basak, C., & Verhaeghen, P. (2011). Aging and switching the focus of attention in working memory: Age differences in item availability but not in item accessibility. *Journal of Gerontology: Psychological Sciences, 66B*(5), 519–526. doi: 10.1093/geronb/gbr028

Becker, J. T. (1988). Working memory and secondary memory deficits in Alzheimer's disease. *Journal of clinical and experimental neuropsychology, 10*(6), 739–753.

Belleville, S., Chertkow, H., & Gauthier, S. (2007). Working memory and control of attention in persons with Alzheimer's disease and mild cognitive impairment. *Neuropsychology, 21*(4), 458.

Bledowski, C., Kaisera, J., & Rahm, B. (2010). Basic operations in working memory: Contributions from functional imaging studies. *Behavioural Brain Research, 214*(2), 172–179. doi: 10.1016/j.bbr.2010.05.041

Bledowski, C., Rahm, B., & Rowe, J. B. (2009). What 'works' in working memory? Separate systems for selection and updating of critical information. *Journal of Neuroscience, 29*(43), 13735–13741. doi: 10.1523/JNEUROSCI.2547–09.2009

Bopp, K. L., & Verhaeghen, P. (2005). Aging and verbal memory span: A meta-analysis. *Journal of Gerontology: Psychological Sciences, 60B*(5), 223–233.

Borlikova, G. G., Trejo, M., Mably, A. J., McDonald, J. M., Frigerio, C. S., Regan, C. M., ... & Walsh, D. M. (2013). Alzheimer brain-derived amyloid β-protein impairs synaptic remodeling and memory consolidation. *Neurobiology of Aging, 34*(5), 1315–1327.

Braver, T. S., & West, R. (2008). Working memory, executive control and aging. In F. I. M. Craik & T. A. Salthouse (Eds.), *The handbook of aging and cognition* (3rd edition, pp. 311–372). Hove: Psychology Press.

Brockmole, J. R., & Logie, R. H. (2013). Age related change in visual working memory: A study of 55,753 participants aged 8 to 75. *Frontiers in Perception Science, 4*(12). doi: 10.3389/fpsyg.2013.00012

Bruno, D., Reiss, P. T., Petkova, E., Sidtis, J. J., & Pomara, N. (2013). Decreased recall of primacy words predicts cognitive decline. *Archives of Clinical Neuropsychology, 28*(2), 95–103.

Budson, A. E., & Kowall, N. W. (Eds.). (2011). *The handbook of Alzheimer's disease and other dementias* (Vol. 7). Oxford, UK: John Wiley & Sons.

Burns, A., & Iliffe, S. (2009). Dementia. *British Medical Journal, 338*, b75. doi: dx.doi.org/10.1136/bmj.b75

Cabeza, R., & Kingstone, A. (2006). *The functional neuroimaging of cognition*. Cambridge, MA: Bradford/MIT Press.

Calderon, J., Perry, R. J., Erzinclioglu, S. W., Berrios, G. E., Dening, T., & Hodges, J. R. (2001). Perception, attention, and working memory are disproportionately impaired in dementia with Lewy bodies compared with Alzheimer's disease. *Journal of Neurology, Neurosurgery & Psychiatry, 70*(2), 157–164.

Chalfonte, B. L., & Johnson, M. K. (1996). Feature memory and binding in young and older adults. *Memory & Cognition, 24*(4), 403–416. doi: 10.1037/70882–7974.15.3.527

Clark, L. R., Stricker, N. H., Libon, D. J., Delano-Wood, L., Salmon, D. P., Delis, D. C., & Bondi, M. W. (2012). Yes/No versus forced-choice recognition memory in mild cognitive impairment and Alzheimer's disease: Patterns of impairment and associations with dementia severity. *The Clinical Neuropsychologist, 26*, 1201–1216.

Colette, F., Hogge, M., Salmon, E., & Van der Linden, M. (2006). Exploration of the neural: Substrates of executive functioning by functional neuroimaging. *Neuroscience, 139*, 209–221.

Coltheart, M. (2004). Brain imaging, connectionism and cognitive neuropsychology. *Cognitive Neuropsychology, 21*, 21–26.

Corkin, S. (2013). *Permanent present tense: The man with no memory, and what he taught the world.* London: Allen Lane/Penguin.

Cowan, N. (1988). Evolving conceptions of memory storage, selective attention, and their mutual constraints within the human information-processing system. *Psychological Bulletin, 104*(2), 163–191. doi.org/10.1037/0033–2909.104.2.163

Cowan, N. (1995). *Attention and memory: An integrated framework.* Oxford Psychology Series #26. New York: Oxford University Press.

Cowan, N. (1999). An embedded-processes model of working memory. In A. Miyake & P. Shah (Eds.), *Models of working memory: Mechanisms of active maintenance and executive control* (pp. 62–101). Cambridge: Cambridge University Press.

Cowan, N. (2001). The magical number 4 in short-term memory: A reconsideration of mental storage capacity. *Behavioral & Brain Sciences, 24*, 87–185.

Cowan, N. (2005). *Working memory capacity.* Hove: Psychology Press.

Craik, F. I. M. (1982). Selective changes in encoding as a function of reduced processing capacity. In F. Klix, J. Hoffman & E. Van der Meer (Eds.), *Cognitive research in psychology* (pp. 152–161). Berlin: Deutscher Verlag der Wissenchaffen.

Craik, F. I. M. (1983). On the transfer of information from temporary to permanent memory. *Philosophical transactions of the Royal Society of London, Series B, 302*, 341–359.

Craik, F. I. M., & Jennings, J. M. (1992). Human memory. In F. I. M. Craik & T. A. Salthouse (Eds.), *The handbook of aging and cognition* (pp. 51–110). Hillsdale, NJ: Erlbaum.

Craik, F. I. M., & Kester, J. D. (2000). Divided attention and memory: Impairment of processing or consolidation? In E. Tulving (Ed.), *Memory consciousness and the brain: The Tallin conference* (pp. 38–51). Philadelphia, PA: Psychology Press.

Craik, F. I. M., & Salthouse, T. A. (2008). *The handbook of aging and cognition* (3rd edition). Hove: Psychology Press.

Dudai, Y. (2004). The neurobiology of consolidations, or, how stable is the engram? *Annual Review of Psychology, 55*, 51–86.

Ebbinghaus, H. (1885/1913). *Memory: A Contribution to Experimental Psychology.* Translated by H. A. Ruger & C. E. Bussenius. New York: Teachers College, Columbia University.

Foster, J. K., & Jelic, M. (1999). *Memory: Systems, process or function?* Oxford: Oxford University Press.

Fozard, J. L., Vercruyssen, M., Reynolds, S. L., Hancock, P. A., & Quilter, R. E. (1994). Age differences and changes in reaction time: The Baltimore longitudinal study of aging. *Journal of Gerontology, 49*, 179–189.

Gagnon, L. G., & Belleville, S. (2011). Working memory in mild cognitive impairment and Alzheimer's disease: Contribution of forgetting and predictive value of complex span tasks. *Neuropsychology, 25*(2), 226.

Goldstein, S., & Naglieri, J. A. (2014). *Handbook of Executive functioning.* New York: Springer.

Goldstein, S., Naglieri, J. A., Princiotta, D., & Otero, T. M. (2014). Introduction: A history of executive functioning as a theoretical and clinical construct. In S. Goldstein & J. A. Naglieri (Eds.), *Handbook of Executive functioning.* New York: Springer.

Gomar, J. J, Bobes-Bascaran, M. T., Conejero-Goldberg, C., Davies, P., & Goldberg, T. E. (2011). Utility of combinations of biomarkers, cognitive markers, and risk factors to predict conversion from mild cognitive impairment to Alzheimer disease in patients in the Alzheimer's disease neuroimaging initiative. *Archives of General Psychiatry, 68*, 961–969.

Gonzalez, C.L.R., Mills, K. J., Genee, I., Li, F., Piquette, N., Rosen, N., & Gibb, R. (2014). Getting the right grasp on executive function. *Frontiers in Psychology, 5*, Article 285. doi: 10.3389/fpsyg.2014.00285

Grady, C. L. (2005). Functional connectivity during memory tasks in healthy aging and dementia. *Cognitive neuroscience of aging: Linking cognitive and cerebral aging* (pp. 286–308). Oxford: Oxford University Press.

Harlow, J. M. (1848). Passage of an iron rod through the head. *Boston Medical & Surgical Journal, 39*, 389–393.

Hartley, T. A. (2004). Does cognitive neuropsychology have a future? *Cognitive Neuropsychology, 21*, 3–16.

Henson, R. (2005). What can functional neuroimaging tell the experimental psychologist? *Quarterly Journal of Experimental Psychology, 58A*, 193–233.

Hertzog, C. (1996). Research design in studies of aging and cognition. In J. E. Birren & K. W. Schaie (Eds.), *Handbook of the psychology of aging* (pp. 24–37). San Diego: Elsevier.

Hoyer, W. J., & Verhaeghen, P. (2006). Memory aging. In J. E. Birren & K. W. Schaie (Eds.), *Handbook of the psychology of aging* (6th edition, pp. 209–232). San Diego: Elsevier.

Hunter, S. J., & Sparrow, E. P. (2012). *Executive function and dysfunction: Identification, assessment and treatment.* Cambridge: Cambridge University Press.

Jack, C. R., & Petersen, R. C. (2000). Structural imaging approaches to Alzheimer's disease. In L. F. M. Scinto & K. R. Daffner (Eds.), *Early diagnosis and treatment of Alzheimer's disease* (pp. 127–148). Totowa, NJ: Human Press.

James, W. (1890). *The principles of psychology.* New York: Henry Holt.

Johnson, M. K., Mitchell, K. J., Raye, C. L., & Greene, E. J. (2004). An age-related deficit in prefrontal cortical function associated with refreshing information. *Psychological Science, 15*(2), 127–132. doi: 10.1111/j.0963–7214.2004.01502009.x

Johnson, M. K., Reeder, J. A., Raye, C. L., & Mitchell, K. J. (2002). Second thoughts versus second looks: An age-related deficit in reflectively refreshing just-activated information. *Psychological Science, 13*(1), 64–67. doi: 10.1111/1467–9280.00411

Johnson, W., Logie, R. H., & Brockmole, J. R. (2010). Working memory tasks differ in factor structure across age cohorts: Implications for dedifferentiation. *Intelligence, 38*, 513–528.

Kerchner, G. A., Racine, C. A., Hale, S., Wilheim, R., Laluz, V., Bruce L., Miller, B. L., & Kramer, J. H. (2012). Cognitive processing speed in older adults: Relationship with white matter integrity. *PLoS ONE, 7*(11), e50425. doi: 10.1371/journal.pone.0050425. doi: 10.1371/journal.pone.0050425

Kilb, A., & Naveh-Benjamin, M. (2015). The reduced attentional resources hypothesis. In R. H. Logie & R. G. Morris (Eds.), *Working memory and ageing* (pp. 48–78). Hove: Psychology Press.

Kolb, B., & Whishaw, I. Q. (2015). *Fundamentals of human neuropsychology* (7th edition). New York: Worth Publishers Inc.

Lange, E. B., & Verhaeghen, P. (2009). No age differences in complex memory search: Older adults search as efficiently as younger adults. *Psychology & Aging, 24*(1), 105–115. doi. org/10.1037/a0013751

Light, L. (2012). Dual process theories of memory in old age: An update. In M. Naveh-Benjamin & N. Ohta (Eds.), *Memory and aging: Current and future directions* (pp. 97–124). New York: Psychology Press.

Logie, R. H. (1995). *Visuo-spatial working memory.* Hove: LEA.

Logie, R. H. (2011). The functional organization and capacity limits of working memory. *Current Directions in Psychological Science, 20*(4), 240–245. doi: 10.1177/ 0963721411415340

Logie, R. H., & Maylor, E. A. (2009). An internet study of prospective memory across adulthood. *Psychology & Aging, 24*, 767–774.

Luria, A. R. (1959). The directive function of speech in development and dissolution, part I. *Word, 15,* 341–352.

Lustig, C., May, C. P., & Hasher, L. (2001). Working memory span and the role of proactive interference. *Journal of Experimental Psychology: General, 130*(2), 199–207.

Lyness, S. A., Lee, A. Y., Zarow, C., Teng, E. L., & Chui, H. C. (2014). 10-minute delayed recall from the modified mini-mental state test predicts Alzheimer's disease pathology. *Journal of Alzheimer's Disease, 39*(3), 575–582.

Mårdh, S., Nägga, K., & Samuelsson, S. (2013). A longitudinal study of semantic memory impairment in patients with Alzheimer's disease. *Cortex, 49,* 528–533.

Marr, D. (1982). *Vision: A computational investigation into the human representation and processing of visual information.* New York: Freeman.

Marvel, C. L., & Desmond, J. E. (2010). Functional topography of the cerebellum in verbal working memory. *Neuropsychology Review, 20*(3), 271–279.

May, C. P., Hasher, L., & Kane, M. J. (1999). The role of interference in memory span. *Memory & Cognition, 27*(5), 759–767.

May, C. P., Zacks, R. T., Hasher, L., & Multhaup, K. S. (1999). Inhibition in the processing of garden-path sentences. *Psychology & Aging, 8*(3), 420–428.

Maylor, E. A., & Logie, R. H. (2010). A large scale comparison of prospective and retrospective memory development from childhood to middle age. *Quarterly Journal of Experimental Psychology, 63,* 442–451.

McClelland, J. L., McNaughton, B. L., & O'Reilly, R. C. (1995). Why there are complimentary learning systems in the hippocampus and neocortex: Insights from the successes and failures of connectionist models of learning and memory. *Psychological Review, 102,* 419–457.

McKhann, G. M., Knopman, D. S., Chertkow, H., Hyman, B. T., Jack Jr., C. R., Kawas, C. H., … & Phelps, C. H. (2011). The diagnosis of dementia due to Alzheimer's disease: Recommendations from the National Institute on Aging-Alzheimer's Association workgroups on diagnostic guidelines for Alzheimer's disease. *Alzheimer's & Dementia, 7*(3), 263–269.

Mitchell, K. J., Johnson, M. K., Raye, C. L., Mather, M., & D'Esposito, M. (2000). Aging and reflective processes of working memory: Binding and test load deficits. *Psychology & Aging, 15*(3), 527–541. doi.org/10.1037/0882-7974.15.3.527

Morris, R. G., & Baddeley, A. D. (1988). Primary and working memory functioning in Alzheimer-type dementia. *Journal of Clinical and Experimental Neuropsychology, 10*(2), 279–296.

Naveh-Benjamin, M. (2000). Adult age differences in memory performance: Tests of an associative deficit hypothesis. *Journal of Experimental Psychology: Learning, Memory, and Cognition, 26*(5), 1170–1187.

Naveh-Benjamin, M. (2012). Age related differences in explicit associative memory: Contributions of effortful-strategic and automatic processes. In M. Naveh-Benjamin & N. Ohta (Eds.), *Memory and aging: Current and future directions* (pp. 71–95). New York: Psychology Press.

Naveh-Benjamin, M., Craik, F. I. M., Guez, J., & Kreuger, S. (2005). Divided attention in younger and older adults: Effects of strategy and relatedness on memory performance and secondary task costs. *Journal of Experimental Psychology: Learning, Memory, and Cognition, 31*(3), 520–537.

Naveh-Benjamin, M., Hussein, Z., Guez, J., & Bar-On, M. (2003). Adult age differences in episodic memory: Further support for an associative deficit hypothesis. *Journal of Experimental Psychology: Learning, Memory, and Cognition, 29*(5), 826–837.

Naveh-Benjamin, M., & Old, S. R. (2008). Aging and memory. In J. H. Byrne, H. Eichenbaum, R. Menzel, H. L. Roediger & D. Sweatt (Eds.), *Learning and memory: A comprehensive reference* (pp. 787–808). Oxford: Elsevier.

Oberauer, K. (2001). Removing irrelevant information from working memory. *Journal of Experimental Psychology: Learning, Memory, and Cognition, 27*(4), 948–957.

Oberauer, K. (2002). Access to information in working memory: Exploring the focus of attention. *Journal of Experimental Psychology: Learning, Memory, and Cognition, 28*(3), 411–421.

Oberauer, K. (2005a). Binding and inhibition in working memory: Individual and age differences in short-term recognition. *Journal of Experimental Psychology: General, 134*(3), 368–387.

Oberauer, K. (2005b). Control of the contents of working memory – a comparison of two paradigms and two age groups. *Journal of Experimental Psychology: Learning, Memory, and Cognition, 31*(4), 714–728.

Oberauer, K., Demmrich, A., Mayr, U., & Kliegl, R. (2001). Dissociating retention and access in working memory: An age-comparative study of mental arithmetic. *Memory & Cognition, 29*, 18–33.

Old, S. R., & Naveh-Benjamin, M. (2008). Differential effects of age on item and associative measures of memory: A meta-analysis. *Psychology & Aging, 23*(1), 104–118. doi: 10.1037/0882-7974.23.1.104

Perry, R. J., & Hodges, J. R. (1999). Attention and executive deficits in Alzheimer's disease: A critical review. *Brain, 122*(3), 383–404.

Poggio, T. (2012). The levels of understanding framework, revised. *Perception, 41*(9), 1017–1023.

Pomara, N., Facelle, T. M., Roth, A. E., Willoughby, L. M., Greenblatt, D. J., & Sidtis, J. J. (2006). Dose-dependent retrograde facilitation of verbal memory in healthy elderly after acute oral lorazepam administration. *Psychopharmacology, 185*(4), 487–494.

Rabbitt, P. (1979). How old and young subjects monitor and control responses for accuracy and speed. *British Journal of Psychology, 70*, 305–311.

Radvansky, G. A. (2005). *Human memory*. London: Pearson.

Raj, A., LoCastro, E., Kuceyeski, A., Tosun, D., Relkin, N., Weiner, M., & Alzheimer's Disease Neuroimaging Initiative (ADNI). (2015). Network Diffusion Model of Progression Predicts Longitudinal Patterns of Atrophy and Metabolism in Alzheimer's Disease. *Cell reports, 10*(3), 359–369.

Rutherford, A., Markopoulos, G., Bruno, D., & Brady-van den Bos, M. (2012). Long-term memory: Encoding to retrieval. In N. Braisby & A. Gellatly (Eds.), *Cognitive Psychology*. Oxford: Oxford University Press.

Salthouse, T. A. (1996). The processing-speed theory of adult age differences in cognition. *Psychological Review, 103*(3), 403–428. doi.org/10.1037/0033-295X.103.3.403

Salthouse, T. A. (2000). Methodological assumptions in cognitive aging research. In F. I. M. Craik & T. A. Salthouse, *The handbook of aging and cognition* (2nd edition., pp. 467–498). Hillsdale, NJ: Lawrence Erlbaum.

Salthouse, T. A. (2005). Relations between cognitive abilities and measures of executive functioning. *Neuropsychology, 19*(4), 532–545.

Salthouse, T. A. (2010). *Major issues in cognitive aging*. Oxford: Oxford University Press.

Salthouse, T. A. (2015). Individual differences in working memory and aging. In R. H. Logie & R. G. Morris (Eds.), *Working memory and ageing* (pp. 1–20). Hove: Psychology Press.

Scoville, W. B., & Milner, B. (1957). Loss of recent memory after bilateral hippocampal lesions. *Journal of Neurology, Neurosurgery & Psychiatry, 20*, 11–21.

Shallice, T., & Warrington, E. K. (1970). Independent functioning of verbal memory stores: A neuropsychological study. *Quarterly Journal of Experimental Psychology, 22*(2), 261–273. doi: 10.1080/00335557043000203

Simons, J. S., Dodson, C. S., Bell, D., & Schacter, D. L. (2004). Specific and partial source memory: Effects of aging. *Psychology and Aging, 19*, 689–694.

Sperling, R. A., Aisen, P. S., Beckett, L. A., Bennett, D. A., Craft, S., Fagan, A. M., . . . & Phelps, C. H. (2011). Toward defining the preclinical stages of Alzheimer's disease: Recommendations from the National Institute on Aging-Alzheimer's Association workgroups on diagnostic guidelines for Alzheimer's disease. *Alzheimer's & Dementia, 7*(3), 280–292.

Stopford, C. L., Snowden, J. S., Thompson, J. C., & Neary, D. (2007). Distinct memory profiles in Alzheimer's disease. *Cortex, 43*(7), 846–857.

Stopford, C. L., Snowden, J. S., Thompson, J. C., & Neary, D. (2008). Variability in cognitive presentation of Alzheimer's disease. *Cortex, 44*(2), 185–195.

Stopford, C. L., Thompson, J. C., Neary, D., Richardson, A. M., & Snowden, J. S. (2012). Working memory, attention, and executive function in Alzheimer's disease and frontotemporal dementia. *Cortex, 48*(4), 429–446.

Stuss, D. T. (2011). Traumatic brain injury: Relation to executive dysfunction. *Current Opinion in Neurology, 24*(6), 584–589. doi: 10.1097/WCO.0b013e32834c7eb9

Stuss, D. T., & Benson, D. F. (1986). *The frontal lobes.* New York: Raven Press.

Surprenant, A. M., & Neath, I. (2009). *Principles of memory.* Hove: Psychology Press.

Tondelli, M., Wilcock, G. K., Nichelli, P., DeJager, C. A., Jenkinson, M., & Zamboni, G. (2012). Structural MRI changes detectable up to ten years before clinical Alzheimer's disease. *Neurobiology of Aging, 33*, 825-e25.

Tulving, E. (1983). *Elements of episodic memory.* Oxford: Clarendon Press.

Turkington, C., & Harris, J. R. (2001). *The encyclopaedia of memory and memory disorders* (2nd edition, pp. 105–106). New York, NY: Facts on File Inc.

Uttal, W. R. (2001). *The new phrenology: The limits of localizing cognitive processes in the brain.* Cambridge, MA: MIT Press.

Uttal, W. R. (2011). *Mind and brain: A critical appraisal of cognitive neuroscience.* Cambridge, MA: MIT Press.

Uttal, W. R. (2013). *Reliability in cognitive neuroscience: A meta-meta-analysis.* Cambridge, MA: MIT Press.

Vaughan, L., Basak, C., Hartmann, M., & Verhaeghen, P. (2008). Aging and working memory inside and outside the focus of attention: Dissociations of availability and accessibility. *Aging, Neuropsychology, & Cognition, 15*(6), 703–724. doi: 10.1080/13825580802061645

Verhaeghen, P. (2012). Working memory still working: Age-related differences in working-memory functioning and cognitive control. In M. Naveh-Benjamin & N. Ohta (Eds.), *Memory and aging: Current issues and future directions* (pp.3–30). Hove: Psychology Press.

Verhaeghen, P., & Basak, C. (2005). Aging and switching of the focus of attention in working memory: Results from a modified N-back task. *Quarterly Journal of Experimental Psychology, 58A*, 134–154.

Verhaeghen, P., & Carella, J. (2002). Aging executive control and attention: A review of meta-analyses. *Neuroscience & Biobehavioral Reviews, 26*, 849–857.

Verhaeghen, P., & Carella, J. (2008). Everything we know about aging and response times: A meta-analytic integration. In S. M. Hofer & D. F. Alwin (Eds.), *The handbook of cognitive aging: Interdisciplinary perspectives* (pp. 134–150). Thousand Oaks, CA: Sage.

Verhaeghen, P., Cerella, J., Bopp, K. L., & Basak, C. (2005). Aging and varieties of cognitive control: A review of meta-analyses on resistance to interference, coordination and task switching, and an experimental exploration of age-sensitivity in the newly identified process of focus switching. In R. W. Engle, G. Sedek, U. Von Hecker & D. N. McIntosh (Eds.), *Cognitive limits in aging and psychopathology: Attention, working memory, and executive functions* (pp. 160–189). New York: Cambridge University Press.

Verhaeghen, P., & De Meersman, L. (1998a). Aging and the Stroop effect: A meta-analysis. *Psychology & Aging, 13*, 120–126.

Verhaeghen, P., & De Meersman, L. (1998b). Aging and negative priming: A meta-analysis. *Psychology & Aging, 13*, 435–444.

Verhaeghen, P., Steitz, D. W., Sliwinski, M. J., & Carella, J. (2003). Aging and dual task performance: A meta-analysis. *Psychology & Aging, 26*, 15–20.

Vygotsky, L. S. (1962/1934). *Thought and language.* Translated by E. Hanfmann & G. Vakar. Cambridge, MA: MIT Press.

Watson, J. B. (1913). Psychology as the behaviourist views it. *Psychological Review, 20*, 158–177.

Wearing, D. (2005). *Forever today: A memoir of love and amnesia.* London: Corgi.

Wixted, J. T. (2004). The psychology and neuroscience of forgetting. *Annual Review of Psychology, 55*, 235–269. doi: 10.1146/annurev.psych.55.090902.141555

Wixted, J. T., & Cai, D. J. (2013). Memory consolidation. In S. Kosslyn & K. Ochsner (Eds.), *Oxford handbook of cognitive neuroscience* (Vol. 2, pp. 436–455). New York: Oxford University Press.

Yonelinas, A. P. (2002). The nature of recollection and familiarity: A review of 30 years of research. *Journal of Memory and Language, 46*, 441–517.

Zacks, R. T., Hasher, L., & Li, K. Z. H. (2000). Human memory. In F. I. M. Craik & T. A. Salthouse (Eds.), *The handbook of aging and cognition* (2nd edition, pp. 293–357). Mahwah, NJ: LEA.

Zelazo, P. D., & Muller, U. (2002). Executive function in typical and atypical development. In U. Goswami (Ed.), *Handbook of childhood cognitive development* (pp. 445–469). Oxford: Blackwell.

2

THE AGING HIPPOCAMPUS

A cross-species examination

Stephanie Leal and Michael Yassa

2.1   Introduction: episodic memory and aging

Memory impairments are a common dysfunction with increasing age. Older adults report memory complaints more frequently than problems in any other cognitive domain (Newson & Kemps, 2006). A large number of studies have shown that episodic memory, or memory for 'events', specifically declines with age in humans (Craik & Simon, 1980; Glisky, 2007; Hedden & Gabrieli, 2004; 2005; Jennings & Jacoby, 1997; Newman & Kaszniak, 2000; Small, Stern, Tang, & Mayeux, 1999). Episodic memory is composed of many components, including object (what), spatial (where), and temporal (when) information. Deficits in both spatial and temporal processing have been reported with aging in animals and humans. Episodic memory has also been classified using a two-process model, which hypothesizes that recollection (specific memory) and familiarity (vague memory) are subserved by different mechanisms. Animal and human data suggest that recollection is selectively impaired by the aging process, while familiarity is relatively spared. Recent data in older rats and humans have also suggested that mnemonic discrimination (dissociating among similar memories) is also compromised with aging. Convergent data from animals and humans suggest that the latter feature is central to the neurocognitive aging process and may explain many of the phenotypes associated with age-related memory decline (e.g., reduced recollection, spatial memory, contextual memory, etc.). Neurobiological evidence suggests that alterations in the medial temporal lobes (hippocampus and surrounding regions) are implicated in these deficits. These recent advances are critical to understanding the nature of age-related memory decline and present novel targets for intervention in reducing or reversing age-related memory deficits. Understanding how the brain changes during normal aging must be investigated before the boundary between normal and pathological conditions can be understood fully (Albert, 2002). In this chapter, we discuss the recently accumulated behavioral and neurobiological evidence for age-related changes in episodic memory, with a particular focus on mnemonic discrimination and its underlying neural computation, pattern separation, and highlight remaining gaps in our understanding and future research directions.

2.2 Memory impairments with aging: a cognitive perspective

2.2.1 Spatial memory impairments with aging

Spatial memory (i.e., memory for spatial configurations and ability to navigate around both familiar and unfamiliar spaces) is one component of episodic memory that has long been known to decline with age (Cohen & Cox, 1977; Gaylord & Marsh, 1975; Perlmutter, Metzger, Nezworski, & Miller, 1981; Salthouse, Mitchell, & Palmon, 1989; Salthouse, Mitchell, Skovronek, & Babcock, 1989). Specifically, older adults have difficulty recalling locations of items (Chalfonte & Johnson, 1996; Uttl & Graf, 1993) or navigating through a recently learned environment (Newman & Kaszniak, 2000; Wilkniss, Jones, Korol, Gold, & Manning, 1997). Age-related changes are accompanied by difficulties in forming and retaining new spatial memories of allocentric relations among locations (Barnes, 1979; Harris & Wolbers, 2012; Head & Isom, 2010; Winocur & Gagnon, 1998). Increasing the similarity between contexts or objects also affects the degree to which memories are retained (Henkel, Johnson, & De Leonardis, 1998).

In rodents, spatial memory has also been known to decline with age (Barnes, 1979; 1988; Gallagher & Pelleymounter, 1988; Gallagher, Burwell, & Burchinal, 1993). The Morris water maze task allows assessment of the rat's ability to learn to navigate to a specific location in a relatively large spatial environment. In this task, rats are placed into a large, circular pool with opaque water in which their goal is to swim to find a hidden platform for safety. Gallagher and colleagues developed a learning index measure that provides information about the spatial distribution of the rat's search during both training and probe trial performance (Gallagher et al., 1993). In their study, aged rats took significantly longer to find the hidden platform across training trials (Figure 2.1a). However, not all aged individuals show memory deficits as a function of chronological age. When examining the learning index scores on the Morris water maze designed to integrate performance over training, Gallagher and colleagues have consistently shown individual differences in aged male outbred Long Evans rats such that some rats aged gracefully (performance on par with the young) and some manifested age-related spatial learning and memory deficits (Figure 2.1b). It is not yet known why this occurs, although many hypotheses have been proposed. For example, some suggest that older adults who do not show age-related declines may have higher 'cognitive reserve', possibly enabling them to be more resilient to brain changes than others (Stern, 2012).

Similar evidence has also been reported in non-human primates (Walker et al., 1988), however, the number of spatial navigation studies in monkeys

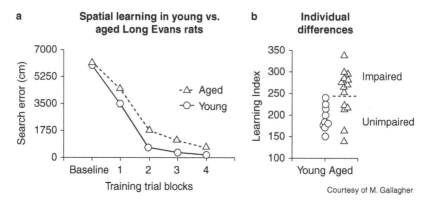

FIGURE 2.1   (a) Amount of time it takes (search error, cm) for rats placed in the Morris water maze to find their way to a hidden platform. Aged rats are slower at finding the platform. (b) Learning index measure based on performance across the training trials suggests that not all aged animals show impairments. A subset of aged animals (Aged Unimpaired) perform just as well as young animals, while a subset of aged animals is impaired (Aged Impaired).

(relative to visuospatial associations or spatial learning) is very limited compared to studies in rodents and humans. In one study, the authors designed a spatial information-processing task in a non-human primate model of cognitive aging, using procedures similar to tasks designed for rats. Monkeys were trained to navigate in a large open field containing eight reward locations. Monkeys rapidly learned to visit each location once per trial. Probe manipulations showed that young animals exhibited 'place learning' and navigated the maze guided by the extra-maze cues (i.e., remembered *where* they went). In contrast, aged monkeys appeared to solve the task using 'response learning', independent of extra-maze spatial information (i.e., remembered a *response*, such as 'turn left') (Rapp, Kansky, & Roberts, 1997). Aged non-human primates have also shown impairments on spatial reversals (rewarded location is reversed compared to initial learning) relative to young adult monkeys (Lai, Moss, Killiany, Rosene, & Herndon, 1995).

2.2.2   Contextual memory and loss of recollection with aging

It has been proposed that recognition memory involves two distinct processes: recollection and familiarity (Wixted, Mickes, & Squire, 2010; Yonelinas, Aly, Wang, & Koen, 2010). The distinction between these two processes can be illustrated by the experience when you recognize and are familiar with a person, but you are not able to recollect who the person is or how you know them. Recollection is associated with recall of specific details, such as location, color, feature or modality of the information (e.g., you remember a person, where you met them, who they are, etc.). Familiarity involves a sense of experience, but lacks any specific details (e.g., you remember the person, but cannot remember where you met them). Such contextual detail recall is diminished in older adults, especially in recently acquired memories (Zacks, Hasher, & Li, 2000). Older adults may attend to salient information but fail to take peripheral detail into account or may fail to integrate contextual aspects of an experience with central content (i.e., a source memory problem) (Glisky, Rubin, & Davidson, 2001).

Both recollection and familiarity can support recognition memory (Yonelinas, 2002); however, the contributions of each to recognition performance may vary according to the type of task used to assess memory. For example, in a yes/no recognition task with targets (repeated items) and foils (completely new items) that share a high level of perceptual overlap (i.e., interference), familiarity alone is not sufficient to guide accurate performance. However, it may be sufficient in a forced-choice recognition paradigm (Westerberg et al., 2006), in which participants are given two items at the same time and asked which one they saw before. Older participants showed a decrease in recollection of unfamiliar faces together with an increase in familiarity and performed better on forced-choice recognition than on yes/no recognition (Bastin & Van der Linden, 2003). This suggests a trade-off in remembering specific information versus more general information in aging.

A signal detection model-based analysis of recognition performance has also been applied to these paradigms using the receiver operating characteristic (ROC) function to plot hit rate (correct item memory) and false alarm rate (incorrect item memory), resulting in a curved graphical depiction of the data. Consistent with the findings discussed above, ROC curve analyses show that older adults exhibit a pattern of impaired recollection and spared familiarity (Daselaar, Fleck, Dobbins, Madden, & Cabeza, 2006; Duverne, Habibi, & Rugg, 2008; Howard, Bessette-Symons, Zhang, & Hoyer, 2006; Prull, Dawes, Martin, Rosenberg, & Light, 2006). In order to provide cross-species evidence of these effects, a similar paradigm that tested odor recognition memory was applied in young and aged rats. Performance was analyzed using an ROC procedure analogous to that used in humans. Young rats appeared to use both recollection and familiarity, while aged rats showed a selective loss of recollection and relative sparing of familiarity, similar to the effects of hippocampal damage and similar to effects previously reported in humans. Furthermore, recollection but not familiarity was correlated with spatial memory; recollection was poorer in spatial memory-impaired aged rats (Robitsek, Fortin, Koh, Gallagher, & Eichenbaum, 2008).

Little work has been done in non-human primates to determine whether aging alters these memory processes. However, recent studies using visual recognition memory tasks in rhesus monkeys suggest that performance is supported by recollection- and familiarity-like processes (Basile & Hampton, 2013; Guderian, Brigham, & Mishkin, 2011). This opens up the possibility of studying these memory processes in aged non-human primates using tasks that are highly analogous to the ones used in humans; however, much more work needs to be done in this area to fully bridge across species.

2.2.3 Susceptibility to interference with aging

Disambiguating similar experiences and overcoming interference is a critical feature of episodic memory (Shapiro & Olton, 1994; Yassa & Stark, 2011). Tasks designed to test this process typically vary the level of perceptual overlap parametrically such that subtle changes in discrimination can be assessed. Across cognitive and behavioral studies in animals and humans, convergent evidence suggests that aging is associated with decreased capacity for novel learning and retention as well as a failure to distinguish between experiences that share common contextual elements, which may be responsible for memory errors. Older adults have difficulty with suppressing irrelevant information, which leads to increased interference in learning new information (Lustig & Hasher, 2001). A number of studies have evaluated young and older adults' ability to discriminate among similar memories (i.e., mnemonic discrimination) across several domains. Below, we describe these results in the object, spatial, temporal, and affective domains.

2.2.3.1 Object domain

The ability of older adults to discriminate among similar object stimuli was tested by Toner and colleagues (2009) as well as Yassa, Lacy, and colleagues (2010) using the same continuous recognition task. Both studies used an identical task design in which young and older adults were shown pictures of everyday objects and asked to indicate for each picture whether it was new, repeated or *similar* to a repeated item. During the task, participants were shown a mixture of new items, repeated items, and items that were similar but not identical to ones previously shown (i.e., lures). Across both studies, the authors reported increases in false alarm rates for similar lures in older adults compared to young adults. Yassa, Lacy et al. (2010) further demonstrated that the discrimination/generalization functions for these stimuli binned according to their mnemonic similarity clearly dissociated young and older adults, but performance on novel and repeated items was indistinguishable between groups.

More recently, a two-phase (incidental study, explicit test) version of the aforementioned object mnemonic discrimination task (Figure 2.2a) was applied to adults ages 18–89 years old, demonstrating that mnemonic discrimination abilities decline as early as the fortieth decade (Stark, Yassa, Lacy, & Stark, 2013). Older adults (age >60) were classified into two groups, aged unimpaired (AU) and aged impaired (AI), based on delayed word recall performance (a standard neuropsychological measure for long-term memory drawn from the Rey Auditory Verbal Learning Task (RAVLT)). The investigators observed impairments in object mnemonic discrimination in the AI group that exceeded the AU group, but no overall impairment in recognition performance across both groups (Figure 2.2d). In contrast, those individuals diagnosed with mild cognitive impairment (MCI) exhibited significantly worse performance on both object discrimination and recognition memory performance (Stark et al., 2013).

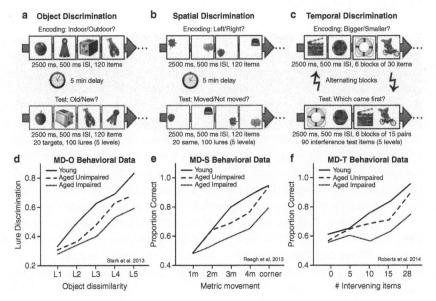

FIGURE 2.2 (a) In the Mnemonic Discrimination Task – Objects Version (MDT-O), participants are shown objects (2500ms, 500ms inter-stimulus interval (ISI)) and asked to respond whether they are indoor or outdoor (encoding phase). After a 5-minute delay, participants are tested on their memory for the items they saw. They are shown repeated items (targets), similar but not identical items (lures), and completely new items (foils) and are asked to perform yes/no recognition. (b) In the Mnemonic Discrimination Task – Spatial Version (MDT-S), participants are shown objects in different locations on the screen (2500ms, 500ms ISI) and are asked to respond whether objects are on the left or right of the screen (encoding phase). After a 5-minute delay, participants are tested on their memory for item locations. They are shown items in the same locations and items that changed locations (lures), which varied in metric distance from the original locations. (c) In the Mnemonic Discrimination Task – Temporal Version (MDT-T), participants are shown objects (2500ms, 500ms ISI) and are asked to indicate whether the current object is bigger or smaller than the previous object (encoding phase); this type of instruction was intended to foster sequential encoding. During the test phase, participants were shown pairs of stimuli on the screen and asked which one came first in the study sequence (i.e., a temporal order judgment). Test item pairs varied in the temporal lag between them during the study phase. (d) Performance measured by lure discrimination (ability to correctly reject similar lures) shows that with increasing object dissimilarity, performance improves across age groups. Older adults were split into aged impaired (AI) and aged unimpaired (AU) groups according to whether or not they were within the young norms on the RAVLT. Both AU and AI adults performed worse than young adults; however, impairment was larger in AI adults. (e) Performance measured by proportion correct shows that with increasing metric movement, performance improves across age groups. AU adults perform on par with young adults in the easiest and hardest conditions, but are impaired in the middle conditions. AI adults perform more poorly than both AU and young adults across all conditions except for the most difficult discrimination, where all three groups approached floor performance. (f) Performance measured by proportion correct shows that with increasing number of intervening items (i.e., temporal lag), performance improves in all age groups. In this case, older adults were split into AI and AU groups based on their performance on a primacy measure (see Roberts, Ly, Murray, & Yassa, 2014, for details). AU adults perform on par with young adults in the easiest and hardest conditions, but are impaired in the middle conditions. AI adults perform more poorly than both AU and young adults across all conditions except for the most difficult discrimination, where all three groups approached floor performance.

In rats and monkeys, similar tasks have been designed in which the perceptual features of objects are slightly altered from the original to test the animals' ability to discriminate these items. One study investigated the ability of young and aged animals to distinguish between objects that shared features. In one study, the investigators trained young and aged rats on performing a spontaneous object recognition task, in which the time taken to investigate a novel object is compared to the time taken to investigate a familiar object (presented during the training phase). Under normal conditions, more time is spent investigating the novel object during the test phase. When the test objects did not share any features (easy perceptual discrimination), both young and aged rats correctly identified the novel object. When the test objects contained overlapping features (similar to lure items as discussed in the human studies), only the young rats showed an exploratory preference for the lure item (Burke et al., 2011). An analogous procedure was used in non-human primates. When the object pairs were dissimilar, both young and aged monkeys learned to select the rewarded object quickly. In contrast, when object pairs contained overlapping features, the aged monkeys took significantly longer than did the young animals to learn to discriminate between the rewarded and the unrewarded object (Burke et al., 2011). Together, these results suggest that discrimination of similar object information is reduced with aging, in a manner that is consistent across species.

2.2.3.2 Spatial domain

Studies evaluating mnemonic discrimination in the spatial domain generally employ a logic based on early work in hippocampal-lesioned rodents (Gilbert, Kesner, & DeCoteau, 1998), which assessed the ability to judge whether stimuli presented during a test phase had moved from locations in which they were originally presented. The difficulty of discrimination is typically tested by systematically varying the metric distance between the study and test phases.

Using this logic, one study (Stark, Yassa, & Stark, 2010) used a spatial discrimination task in which individuals studied pairs of unfamiliar scenes presented concurrently on the screen in randomly assigned positions. During the test phase, participants were asked to indicate if the image pair was in the same location as during the study phase, or if one of the images moved. The difficulty of the discrimination was manipulated according to the exact metric distance of the image moved. Older adults were found to perform on par with young adults in general on the task; however, their performance on the task correlated with their performance on a word list recall test (RAVLT). When the RAVLT was used to divide the older adults into AU and AI groups, the AI group was significantly impaired on the task compared to both AU and young adult groups.

Another study (Holden & Gilbert, 2012) used a delayed-match-to-sample discrimination task in which during the sample phase (study), a circle briefly appeared in a specific location on a computer screen. During the choice phase (test), two circles were displayed simultaneously, and the participant was asked to indicate which circle was in the same location as the one shown during the sample phase. Performance increased as a function of increased metric distance between study and test phases in both young and older adults. However, young adults outperformed older adults on the task overall, possibly indicating a failure of discrimination abilities in older adults.

Finally, a recent study (Reagh et al., 2013) used a spatial discrimination task with single objects presented in one of 35 grid locations on the screen during the study phase (Figure 2.2b). During the test phase, subjects were asked if the object currently viewed was presented in the same location or a different location from study. Difficulty was manipulated using the number of grid spaces moved, which varied from 0–4 spaces. Also included was a control condition that did not require fine-level discrimination, in which objects moved from one corner to the diagonal corner. Overall, older adults showed a general deficit on the task compared to young adults. When older adults were split into AI and AU groups according to the RAVLT, AI individuals were found to be impaired at every interference level, including trials with minimal interference (corner moves) (Figure 2.2e). AU individuals, on the other hand, were not impaired at the highest and lowest interference bins compared to young adults. The results suggest that when discrimination is too difficult or when it is not required, there is no significant age-related deficit. On trials that require interference reduction and the discrimination is not too difficult, there is a significant age-related deficit that is more severe in some individuals than others.

Collectively, the cognitive studies evaluating spatial discrimination in older adults strongly suggest that spatial discrimination is impaired in at least a subset of older adults, with some expressing performance on par with young adults under most testing conditions.

2.2.3.3 Temporal domain

Studies evaluating mnemonic discrimination in the temporal domain are based on the notion that experiences that are presented in close temporal proximity will be more difficult to disambiguate than experiences that are presented farther apart in time. Thus, the time between study items presented is the critical variable used to manipulate temporal interference.

Perlmutter and colleagues (1981) investigated temporal order memory in older adults by showing them a sequence of drawings on paper. After viewing the sequence of drawings, they were shown pairs of drawings from the sequence and asked to determine which of the objects appeared earlier in the original sequence. The study found no differences between young adults and older adults with respect to the number of correct responses; however, the authors noted that older adults took more time with the task. In a more recent investigation (Tolentino, Pirogovsky, Luu, Toner, & Gilbert, 2012), which was modeled after temporal discrimination tasks in rodents (Gilbert, Kesner, & Lee, 2001), participants were shown a digital representation of an overhead view of an eight-arm radial maze. A dot appeared at the end of each of the arms for 2 seconds followed by 2 seconds between stimuli, creating a sequence of eight events. In the test phase, two dots simultaneously appeared at the ends of two arms and the participants were asked to indicate in which arm the dot appeared earlier in the original sequence. In contrast to Perlmutter et al. (1981), the authors found that older adults were impaired relative to young adults, which they suggested might be attributed to a deficit in discrimination of temporal information in aging.

Finally, a recent study examining temporal discrimination in young and older adults used study-test blocks that were composed of sequences of 30 stimuli (Figure 2.2c). Subjects were shown objects one at a time and asked to indicate whether the object was bigger or smaller than the prior object to foster sequential relational encoding. During the test phase, subjects were presented with two previously presented stimuli side-by-side and asked to indicate which one came first in the sequence. Paired objects varied in the amount of temporal lag between their study presentations. Older adults were impaired relative to young adults at moderate and high temporal lags (Roberts et al., 2014), but not at low lags (where performance approached floor). Older adults' ability to benefit from primacy, defined in this task as an enhanced performance for order judgment on the first few items of any given sequence, was used to split older adults into AI and AU groups, with the AU group's primacy performance on par with young adults. Temporal discrimination performance in AU adults was similar to young adults at the highest and lowest lags with a marked change in the middle bins, whereas AI adults were consistently impaired across all bins except the most difficult one, in which performance approached floor. The latter is consistent with a generalized temporal processing deficit (Figure 2.2f).

Little work has been done in animals to determine whether aging alters these temporal discrimination processes. However, tasks such as the one used by Gilbert and colleagues (2001) can be used to test temporal discrimination in rodents. To assess spatial temporal order memory, rats were allowed to visit each arm of a radial eight-arm maze once in a randomly determined sequence. The rats were then presented with two arms and were required to choose the arm that occurred earliest in the sequence. The choice arms varied according to temporal separation (0, 2, 4 or 6) or the number of arms that occurred between the two choice arms in the sample phase sequence (Gilbert et al., 2001). These paradigms open up the possibility of studying the neural mechanisms of temporal memory in aged animals, where much more work needs to be done.

2.2.3.4   Affective domain

While episodic memory deficits are a hallmark characteristic of aging, emotion's modulatory influence on memory remains less well characterized in aging. Decades of research in healthy young animals have shown that emotional (or affective) experiences are better remembered than non-emotional experiences (LeDoux, 2007; McGaugh, 2004). Many human studies have shown that memory for emotional experiences is preserved with age (Denburg, Buchanan, Tranel, & Adolphs, 2003; Kensinger, Brierley, Medford, Growdon, & Corkin, 2002). However, not all aspects of an emotional event are remembered better. Emotional arousal can enhance memory for the general theme or 'gist-based' information but impair memory for detailed information (Adolphs, Denburg, & Tranel, 2001; Kensinger, 2009). This trade-off likely plays a critical role in the storage of long-lasting memories and distinguishes the aspects of those memories that are remembered with better accuracy. Additionally, some have suggested that there is a 'positivity effect', where older adults may be more likely to attend to positive information in the environment (Mather & Carstensen, 2005; Wong et al., 2012). In contrast, some have suggested that memory for detailed information in older adults reveals no such positivity effect and may actually be biased towards remembering negative details (Kensinger, Garoff-Eaton, & Schacter, 2007). Very few studies have further investigated these potential alterations in emotional mnemonic discrimination in aging.

Only one study to our knowledge (Leal & Yassa, 2014) used an emotional interference paradigm to examine affective discrimination in young and older adults. Participants were shown scenes that varied in emotional valence (negative, positive or neutral) during the study phase. During the test phase, participants were shown some of the same scenes they saw before, similar but not identical scenes (lures), and completely new scenes and were asked to make an old or new judgment. While young adults showed reduced emotional compared to neutral discrimination of similar items, the pattern was reversed in older adults. The shift in emotional modulation could be due to at least two possible explanations: 1) a compensatory effect such that emotional arousal can boost discrimination performance on similar items and help increase memory for more important emotional events, or 2) an aberration of emotional-mnemonic processing in older adults such that the boost in emotional discrimination is actually maladaptive, since it would be better to remember the gist for emotional events rather than the details. Young adults' discrimination (ability to suppress false recognition) was enhanced on neutral items compared to emotional items, presumably due to a trade-off between gist and detail. Thus, it may be more adaptive to forget minute details of emotional experiences in favor of retaining the bigger picture (Adolphs et al., 2001; Kensinger, 2009; Loftus, Loftus, & Messo, 1987). Older adults, on the other hand, appear to suppress false alarms better for emotional items, suggesting that they may be engaging in a more costly mnemonic operation without clear adaptive value.

Although slightly different from emotional modulation, discrimination of reward value (Gilbert & Kesner, 2002) has been tested in hippocampal-lesioned rats, but has yet to be applied to aged animals. Further developing such discrimination tasks in animal models will aid in our understanding of emotion- and valence-based mnemonic discrimination and how these processes change with age.

2.3 Memory impairments with aging: a neurobiological perspective

2.3.1 Medial temporal lobe anatomy

The medial temporal lobe (MTL), which consists of the hippocampus and surrounding structures, has a well-established role in memory processing (Milner, Squire, & Kandel, 1998; Squire, Stark, & Clark, 2004) and is particularly vulnerable to the effects of advancing age (Burke & Barnes, 2006; Chee et al., 2006; Murty et al., 2009; Raz et al., 2005; Sperling, 2007; Wilson, Gallagher, Eichenbaum, & Tanila, 2006). In this section, we attempt to synthesize recent neurobiological, neurophysiological, and neuroimaging findings across species on the changes associated with aging, focusing in particular on the hippocampal system.

The MTL network is made up of multiple structures, including the hippocampus (which includes CA1–4 (*cornu ammonis*) and the dentate gyrus (DG)), subiculum, presubiculum, parasubiculum, perirhinal cortex (PRC), parahippocampal cortex (PHC), entorhinal cortex (EC), and the amygdala (Figure 2.3). Each structure has multiple input and output pathways and is part of an extensive neural network with intricate connectivity. There are multiple levels of associative processing in the MTL, with the type of information processed becoming more complex from cortical structures to hippocampus (Lavenex & Amaral, 2000).

Briefly, the PRC and PHC receive sensory input from association cortices. This information projects to the EC, in which EC layer II neurons project to the DG and CA3 subregions of the hippocampus (via the perforant path). Granule cells in the DG project to CA3 via the mossy fiber pathway. Pyramidal cells in CA3 project to CA1 via Schaffer collaterals. Additionally, CA3 pyramidal cells heavily project back onto themselves, creating a recurrent collateral network. Pyramidal cells in CA1 project to the subiculum. Both CA1 and subiculum project to the deep layers of the EC (layers IV and V). This is the major output pathway from the hippocampus to cortical structures, including back to PRC and PHC, which project back to neocortical regions.

This description of hippocampal connectivity and processing is overly simplified, but encompasses the major studied pathways of the hippocampal 'trisynaptic circuit' (EC→DG→CA3→CA1) (Amaral, Scharfman, & Lavenex, 2007; Lavenex & Amaral, 2000; Squire et al., 2004). The hippocampus is also under modulatory control from several sources: 1) the DG, CA1, and the CA3 receive cholinergic input from the medial septum, and 2) the DG receives noradrenergic input from the locus coeruleus, serotonergic input from the Raphe nuclei, and dopaminergic input from the ventral tegmental area (Figure 2.3).

This network of brain regions that make up the MTL are intricately connected and project widely to the rest of the brain. The same network is also highly susceptible to age-related changes in functional and representational capacity, plasticity, modulatory and inhibitory tone, and adult neurogenesis. We discuss these changes in detail in the following sections.

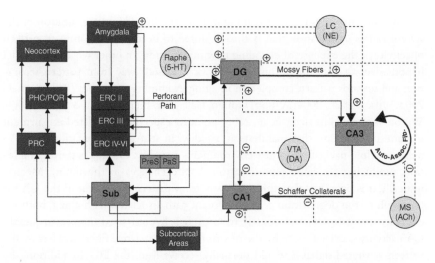

FIGURE 2.3 A schematic representation of the medial temporal lobe anatomical connections. Entorhinal cortex (ERC) layer II projects to the hippocampus (medium grey boxes), specifically the dentate gyrus (DG) subregion via the perforant path, which then projects to CA3 via mossy fibers, then to CA1 via Schaffer collaterals, then to the subiculum, and back to ERC IV-VI. The ERC receives reciprocal connections from surrounding medial temporal lobe regions such as the perirhinal cortex (PRC), parahippocampal cortex (PHC, or postrhinal in the rat (POR)), amygdala, and neocortex (dark grey boxes). Acetylcholine (ACh) from the medial septum (MS), dopamine (DA) from the ventral tegmental area (VTA), norepinephrine (NE) from the locus coeruleus (LC), and serotonin (5-HT) from the Raphe nucleus (light grey circles) can provide modulatory input into the hippocampus at various subregions of the hippocampus and alter hippocampal functioning.

2.3.2   Reduced pattern separation in the aging hippocampus

The hippocampus has been proposed to be involved in two key computations: pattern separation and pattern completion. Pattern separation is the process of reducing interference among similar inputs by using non-overlapping representations and is thought to rely on hippocampal DG. Pattern completion is the process by which representations can be retrieved when given partial or degraded input and is ascribed to hippocampal CA3, where the region's recurrent collaterals may act as an auto-associative network (Marr, 1971; McClelland, McNaughton, & O'Reilly, 1995; Treves & Rolls, 1994; Yassa & Stark, 2011). These computations are thought to underlie the behavioral phenomenon of mnemonic discrimination and give rise to our rich episodic memories.

In 2006, Wilson and colleagues proposed a model of neurocognitive aging (Wilson et al., 2006), suggesting that small concurrent changes during aging strengthen the auto-associative network of the CA3 subregion of the hippocampus at the cost of processing new information coming in from the EC. This reorganization of the system causes information that is already stored to become the dominant pattern of activity at the expense of encoding new information. In other words, the model hypothesizes that the hippocampal network is biased away from pattern separation and towards pattern completion in aging. A number of studies (Wilson et al., 2003; Wilson et al., 2004; Wilson, Ikonen, Gallagher, Eichenbaum, & Tanila, 2005; Wilson, Ikonen, Gurevicius et al., 2005) point to a specific age-related impairment in pattern separation that manifests as 'rigidity' in spatial representations in CA3 neurons while navigating similar environments (i.e., bias towards pattern completion, producing the same representation despite changes in the input). Mechanistically, it is proposed that this shift away from pattern separation in the CA3 is the result of the degradation of the perforant path associated with aging, both via degraded input to DG and directly to CA3. It is hypothesized that, consequently, CA3 activity is driven more by the recurrent auto-associative fibers and less by the pattern-separated signal it would normally receive from the DG. In addition, the model proposes that hyperactivity in CA3's auto-associative network is the result of attenuated cholinergic modulation of the hippocampus and concomitant reduction in inhibitory interneuron activity, which we discuss in later sections.

Notably, these age-related deficits are only found in a subset of aged rats. As previously mentioned, some aged rats are completely unimpaired in spatial learning and behave just like young rats (Gallagher et al., 1993; Figure 2.1b). AU rats are intact in terms of neuron number, hippocampal synaptic density (Rapp & Gallagher, 1996; Smith, Adams, Gallagher, Morrison, & Rapp, 2000), and cholinergic signaling mechanisms (Chouinard, Gallagher, Yasuda, Wolfe, & McKinney, 1995; Nicolle, Gallagher, & McKinney, 2001; Zhang, Lin, & Nicolelis, 2010). There is some evidence, however, that AU rats shift synaptic plasticity mechanisms in order to rescue performance (Boric, Muñoz, Gallagher, & Kirkwood, 2008; Lee, Min, Gallagher, & Kirkwood, 2005). Together, these findings suggest that age-related learning deficits are due to an inability to overcome interference from previously stored information (a bias towards pattern completion), which weakens the processing of new information.

The above model was extended to older humans using high-resolution (1.5 mm isotropic) functional magnetic resonance imaging (fMRI), capable of resolving hippocampal subfields (although DG and CA3 are combined into a single subregion). During an object mnemonic discrimination task (described earlier), older adults were found to exhibit 'representational rigidity' in the DG/CA3 region, which manifested as a diminished novelty response to similar but not identical items (Yassa, Mattfeld, Stark, & Stark, 2011). Compared to young adults, their performance on the object mnemonic discrimination task was impaired, and the extent of the impairment correlated with the extent of their fMRI activity rigidity. Using ultrahigh-resolution diffusion imaging, which measures microstructural features of white matter, the study also quantified both the integrity of the perforant path (input pathway to the hippocampus) as well as DG/CA3 dendritic integrity and found that both were correlated with DG/CA3 representational rigidity. Overall, these results provide strong cross-species support for the model proposed by Wilson and colleagues (2006).

In contrast to these results, a recent study using zif268/egr1 as a marker of cellular activity showed that the DG in older animals was more likely to recruit distinct granule cell populations during two visits to highly similar (or even the same) environments. However, if two highly distinct environments are visited, this age-related change is no longer apparent (Marrone, Adams, & Satvat, 2011). The authors interpret this as an increase in pattern separation with aging. One potential alternative interpretation of these data, however, is that the stability of DG representations is compromised with age, which may phenocopy a pattern separation enhancement but be the result of instability rather than increased sparsity. Consistent with this alternative, the authors show that this change in DG firing patterns correlates with decline in the ability of aged animals to disambiguate similar contexts in a sequential spatial recognition task. Whether the signals reported here are evidence for a more efficient pattern separation process or evidence for age-related instability requires further studies, which must also consider other age-related changes in the hippocampal network such as changes in neurogenesis.

2.3.3   Reduced EC input to hippocampal DG and CA3

Reductions in hippocampal volume, measured using MRI, have been reported in typical aging, the extent of which predicts declining memory performance (Golomb et al., 1996). High-resolution MRI studies have suggested that this volume loss is specific to CA1 and the DG/CA3 subregions (Mueller & Weiner, 2009). While earlier rodent studies suggested that the volume reduction seen in the hippocampus of aged animals was due to neuronal cell loss (Scheibel, Lindsay, Tomiyasu, & Scheibel, 1976), more recent studies using unbiased stereological techniques (Rapp & Gallagher, 1996) reliably demonstrated that this was not the case. The primary cause underlying volume reductions in the hippocampus appears to be synapse loss (Burke & Barnes, 2006). This synapse loss appears to be highly specific to the cortical inputs into the hippocampus (e.g., the perforant path). In aged rats, the DG receives approximately one-third fewer synaptic connections from EC layer II than in young rats (Geinisman, de Toledo-Morrell, Morrell, Persina, & Rossi, 1992; Smith et al., 2000). The amount of synaptic reduction of the perforant path correlates with the degree of spatial memory impairment in aged rats (Smith et al., 2000). Electrophysiological studies have shown that stimulating the perforant path generates less excitation of the DG in aged rats compared to young rats (Burke & Barnes, 2006).

Studies in humans using diffusion tensor imaging (DTI), which measures microstructural features of white matter, have found changes in the parahippocampal region in normal aging (Jahng et al., 2011). Recent studies using DTI at ultrahigh in-plane resolution (0.7 mm) revealed evidence of age-related perforant path degradation in humans *in vivo* (Yassa, Lacy et al., 2010; Yassa et al., 2011). This degradation was pathway specific, as there was no loss found in the alveus. This pathway is also part of the MTL and was used as a control pathway, since age-related changes do not occur in the alveus. Overall, these results suggest that pathway degradation is not a feature of global decline with age, but rather is specific to particular pathways that are vulnerable to the aging process. Importantly, the extent of perforant path reduction in older adults correlated with performance on object mnemonic discrimination tasks and the RAVLT, which confirms that perforant path integrity is related to memory impairment (Yassa et al., 2011; Yassa, Stark et al., 2010). Overall, these findings suggest that a major change in neurocognitive aging is the loss of input from the EC to the DG and CA3 subregions of the hippocampus in both animal models of neurocognitive aging and normal aging humans.

2.3.4 Hyperexcitability and reduced inhibitory tone in the aging hippocampus

The largest source of input to the hippocampal CA3 region is itself. With its massive recurrent collateral network, the CA3 network is typically kept under tight inhibitory control, which plays a role in preventing runaway excitation that can lead to seizure activity and instability of information processing. Data from Wilson, Ikonen, Gallagher, Eichenbaum, and Tanila (2005) demonstrate that place cells in aged rodents' CA3 region exhibit abnormally elevated firing rates. This is perhaps due to the loss of inhibition that occurs with age, which may reinforce the CA3 recurrent collateral network, simultaneously leading to hyperactivity and to a shift in the balance between excitation and inhibition (Hasselmo, 2006; Vela, Gutierrez, Vitorica, & Ruano, 2003), which may then lead to a shift in computational processing from pattern separation to pattern completion (Wilson et al., 2006).

CA3 gamma oscillations (20–80 Hz) in mouse hippocampal slices exhibit age-related changes. For example, induced gamma oscillations were decreased in aged mice relative to young mice, a change that was associated with reduced activity in CA3 inhibitory interneurons (Vreugdenhil & Toescu, 2005). Recently, intracranial recordings in freely moving animals and extracellular recordings in hippocampal slices both revealed frequent spikes in the CA3 of aged mice, while these spikes occurred only occasionally in the CA3 of young mice. Spontaneous field potentials with large amplitudes, originating from CA3, were also frequently observed in hippocampal slices of aged mice but rarely in slices from young adults (El-Hayek et al., 2013). In AI rats, a reduction in the expression of genes underlying synaptic inhibition was found, as measured by performance on the Morris water maze task, which is consistent with increased neuronal firing rates recorded from principal CA3 pyramidal cells (Haberman, Colantuoni, Koh, & Gallagher, 2013).

Consistent with animal studies, human studies using fMRI to examine activity in the hippocampus during memory task performance have also demonstrated similar evidence of hyperactivity. Using a face-name association task, elevated activity in the hippocampus was found in low-performing older adults (Miller et al.,

2008). More recently, high-resolution fMRI was used to specifically test whether the DG/CA3 selectively expressed such hyperactivity. Using the object mnemonic discrimination task that is intended to assess the capacity for pattern separation in hippocampal subfields, Yassa, Lacy, and colleagues (2010) found that older adults exhibited elevated activation levels selectively in the DG/CA3 region during task performance, the extent of which predicted performance impairments. Evidence of a more dramatic version of this hyperactivity was also reported in individuals with MCI, a prodrome for Alzheimer's disease (Yassa, Stark et al., 2010).

One important aspect of the hippocampal network are the numerous interneurons that are involved in inhibition, which is important for keeping the system from becoming over excited (i.e., hyperactivity). The density of interneurons positive for the gamma-aminobutyric acid (GABA)-synthesizing enzyme glutamate decarboxylase-67 (GAD-67) declines as a function of age in area CA1 of the hippocampus (Shetty & Turner, 1998; Shi, Argenta, Winseck, & Brunso-Bechtold, 2004; Stanley & Shetty, 2004; Vela et al., 2003). The density of interneurons positive for somatostatin (SOM), calbindin, and neuropeptide Y (NPY) decreases with aging (Cadiacio, Milner, Gallagher, & Pierce, 2003; Vela et al., 2003). Specific losses have been found for interneurons in the hilus that express NPY (Cadiacio et al., 2003). Numbers of GAD67- and SOM-positive interneurons decline with age across multiple fields of the hippocampus; however, alterations specifically related to cognitive performance in aged animals were observed exclusively in the hilus of the DG. The total number of NeuN-immunoreactive hilar neurons was unaffected, suggesting the decline observed with other markers likely reflects a loss of target protein rather than neuron death (Spiegel, Koh, Vogt, Rapp, & Gallagher, 2013). Stereological quantification of SOM-immunoreactive neurons in the DG hilus of diversity outbred mice showed that high-performing young and AU mice had similar numbers of SOM-positive interneurons, while aged mice that were impaired in the Morris water maze task had significantly fewer such neurons (Koh, Spiegel, & Gallagher, 2014).

Across species, the data suggest that hyperactivity is an index of network dysfunction and disinhibition and not evidence of adaptive compensation. This elevation in activity can be targeted with inhibitory pharmacological manipulations that reduce excitation (levetiracetam, an anti-epileptic) or enhance inhibition (NPY enhancement) (Koh, Haberman, Foti, McCown, & Gallagher, 2010), reversing memory deficits in treated animals. When treated with the levetiracetam, hilar SOM expression was fully restored in AI rats, suggesting that this is a pharmacologically modifiable target (Spiegel et al., 2013).

The remarkable consistency across animal and human studies here was used recently to leverage translational work in a clinical trial with low-dose levetiracetam in individuals with MCI. The proof-of-concept trial reported positive results in which levetiracetam successfully reduced DG/CA3 hyperactivity and reversed deficits on the object mnemonic discrimination task (Bakker et al., 2012). This approach may have strong therapeutic potential, contingent on successful Phase III clinical trials in individuals with MCI and age-related memory impairment.

2.3.5   Reduced modulatory input to the aging hippocampus

Aging is associated with decreases in modulatory inputs to the hippocampus, which could alter the balance between excitation and inhibition of hippocampal subregions, leading to hippocampal dysregulation and interacting with the afore-mentioned deficits in inhibition. Below we describe these changes in specific neu-rotransmitter systems.

2.3.5.1   Cholinergic modulation

In what are now considered to be classic studies, young human subjects who were given scopolamine, a cholinergic antagonist, showed memory impairments that were very similar to the memory impairments reported in aged individuals (Drach-man & Leavitt, 1974). The assumed mechanism implicated cholinergic neurons of the basal forebrain, since these cells exhibited neurodegeneration in AD (Davies & Maloney, 1976; Whitehouse, Price, Clark, Coyle, & DeLong, 1981). The basal fore-brain cholinergic system modulates cortical and limbic structures and can alter learning and memory mechanisms. Experimentally reducing cholinergic input replicates the age-related learning deficits (Ikonen, McMahan, Gallagher, Eichen-baum, & Tanila, 2002), while activating the medial septum using a cholinergic ago-nist reverses them (Sava & Markus, 2008). A recent study administered a single dose of a muscarinic receptor antagonist before and after healthy older adults performed a delayed recall task and measured hippocampus and basal forebrain volumes. They found that higher doses of the muscarinic antagonist reduced delayed recall per-formance and was related to an uncoupling of the association of task performance with cholinergic basal forebrain and hippocampal volumes (Teipel, Bruno, Grothe, Nierenberg, & Pomara, 2015). Increases in cholinergic activity are thought to bias the hippocampus towards learning new information, whereas decreased cholinergic modulation is thought to favor the reactivation of previously stored information (Hasselmo & Schnell, 1994; Hasselmo & Wyble, 1997). Investigations of choliner-gic modulation in aged rodents demonstrated a depletion of cholinergic tone, the extent of which correlated with the degree of memory impairment (Chouinard et al., 1995; Nicolle et al., 2001; Sugaya et al., 1998). Reduced cholinergic input in aging may also decrease inhibition in the CA3 auto-associative network (Hasselmo, Schnell, & Barkai, 1995; Wilson et al., 2006), contributing to an overactive CA3 (discussed earlier).

2.3.5.2   Dopaminergic modulation

Dopaminergic (DA) neurons also have a modulatory influence on memory process-ing (Taghzouti, Louilot, Herman, Le Moal, & Simon, 1985). Studies have reported an age-dependent degeneration of substantia nigra/ventral tegmental area dopamine neurons in aging (Bäckman et al., 2006; Fearnley & Lees, 1991), which may affect the hippocampus's ability to consolidate memories (Chowdhury, Guitart-Masip,

Bunzeck, Dolan, & Duzel, 2012). Loss of dopaminergic neurons that specifically project to CA1 has been reported, which may contribute to impairments in synaptic plasticity (Lisman & Grace, 2005; Siddiqi, Kemper, & Killiany, 1999). A recent study conducted in healthy older adults suggested that administering levodopa (a DA precursor) within a narrow dose range to older adults enhances scene recollection, a benefit that appears to influence consolidation mechanisms rather than encoding (Chowdhury et al., 2012). Evidence from studies using positron emission topography (PET), in which tracers are injected to allow visualization of certain compounds in the brain, link DA receptor density to cognitive performance. Specifically, DA binding in the hippocampus was found to be correlated with immediate recall (Cervenka, Bäckman, Cselényi, Halldin, & Farde, 2008; Takahashi et al., 2007). Importantly, DA loss with age of both D2 receptors and dopamine transporter appears to mediate age-related episodic memory deficits (Bäckman et al., 2000; Erixon-Lindroth et al., 2005). Overall, this suggests that there are alterations in dopamine input to the hippocampus, which may result in changes in hippocampal function (such as memory dysfunction).

2.3.5.3 Noradrenergic modulation

The locus coeruleus is the principal site for the synthesis for noradrenaline (or norepinephrine, NE). These neurons project widely to several brain regions, including the hippocampus and amygdala (Bass, Nizam, Partain, Wang, & Manns, 2014; Hu et al., 2007). A reduction of NE input to the hippocampus (Kubanis & Zornetzer, 1981) as well as changes in peripheral epinephrine levels (Sternberg, Martinez, Gold, & McGaugh, 1985) have been reported in animal models of aging. Aged rats that were impaired on Morris water maze task performance had a global decrease in NE concentrations throughout the hippocampus. The extent of NE depletion in dorsal hippocampus was associated with the extent of memory deficits in aged animals (Stemmelin, Lazarus, Cassel, Kelche, & Cassel, 2000).

In humans, it has been shown that the locus coeruleus develops fully formed neurofibrillary tangles (hyperphosphorylated tau) and their precursors in the course of normal aging, but these abnormalities become significantly more prominent in MCI and early Alzheimer's disease. The extent of this locus coeruleus pathology is correlated with overall cognitive state as measured by the Mini Mental State Examination (a test for general cognitive functioning), suggesting that noradrenergic dysfunction may be among the numerous factors mediating the onset of cognitive impairments in the aging-MCI-AD continuum (Grudzien et al., 2007).

2.3.5.4 Serotonergic modulation

Serotonin (5-HT) neurons are primarily located in the Raphe nucleus in the brainstem. There are limited and conflicting data in the literature regarding changes in the 5-HT system in normal aging. Several post mortem human studies have reported a reduction in the number of serotonin binding sites with age in frontal lobe, occipital lobe, and hippocampus. A decline in 5-HT function with aging is consistent with observations of age-related changes in behaviors, such as sleep, that are linked to serotonergic function (Meltzer et al., 1998). However, some analyses of post mortem human and animal brains fail to demonstrate a decline with age in the concentrations of 5-HT or its primary metabolite. In some instances, there is an age-related increase in the brain content of these compounds (McEntee & Crook, 1991). Thus, the state of the evidence regarding serotonergic modulation in the aging brain is conflicting and requires further investigation.

2.4   Reduced adult neurogenesis in the aging DG

There is extensive evidence that new neurons are generated in the DG during adulthood, with a subset of these new neurons becoming functional mature granule cells that are incorporated into the DG (van Praag et al., 2002). The exact role of adult neurogenesis in modulating learning and memory mechanisms is not well understood. Several studies have reported that factors that improve memory, such as exercise (see Chapter 9) and enriched environments, can also increase neurogenesis (Fabel et al., 2009; Gould, Beylin, Tanapat, Reeves, & Shors,1999; van Praag, 2009). Likewise, factors that impair memory, such as aging, stress, and other diseases, are associated with lower neurogenesis levels (Jessberger & Gage, 2008; Warner-Schmidt & Duman, 2006). It has been suggested that neurogenesis may play an important role in pattern separation. When DG neurogenesis was knocked down by focal x-irradiation, deficits were seen in a touchscreen task that relies on fine discrimination (Clelland et al., 2009). Several studies have also demonstrated that enhancement of neurogenesis via exercise (Creer, Romberg, Saksida, van Praag, & Bussey, 2010) as well as genetically enhancing the survivability of newborn granule cells (Sahay et al., 2011) improved discrimination performance, which is thought to rely on pattern separation mechanisms.

Interestingly, newborn granule cells receive preferential innervation from the lateral entorhinal cortex (LEC) and not the medial entorhinal cortex (MEC) (Vivar et al., 2012; Vivar & van Praag, 2013), which may have implications for learning mechanisms, as the predominant view is that the LEC selectively provides external sensory input to the hippocampus, with the PHC and MEC providing internally generated self-motion for path integration (Knierim, Neunuebel, & Deshmukh, 2014). This may be partially responsible for the failure to learn new information that is common with aging.

Although neurogenesis continues throughout life, its rate declines with increasing age (Czéh & Lucassen, 2007; Gould et al., 1999; Kempermann, 2002; Kuhn, Dickinson-Anson, & Gage, 1996; Seki & Arai, 1995). In aged rats, the proliferation rate of neural progenitor stem cells in the DG is reduced by 80% (Jin et al., 2003). The age-associated reduction in adult neurogenesis may be associated with changes in responsiveness to environmental cues (Lichtenwalner et al., 2001). Repeated social stress significantly decreased the rate of neural progenitor stem cell proliferation in mice (Mitra, Sundlass, Parker, Schatzberg, & Lyons, 2006), while environmental enrichment reversed these effects (Kempermann, 2002; van Praag, Kempermann, & Gage, 1999). Thus, environmental conditions may have a crucial role in the modulation of neurogenesis during aging. It has been proposed that the age-related decline in neurogenesis may underlie memory deficits and could contribute to pathological conditions such as Alzheimer's disease (Donovan et al., 2006; Haughey, Liu, Nath, Borchard, & Mattson, 2002; Haughey, Nath et al., 2002). While neurogenesis may contribute to DG function, neurogenesis alone is not sufficient to preserve function during normal aging (Galvan & Jin, 2007). Furthermore, while neurogenesis clearly declines in aged animals, the extent to which it is linked to age-related memory deficits is unclear (e.g. see Bizon & Gallagher, 2003).

A recent study assessing the generation of hippocampal cells in humans by measuring the concentration of nuclear-bomb-test-derived 14C in genomic DNA found that neurons are generated throughout adulthood and that the rates are comparable in middle-aged humans and mice, with only a modest decline during aging (Spalding et al., 2013). Thus, although neurogenesis declines with age in both humans and rodents, the relative decline during adulthood appears smaller in humans than in rodents. While assessing neurogenesis *in vivo* in humans has remained a significant challenge (Ho, Hooker, Sahay, Holt, & Roffman, 2013), some studies have provided evidence consistent with the notion that adult neurogenesis in humans is a modifiable target. For example, Pereira et al. (2007) used gadolinium-enhanced high-resolution perfusion imaging to show that cerebral blood volume (CBV) in the human DG increases as a function of exercise, which is hypothesized to target newborn granule cells (although this relationship is certainly not exclusive, and may be indirect). It is more likely that this marker is an index of healthy synaptic function in the region, rather than a specific marker for neurogenesis. It is worth noting that high-resolution CBV perfusion was used in a recent interventional trial of flavanol treatment, demonstrating enhanced DG function in older adults who consumed the high flavanol diet for three months (Brickman et al., 2014), thus it appears to be a sensitive measure of DG integrity.

Assessing the role of declining neurogenesis in age-related memory impairment requires the development of sensitive techniques that are capable of assessing the state of newborn granule cells *in vivo*, for example using neuroimaging techniques. Such attempts have been made but, unfortunately, the specificity of these techniques has yet to be determined. For example, Manganas et al. (2007) used proton nuclear magnetic resonance spectroscopy to derive a biomarker signal unique to neural and stem cell progenitor cells. This spectroscopic signal was a prominent peak at the frequency of 1.28 parts per million (ppm), which was not observed in other cell types. The amplitude of the 1.28-ppm signal on the 1H-NMR spectra was proportional to the number of NPCs taken for analysis, which opened up the possibility of quantitatively assessing NPCs based on the amount of the 1.28-ppm 1H-NMR signal. However, these results and the approaches used for analyses have been called into serious question (Friedman, 2008; Hoch, Maciejewski, & Gryk, 2008; Jansen, Gearhart, & Bulte, 2008) and the results still remain to be replicated. Thus, its utility for examining age-related changes in neurogenesis is currently unknown. A critical avenue for future research is to develop novel tools to dynamically assess and track neurogenesis in humans *in vivo*, such that the contributions of neurogenesis to memory and cognition in humans can be evaluated, and the impact of therapeutic interventions aimed to reverse age-related cognitive decline.

2.5 Conclusions: A cross-species synthesis

Despite differences in procedures and approaches across studies in both animals and humans, a cross-species consensus begins to emerge with respect to the mechanisms for episodic memory deficits associated with the aging hippocampus. The general findings that contribute to this consensus and the conclusions associated with them are summarized point by point below.

1   Input to the DG/CA3 network through the perforant path appears to degrade with age. Both rodent and human studies have demonstrated this phenomenon and demonstrated that the extent of such degradation is linked to behavioral deficits.
2   Adult neurogenesis in the DG declines with age in both animals and humans, although the extent to which neurogenesis alterations contribute to age-related memory loss is not clear. New tools for monitoring neurogenesis *in vivo* are required to understand these relationships better.
3   The DG/CA3 network exhibits several age-related structural and functional features that include reduced inhibitory tone and reduced modulatory inputs from various neurotransmitter systems.
4   The above changes may work synergistically to contribute to elevated firing rates and hyperexcitability in the CA3 region, which can be observed in animals and humans, and is likely the culprit for rigidity in place cell firing and fMRI activity, consistent with a shift in computational bias from pattern separation to pattern completion.
5   The cognitive/behavioral consequence of changes 1–4 above manifest as deficits in mnemonic discrimination of similar experiences, which spans several domains that include but are likely not limited to object, spatial, temporal, and affective memories.
6   These age-related deficits in discrimination task performance and their underlying neural bases provide a mechanistic explanation for many of the previously reported episodic memory changes with age, such as loss of contextual memory and recollection with a relative sparing of familiarity.

References

Adolphs, R., Denburg, N.L., & Tranel, D. (2001). The amygdala's role in long-term declarative memory for gist and detail. *Behavioral Neuroscience, 115*, 983–992.
Albert, M.S. (2002). Memory decline: The boundary between aging and age-related disease. *Annals of Neurology, 51*(3), 282–284.

Amaral, D.G., Scharfman, H.E., & Lavenex, P. (2007). *The dentate gyrus: A comprehensive guide to structure, function, and clinical implications. Progress in brain research* (Vol. 163, pp. 3–22). Amsterdam, The Netherlands: Elsevier.

Bäckman, C.M., Malik, N., Zhang, Y., Shan, L., Grinberg, A., Hoffer, B.J., ... Tomac, A.C. (2006). Characterization of a mouse strain expressing Cre recombinase from the 3' untranslated region of the dopamine transporter locus. *Genesis, 44*(8), 383–390.

Bäckman, L., Ginovart, N., Dixon, R.A., Wahlin, T.B.R., Wahlin, Å., Halldin, C., & Farde, L. (2000). Age-related cognitive deficits mediated by changes in the striatal dopamine system. *American Journal of Psychiatry, 157*, 635–637.

Bakker, A., Krauss, G.L., Albert, M.S., Speck, C.L., Jones, L.R., Stark, C.E., ... Gallagher, M. (2012). Reduction of hippocampal hyperactivity improves cognition in amnestic mild cognitive impairment. *Neuron, 74*(3), 467–474.

Barnes, C.A. (1979). Memory deficits associated with senescence: A neurophysiological and behavioral study in the rat. *Journal of Comparative and Physiological Psychology, 93*(1), 74–104.

Barnes, C.A. (1988). Neurological and behavioral investigations of memory failure in aging animals. *International Journal of Neurology, 21–22*, 130–136.

Basile, B.M., & Hampton, R.R. (2013). Recognition errors suggest fast familiarity and slow recollection in rhesus monkeys. *Learning & Memory, 20*(8), 431–437.

Bass, D.I., Nizam, Z.G., Partain, K.N., Wang, A., & Manns, J.R. (2014). Amygdala-mediated enhancement of memory for specific events depends on the hippocampus. *Neurobiology of Learning and Memory, 107*, 37–41.

Bastin, C., & Van der Linden, M. (2003). The contribution of recollection and familiarity to recognition memory: A study of the effects of test format and aging. *Neuropsychology, 17*(1), 14–24.

Bizon, J.L., & Gallagher, M. (2003). Production of new cells in the rat dentate gyrus over the lifespan: Relation to cognitive decline. *The European Journal of Neuroscience, 18*(1), 215–219.

Boric, K., Muñoz, P., Gallagher, M., & Kirkwood, A. (2008). Potential adaptive function for altered long-term potentiation mechanisms in aging hippocampus. *The Journal of Neuroscience, 28*(32), 8034–8039.

Brickman, A. M., Khan, U.A., Provenzano, F.A., Yeung, L.-K., Suzuki, W., Schroeter, H., ... Small, S.A. (2014). Enhancing dentate gyrus function with dietary flavanols improves cognition in older adults. *Nature Neuroscience, 17*(12), 1798–1803.

Burke, S. N., & Barnes, C. A. (2006). Neural plasticity in the ageing brain. *Nature Reviews Neuroscience, 7*(1), 30–40.

Burke, Sarah N., Wallace, J.L., Hartzell, A.L., Nematollahi, S., Plange, K., & Barnes, C.A. (2011). Age-associated deficits in pattern separation functions of the perirhinal cortex: A cross-species consensus. *Behavioral Neuroscience, 125*(6), 836–847.

Cadiacio, C.L., Milner, T.A., Gallagher, M., & Pierce, J.P. (2003). Hilar neuropeptide Y interneuron loss in the aged rat hippocampal formation. *Experimental Neurology, 183*, 147–158.

Cervenka, S., Bäckman, L., Cselényi, Z., Halldin, C., & Farde, L. (2008). Associations between dopamine D2-receptor binding and cognitive performance indicate functional compartmentalization of the human striatum. *NeuroImage, 40*(3), 1287–1295.

Chalfonte, B.L., & Johnson, M.K. (1996). Feature memory and binding in young and older adults. *Memory & Cognition, 24*, 403–416.

Chee, M.W.L., Goh, J.O.S., Venkatraman, V., Tan, J.C., Gutchess, A., Sutton, B., ... Park, D. (2006). Age-related changes in object processing and contextual binding revealed using fMR adaptation. *Journal of Cognitive Neuroscience, 18*, 495–507.

Chouinard, M.L., Gallagher, M., Yasuda, R.P., Wolfe, B.B., & McKinney, M. (1995). Hippocampal muscarinic receptor function in spatial learning-impaired aged rats. *Neurobiology of Aging, 16*(6), 955–963.

Chowdhury, R., Guitart-Masip, M., Bunzeck, N., Dolan, R.J., & Duzel, E. (2012). Dopamine modulates episodic memory persistence in old age. *Journal of Neuroscience, 32*(41), 14193–14204.

Clelland, C.D., Choi, M., Romberg, C., Clemenson, G.D., Fragniere, A., Tyers, P., . . . Bussey, T.J. (2009). A functional role for adult hippocampal neurogenesis in spatial pattern separation. *Science, 325*, 210–213.

Cohen, D., & Cox, G. (1977). Memory for a geometrical configuration in the cognitively impaired elderly. *Experimental Aging Research, 3*(4–6), 245–251.

Craik, F.I.M., & Simon, E. (1980). Age differences in memory: The roles of attention and depth of processing. *New Directions in Memory and Aging,* 95–112.

Creer, D.J., Romberg, C., Saksida, L.M., van Praag, H., & Bussey, T.J. (2010). Running enhances spatial pattern separation in mice. *PNAS, 107*(5), 2367–2372.

Czéh, B., & Lucassen, P.J. (2007). What causes the hippocampal volume decrease in depression? Are neurogenesis, glial changes and apoptosis implicated? *European Archives of Psychiatry and Clinical Neuroscience, 257*(5), 250–260.

Daselaar, S.M., Fleck, M.S., Dobbins, I.G., Madden, D.J., & Cabeza, R. (2006). Effects of healthy aging on hippocampal and rhinal memory functions: An event-related fMRI study. *Cerebral Cortex, 16*(12), 1771–1782.

Davies, P., & Maloney, A.J. (1976). Selective loss of central cholinergic neurons in Alzheimer's disease. *Lancet, 2*(8000), 1403.

Denburg, N.L., Buchanan, T.W., Tranel, D., & Adolphs, R. (2003). Evidence for preserved emotional memory in normal older persons. *Emotion, 3*, 239–253.

Donovan, M.H., Yazdani, U., Norris, R.D., Games, D., German, D. C., & Eisch, A.J. (2006). Decreased adult hippocampal neurogenesis in the PDAPP mouse model of Alzheimer's disease. *The Journal of Comparative Neurology, 495*(1), 70–83.

Drachman, D.A., & Leavitt, J. (1974). Human memory and the cholinergic system. A relationship to aging? *Archives of Neurology, 30*(2), 113–121.

Duverne, S., Habibi, A., & Rugg, M.D. (2008). Regional specificity of age effects on the neural correlates of episodic retrieval. *Neurobiology of Aging, 29*(12), 1902–1916.

El-Hayek, Y.H., Wu, C., Ye, H., Wang, J., Carlen, P.L., & Zhang, L. (2013). Hippocampal excitability is increased in aged mice. *Experimental Neurology, 247*, 710–719.

Erixon-Lindroth, N., Farde, L., Wahlin, T.B.R., Sovago, J., Halldin, C., & Backman, L. (2005). The role of the striatal dopamine transporter in cognitive aging. *Psychiatry Research-Neuroimaging, 138*, 1–12.

Fabel, K., Wolf, S.A., Ehninger, D., Babu, H., Leal-Galicia, P., & Kempermann, G. (2009). Additive effects of physical exercise and environmental enrichment on adult hippocampal neurogenesis in mice. *Frontiers in Neuroscience, 3*, 50.

Fearnley, J.M., & Lees, A.J. (1991). Ageing and Parkinson's disease: Substantia nigra regional selectivity. *Brain: A Journal of Neurology, 114*(5), 2283–2301.

Friedman, S.D. (2008). Comment on "Magnetic resonance spectroscopy identifies neural progenitor cells in the live human brain". *Science, 321*(5889), 640; author reply 640.

Gallagher, M., Burwell, R., & Burchinal, M. (1993). Severity of spatial learning impairment in aging: development of a learning index for performance in the Morris water maze. *Behavioral Neuroscience, 107*(4), 618–626.

Gallagher, M., & Pelleymounter, M. A. (1988). Spatial learning deficits in old rats: A model for memory decline in the aged. *Neurobiology of Aging, 9*(5–6), 549–556.

Galvan, V., & Jin, K. (2007). Neurogenesis in the aging brain. *Clinical Interventions in Aging, 2*(4), 605–610.

Gaylord, S.A., & Marsh, G.R. (1975). Age differences in the speed of a spatial cognitive process. *Journal of Gerontology, 30*(6), 674–678.

Geinisman, Y., de Toledo-Morrell, L., Morrell, F., Persina, I.S., & Rossi, M. (1992). Structural synaptic plasticity associated with the induction of long-term potentiation is preserved in the dentate gyrus of aged rats. *Hippocampus, 2*, 445–456.

Gilbert, P. E., & Kesner, R. P. (2002). The amygdala but not the hippocampus is involved in pattern separation based on reward value. *Neurobiology of Learning and Memory, 77*, 338–353.

Gilbert, P. E., Kesner, R.P., & DeCoteau, W.E. (1998). Memory for spatial location: Role of the hippocampus in mediating spatial pattern separation. *The Journal of Neuroscience, 18*, 804–810.

Gilbert, P. E., Kesner, R. P., & Lee, I. (2001). Dissociating hippocampal subregions: Double dissociation between dentate gyrus and CA1. *Hippocampus, 11*, 626–636.

Glisky, E. (2007). Changes in cognitive function in human aging. In D. Riddle (Ed.), *Brain aging: Models, methods, and mechanisms* (pp. 1–10). Boca Raton: CRC Press.

Glisky, E.L., Rubin, S.R., & Davidson, P.S. (2001). Source memory in older adults: An encoding or retrieval problem? *Journal of Experimental Psychology. Learning, Memory, and Cognition, 27*, 1131–1146.

Golomb, J., Kluger, A., de Leon, M.J., Ferris, S.H., Mittelman, M.P., Cohen, J., & George, A.E. (1996). Hippocampal formation size predicts declining memory performance in normal aging. *Neurology, 47*(3), 810–813.

Gould, E., Beylin, A., Tanapat, P., Reeves, A., & Shors, T.J. (1999). Learning enhances adult neurogenesis in the hippocampal formation. *Nature Neuroscience, 2*(3), 260–265.

Grudzien, A., Shaw, P., Weintraub, S., Bigio, E., Mash, D. C., & Mesulam, M.M. (2007). Locus coeruleus neurofibrillary degeneration in aging, mild cognitive impairment and early Alzheimer's disease. *Neurobiology of Aging, 28*(3), 327–335.

Guderian, S., Brigham, D., & Mishkin, M. (2011). Two processes support visual recognition memory in rhesus monkeys. *PNAS, 108*(48), 19425–19430.

Haberman, R.P., Colantuoni, C., Koh, M.T., & Gallagher, M. (2013). Behaviorally activated mRNA expression profiles produce signatures of learning and enhanced inhibition in aged rats with preserved memory. *PloS One, 8*(12), e83674.

Harris, M.A., & Wolbers, T. (2012). Ageing effects on path integration and landmark navigation. *Hippocampus, 22*, 1770–1780.

Hasselmo, M. E. (2006). The role of acetylcholine in learning and memory. *Current Opinion in Neurobiology, 16*(6), 710–715.

Hasselmo, M. E., & Schnell, E. (1994). Laminar selectivity of the cholinergic suppression of synaptic transmission in rat hippocampal region CA1: Computational modeling and brain slice physiology. *The Journal of Neuroscience, 14*, 3898–3914.

Hasselmo, M. E., Schnell, E., & Barkai, E. (1995). Dynamics of learning and recall at excitatory recurrent synapses and cholinergic modulation in rat hippocampal region CA3. *The Journal of Neuroscience, 15*, 5249–5262.

Hasselmo, M. E., & Wyble, B.P. (1997). Free recall and recognition in a network model of the hippocampus: Simulating effects of scopolamine on human memory function. *Behavioural Brain Research, 89*, 1–34.

Haughey, N.J., Liu, D., Nath, A., Borchard, A.C., & Mattson, M.P. (2002). Disruption of neurogenesis in the subventricular zone of adult mice, and in human cortical neuronal precursor cells in culture, by amyloid beta-peptide: implications for the pathogenesis of Alzheimer's disease. *Neuromolecular Medicine, 1*(2), 125–135.

Haughey, N.J., Nath, A., Chan, S.L., Borchard, A.C., Rao, M.S., & Mattson, M.P. (2002). Disruption of neurogenesis by amyloid beta-peptide, and perturbed neural progenitor cell homeostasis, in models of Alzheimer's disease. *Journal of Neurochemistry, 83*(6), 1509–1524.

Head, D., & Isom, M. (2010). Age effects on wayfinding and route learning skills. *Behavioural Brain Research, 209*(1), 49–58.

Hedden, T., & Gabrieli, J.D.E. (2004). Insights into the ageing mind: A view from cognitive neuroscience. *Nature Reviews Neuroscience, 5*(2), 87–96.

Hedden, T., & Gabrieli, J.D.E. (2005). Healthy and pathological processes in adult development: new evidence from neuroimaging of the aging brain. *Current Opinion in Neurology, 18*(6), 740–747.

Henkel, L.A., Johnson, M.K., & De Leonardis, D.M. (1998). Aging and source monitoring: Cognitive processes and neuropsychological correlates. *Journal of Experimental Psychology: General, 127*, 251–268.

Ho, N.F., Hooker, J.M., Sahay, A., Holt, D.J., & Roffman, J.L. (2013). In vivo imaging of adult human hippocampal neurogenesis: Progress, pitfalls and promise. *Molecular Psychiatry, 18*(4), 404–416.

Hoch, J.C., Maciejewski, M.W., & Gryk, M.R. (2008). Comment on "magnetic resonance spectroscopy identifies neural progenitor cells in the live human brain". *Science, 321*(5889), 640; author reply 640.

Holden, H.M., & Gilbert, P.E. (2012). Less efficient pattern separation may contribute to age-related spatial memory deficits. *Frontiers in Aging Neuroscience, 4*, 9.

Howard, M.W., Bessette-Symons, B., Zhang, Y., & Hoyer, W.J. (2006). Aging selectively impairs recollection in recognition memory for pictures: Evidence from modeling and receiver operating characteristic curves. *Psychology and Aging, 21*(1), 96–106.

Hu, H., Real, E., Takamiya, K., Kang, M.-G., Ledoux, J., Huganir, R.L., & Malinow, R. (2007). Emotion enhances learning via norepinephrine regulation of AMPA-receptor trafficking. *Cell, 131*(1), 160–173.

Ikonen, S., McMahan, R., Gallagher, M., Eichenbaum, H., & Tanila, H. (2002). Cholinergic system regulation of spatial representation by the hippocampus. *Hippocampus, 12*(3), 386–397.

Jahng, G.-H., Xu, S., Weiner, M.W., Meyerhoff, D.J., Park, S., & Schuff, N. (2011). DTI studies in patients with Alzheimer's disease, mild cognitive impairment, or normal cognition with evaluation of the intrinsic background gradients. *Neuroradiology, 53*(10), 749–762.

Jansen, J.F.A., Gearhart, J.D., & Bulte, J.W.M. (2008). Comment on "Magnetic resonance spectroscopy identifies neural progenitor cells in the live human brain". *Science, 321*(5889), 640; author reply 640.

Jennings, J.M., & Jacoby, L.L. (1997). An opposition procedure for detecting age-related deficits in recollection: Telling effects of repetition. *Psychology and Aging, 12*(2), 352–361.

Jessberger, S., & Gage, F.H. (2008). Stem-cell-associated structural and functional plasticity in the aging hippocampus. *Psychology and Aging, 23*, 684–691.

Jin, K., Sun, Y., Xie, L., Batteur, S., Mao, X.O., Smelick, C., . . . Greenberg, D.A. (2003). Neurogenesis and aging: FGF-2 and HB-EGF restore neurogenesis in hippocampus and subventricular zone of aged mice. *Aging Cell, 2*(3), 175–183.

Kempermann, G. (2002). Why new neurons? Possible functions for adult hippocampal. *The Journal of Neuroscience, 22*(3), 635–638.

Kensinger, E.A. (2009). Remembering the details: Effects of emotion. *Emotion Review, 1*(2), 99–113.

Kensinger, E.A., Brierley, B., Medford, N., Growdon, J.H., & Corkin, S. (2002). Effects of normal aging and Alzheimer's disease on emotional memory. *Emotion, 2*, 118–134.

Kensinger, E.A., Garoff-Eaton, R.J., & Schacter, D.L. (2007). Effects of emotion on memory specificity in young and older adults. *The Journals of Gerontology Series B Psychological Sciences and Social Sciences, 62*, P208–215.

Knierim, J.J., Neunuebel, J.P., & Deshmukh, S.S. (2014). Functional correlates of the lateral and medial entorhinal cortex: Objects, path integration and local-global reference frames. *Philosophical Transactions of the Royal Society of London. Series B, Biological Sciences, 369*(1635). doi:10.1098/rstb.2013.0369

Koh, M.T., Haberman, R.P., Foti, S., McCown, T.J., & Gallagher, M. (2010). Treatment strategies targeting excess hippocampal activity benefit aged rats with cognitive impairment. *Neuropsychopharmacology: Official publication of the American College of Neuropsychopharmacology, 35*(4), 1016–1025.

Koh, M.T., Spiegel, A. M., & Gallagher, M. (2014). Age-associated changes in hippocampal-dependent cognition in Diversity Outbred mice. *Hippocampus, 24*(11), 1300–1307.

Kubanis, P., & Zornetzer, S.F. (1981). Age-related behavioral and neurobiological changes: A review with an emphasis on memory. *Behavioral and Neural Biology, 31*(2), 115–172.

Kuhn, H.G., Dickinson-Anson, H., & Gage, F.H. (1996). Neurogenesis in the dentate gyrus of the adult rat: Age-related decrease of neuronal progenitor proliferation. *The Journal of Neuroscience: The Official Journal of the Society for Neuroscience, 16*(6), 2027–2033.

Lai, Z.C., Moss, M.B., Killiany, R.J., Rosene, D.L., & Herndon, J.G. (1995). Executive system dysfunction in the aged monkey: Spatial and object reversal learning. *Neurobiology of Aging, 16,* 947–954.

Lavenex, P., & Amaral, D.G. (2000). Hippocampal-neocortical interaction: A hierarchy of associativity. *Hippocampus, 10*(4), 420–430.

Leal, S. L., & Yassa, M. A. (2014). Effect of aging on mnemonic discrimination of emotional information. *Behavioral Neuroscience, 128*(5), 539–547.

LeDoux, J. (2007). The amygdala. *Current Biology, 17,* 868–874.

Lee, H.-K., Min, S.S., Gallagher, M., & Kirkwood, A. (2005). NMDA receptor-independent long-term depression correlates with successful aging in rats. *Nature Neuroscience, 8*(12), 1657–1659.

Lichtenwalner, R.J., Forbes, M.E., Bennett, S.A., Lynch, C.D., Sonntag, W.E., & Riddle, D.R. (2001). Intracerebroventricular infusion of insulin-like growth factor-I ameliorates the age-related decline in hippocampal neurogenesis. *Neuroscience, 107*(4), 603–613.

Lisman, J.E., & Grace, A. A. (2005). The hippocampal-VTA loop: Controlling the entry of information into long-term memory. *Neuron, 46*(5), 703–713.

Loftus, E.F., Loftus, G.R., & Messo, J. (1987). Some facts about "weapon focus". *Law and Human Behavior, 11,* 55–62.

Lustig, C., & Hasher, L. (2001). Implicit memory is vulnerable to proactive interference. *Psychological Science: A Journal of the American Psychological Society, 12,* 408–412.

Manganas, L.N., Zhang, X., Li, Y., Hazel, R.D., Smith, S.D., Wagshul, M.E., . . . Maletic-Savatic, M. (2007). Magnetic resonance spectroscopy identifies neural progenitor cells in the live human brain. *Science, 318*(5852), 980–985.

Marr, D. (1971). Simple memory: A theory for archicortex. *Philosophical Transactions of the Royal Society of London Series B Biological Sciences, 262,* 23–81.

Marrone, D.F., Adams, A.A., & Satvat, E. (2011). Increased pattern separation in the aged fascia dentata. *Neurobiology of Aging, 32*(12), 2317.e23–2317.e32.

Mather, M., & Carstensen, L.L. (2005). Aging and motivated cognition: The positivity effect in attention and memory. *Trends in Cognitive Sciences, 9,* 496–502.

McClelland, J.L., McNaughton, B.L., & O'Reilly, R.C. (1995). Why there are complementary learning systems in the hippocampus and neocortex: Insights from the successes and failures of connectionist models of learning and memory. *Psychological Review, 102*(3), 419–457.

McEntee, W., & Crook, T. (1991). Serotonin, memory, and the aging brain. *Psychopharmacology, 103,* 143–149.

McGaugh, J.L. (2004). The amygdala modulates the consolidation of memories of emotionally arousing experiences. *Annual Review of Neuroscience, 27,* 1–28.

Meltzer, C.C., Smith, G., DeKosky, S.T., Pollock, B.G., Mathis, C.A., Moore, R.Y., . . . Reynolds, C.F. (1998). Serotonin in Aging, Late-Life Depression, and Alzheimer's Disease: The Emerging Role of Functional Imaging. *Neuropsychopharmacology, 18*(6), 407–430.

Miller, S. L., Celone, K., DePeau, K., Diamond, E., Dickerson, B. C., Rentz, D., . . . Sperling, R. A. (2008). Age-related memory impairment associated with loss of parietal deactivation but preserved hippocampal activation. *Proceedings of the National Academy of Sciences of the United States of America, 105*(6), 2181–2186.

Milner, B., Squire, L.R., & Kandel, E.R. (1998). Cognitive neuroscience and the study of memory, *Neuron, 20*, 445–468.

Mitra, R., Sundlass, K., Parker, K.J., Schatzberg, A.F., & Lyons, D.M. (2006). Social stress-related behavior affects hippocampal cell proliferation in mice. *Physiology & Behavior, 89*(2), 123–127.

Mueller, S.G., & Weiner, M.W. (2009). Selective effect of age, Apo e4, and Alzheimer's disease on hippocampal subfields. *Hippocampus, 19*(6), 558–564.

Murty, V.P., Sambataro, F., Das, S., Tan, H.-Y., Callicott, J.H., Goldberg, T.E., . . . Mattay, V.S. (2009). Age-related alterations in simple declarative memory and the effect of negative stimulus valence. *Journal of Cognitive Neuroscience, 21*(10), 1920–1933.

Newman, M. C., & Kaszniak, A. W. (2000) Spatial memory and aging: Performance on a human analog of the morris water maze. *Aging, Neuropsychology, and Cognition, 7*(2), 86–93.

Newson, R.S., & Kemps, E.B. (2006). The nature of subjective cognitive complaints of older adults. *International Journal of Aging & Human Development, 63*(2), 139–151.

Nicolle, M.M., Gallagher, M., & McKinney, M. (2001). Visualization of muscarinic receptor-mediated phosphoinositide turnover in the hippocampus of young and aged, learning-impaired Long Evans rats. *Hippocampus, 11*(6), 741–746.

Pereira, A.C., Huddleston, D.E., Brickman, A. M., Sosunov, A.A., Hen, R., McKhann, G.M., . . . Small, S.A. (2007). An in vivo correlate of exercise-induced neurogenesis in the adult dentate gyrus. *PNAS, 104*(13), 5638–5643.

Perlmutter, M., Metzger, R., Nezworski, T., & Miller, K. (1981). Spatial and temporal memory in 20 to 60 year olds. *Journal of Gerontology, 36*(1), 59–65.

Prull, M.W., Dawes, L.L.C., Martin, A. M., Rosenberg, H.F., & Light, L.L. (2006). Recollection and familiarity in recognition memory: Adult age differences and neuropsychological test correlates. *Psychology and Aging, 21*(1), 107–118.

Rapp, P.R., & Gallagher, M. (1996). Preserved neuron number in the hippocampus of aged rats with spatial learning deficits. *PNAS, 93*, 9926–9930.

Rapp, P.R., Kansky, M.T., & Roberts, J.A. (1997). Impaired spatial information processing in aged monkeys with preserved recognition memory. *Neuroreport, 8*, 1923–1928.

Raz, N., Lindenberger, U., Rodrigue, K.M., Kennedy, K.M., Head, D., Williamson, A., . . . Acker, J.D. (2005). Regional brain changes in aging healthy adults: General trends, individual differences and modifiers. *Cerebral Cortex, 15*(11), 1676–1689.

Reagh, Z.M., Roberts, J.M., Ly, M., Diprospero, N., Murray, E., & Yassa, M.A. (2013). Spatial discrimination deficits as a function of mnemonic interference in aged adults with and without memory impairment. *Hippocampus, 24*(3), 303–314.

Roberts, J.M., Ly, M., Murray, E., & Yassa, M.A. (2014). Temporal discrimination deficits as a function of lag interference in older adults. *Hippocampus, 24*(10), 1189–1196.

Robitsek, R.J., Fortin, N.J., Koh, M.T., Gallagher, M., & Eichenbaum, H. (2008). Cognitive aging: A common decline of episodic recollection and spatial memory in rats. *The Journal of Neuroscience, 28*(36), 8945–8954.

Sahay, A., Scobie, K.N., Hill, A.S., O'Carroll, C.M., Kheirbek, M. A., Burghardt, N.S., . . . Hen, R. (2011). Increasing adult hippocampal neurogenesis is sufficient to improve pattern separation. *Nature, 472*(7344), 466–470.

Salthouse, T.A., Mitchell, D.R., & Palmon, R. (1989). Memory and age differences in spatial manipulation ability. *Psychology and Aging, 4*(4), 480–486.

Salthouse, T.A., Mitchell, D.R., Skovronek, E., & Babcock, R.L. (1989). Effects of adult age and working memory on reasoning and spatial abilities. *Journal of Experimental Psychology: Learning, Memory, and Cognition, 15*(3), 507–516.

Sava, S., & Markus, E.J. (2008). Activation of the medial septum reverses age-related hippocampal encoding deficits: A place field analysis. *The Journal of Neuroscience, 28*, 1841–1853.

Scheibel, M.E., Lindsay, R.D., Tomiyasu, U., & Scheibel, A.B. (1976). Progressive dendritic changes in the aging human limbic system. *Experimental Neurology, 53*(2), 420–430.

Seki, T., & Arai, Y. (1995). Age-related production of new granule cells in the adult dentate gyrus. *Neuroreport, 6*(18), 2479–2482.

Shapiro, M. L., & Olton, D. (1994). Hippocampal function and interference. In D. Schacter & E. Tulving (Eds.), *Memory Systems 1994* (pp. 87–117). Cambridge, MA: MIT Press.

Shetty, A.K., & Turner, D.A. (1998). Hippocampal interneurons expressing glutamic acid decarboxylase and calcium-binding proteins decrease with aging in Fischer 344 rats. *Journal of Comparative Neurology, 394*, 252–269.

Shi, L., Argenta, A.E., Winseck, A.K., & Brunso-Bechtold, J.K. (2004). Stereological quantification of GAD-67-immunoreactive neurons and boutons in the hippocampus of middle-aged and old Fischer 344 x Brown Norway rats. *Journal of Comparative Neurology, 478*(3), 282–291.

Siddiqi, Z., Kemper, T.L., & Killiany, R. (1999). Age-related neuronal loss from the substantia nigra-pars compacta and ventral tegmental area of the rhesus monkey. *Journal of Neuropathology and Experimental Neurology, 58*(9), 959–971.

Small, S.A., Stern, Y., Tang, M., & Mayeux, R. (1999). Selective decline in memory function among healthy elderly. *Neurology, 52*(7), 1392–1392.

Smith, T.D., Adams, M.M., Gallagher, M., Morrison, J.H., & Rapp, P.R. (2000). Circuit-specific alterations in hippocampal synaptophysin immunoreactivity predict spatial learning impairment in aged rats. *The Journal of Neuroscience, 20*(17), 6587–6593.

Spalding, K.L., Bergmann, O., Alkass, K., Bernard, S., Salehpour, M., Huttner, H.B., . . . Frisén, J. (2013). Dynamics of hippocampal neurogenesis in adult humans. *Cell, 153*(6), 1219–1227.

Sperling, R. (2007). Functional MRI studies of associative encoding in normal aging, mild cognitive impairment, and Alzheimer's disease. *Annals of the New York Academy of Sciences, 1097*, 146–155.

Spiegel, A. M., Koh, M.T., Vogt, N.M., Rapp, P.R., & Gallagher, M. (2013). Hilar interneuron vulnerability distinguishes aged rats with memory impairment. *Journal of Comparative Neurology, 521*, 3508–3523.

Squire, L.R., Stark, C.E.L., & Clark, R.E. (2004). The medial temporal lobe. *Annual Review of Neuroscience, 27*, 279–306.

Stanley, D.P., & Shetty, A.K. (2004). Aging in the rat hippocampus is associated with widespread reductions in the number of glutamate decarboxylase-67 positive interneurons but not interneuron degeneration. *Journal of Neurochemistry, 89*, 204–216.

Stark, S.M., Yassa, M.A., Lacy, J.W., & Stark, C.E.L. (2013). A task to assess behavioral pattern separation (BPS) in humans: Data from healthy aging and mild cognitive impairment. *Neuropsychologia*, 1–8.

Stark, S.M., Yassa, M.A., & Stark, C.E.L. (2010). Individual differences in spatial pattern separation performance associated with healthy aging in humans. *Learning & Memory, 17*(6), 284–288.

Stemmelin, J., Lazarus, C., Cassel, S., Kelche, C., & Cassel, J.C. (2000). Immunohistochemical and neurochemical correlates of learning deficits in aged rats. *Neuroscience, 96*, 275–289.

Stern, Y. (2012). Cognitive reserve in ageing and Alzheimer's disease. *Lancet Neurology, 11*(11), 1006–1012.

Sternberg, D.B., Martinez, J.L., Gold, P.E., & McGaugh, J.L. (1985). Age-related memory deficits in rats and mice: Enhancement with peripheral injections of epinephrine. *Behavioral and Neural Biology, 44*(2), 213–220.

Sugaya, K., Greene, R., Personett, D., Robbins, M., Kent, C., Bryan, D., . . . Mckinney, M. (1998). Septo-hippocampal cholinergic and neurotrophin markers in age-induced cognitive decline. *Neurobiology of Aging, 19*, 351–361.

Suzuki, W.A., Zola-Morgan, S., Squire, L.R., & Amaral, D.G. (1993). Lesions of the perirhinal and parahippocampal cortices in the monkey produce long-lasting memory impairment in the visual and tactual modalities. *The Journal of Neuroscience, 13*(6), 2430–2451.

Taghzouti, K., Louilot, A., Herman, J.P., Le Moal, M., & Simon, H. (1985). Alternation behavior, spatial discrimination, and reversal disturbances following 6-hydroxydopamine lesions in the nucleus accumbens of the rat. *Behavioral and Neural Biology, 44*, 354–363.

Takahashi, H., Kato, M., Hayashi, M., Okubo, Y., Takano, A., Ito, H., & Suhara, T. (2007). Memory and frontal lobe functions: Possible relations with dopamine D2 receptors in the hippocampus. *NeuroImage, 34*(4), 1643–1649.

Teipel, S.J., Bruno, D., Grothe, M.J., Nierenberg, J., & Pomara, N. (2015). Hippocampus and basal forebrain volumes modulate effects of anticholinergic treatment on delayed recall in healthy older adults. *Alzheimer's & Dementia: Diagnosis, Assessment and Disease Monitoring, 1*(2), 216–219.

Tolentino, J. C., Pirogovsky, E., Luu, T., Toner, C. K., & Gilbert, P. E. (2012). The effect of interference on temporal order memory for random and fixed sequences in nondemented older adults. *Learning & Memory, 19*(6), 251–255.

Toner, C.K., Pirogovsky, E., Kirwan, C.B., & Gilbert, P.E. (2009). Visual object pattern separation deficits in nondemented older adults. *Learning & Memory, 16*(5), 338–342.

Treves, A., & Rolls, E.T. (1994). Computational analysis of the role of the hippocampus in memory. *Hippocampus, 4*(3), 374–391.

Uttl, B., & Graf, P. (1993). Episodic spatial memory in adulthood. *Psychology and Aging, 8*, 257–273.

Van Praag, H. (2009). Exercise and the brain: Something to chew on. *Trends in Neurosciences, 32*(5), 283–290.

Van Praag, H., Kempermann, G., & Gage, F.H. (1999). Running increases cell proliferation and neurogenesis in the adult mouse dentate gyrus. *Nature Neuroscience, 2*(3), 266–270.

Van Praag, H., Schinder, A.F., Christie, B.R., Toni, N., Palmer, T.D., & Gage, F.H. (2002). Functional neurogenesis in the adult hippocampus. *Nature, 415*, 1030–1034.

Vela, J., Gutierrez, A., Vitorica, J., & Ruano, D. (2003). Rat hippocampal GABAergic molecular markers are differentially affected by ageing. *Journal of Neurochemistry, 85*, 368–377.

Vivar, C., Potter, M.C., Choi, J., Lee, J., Stringer, T.P., Callaway, E.M., . . . van Praag, H. (2012). Monosynaptic inputs to new neurons in the dentate gyrus. *Nature Communications, 3*, 1107. doi:10.1038/ncomms2101

Vivar, C., & van Praag, H. (2013). Functional circuits of new neurons in the dentate gyrus. *Frontiers in Neural Circuits, 7*, 15.

Vreugdenhil, M., & Toescu, E.C. (2005). Age-dependent reduction of gamma oscillations in the mouse hippocampus in vitro. *Neuroscience, 132*(4), 1151–1157.

Walker, L.C., Kitt, C.A., Struble, R.G., Wagster, M.V, Price, D.L., & Cork, L.C. (1988). The neural basis of memory decline in aged monkeys. *Neurobiology of Aging, 9*(5–6), 657–666.

Warner-Schmidt, J.L., & Duman, R.S. (2006). Hippocampal neurogenesis: Opposing effects of stress and antidepressant treatment. *Hippocampus, 16*, 239–249.

Westerberg, C.E., Paller, K. A., Weintraub, S., Mesulam, M.-M., Holdstock, J.S., Mayes, A.R., & Reber, P.J. (2006). When memory does not fail: Familiarity-based recognition in mild cognitive impairment and Alzheimer's disease. *Neuropsychology*, *20*(2), 193–205.

Whitehouse, P.J., Price, D.L., Clark, A.W., Coyle, J.T., & DeLong, M.R. (1981). Alzheimer disease: Evidence for selective loss of cholinergic neurons in the nucleus basalis. *Annals of Neurology*, *10*, 122–126.

Wilkniss, S.M., Jones, M.G., Korol, D.L., Gold, P.E., & Manning, C.A. (1997). Age-related differences in an ecologically based study of route learning. *Psychology and Aging*, *12*, 372–375.

Wilson, I.A., Gallagher, M., Eichenbaum, H., & Tanila, H. (2006). Neurocognitive aging: Prior memories hinder new hippocampal encoding. *Trends in Neurosciences*, *29*(12), 662–670.

Wilson, I.A., Ikonen, S., Gallagher, M., Eichenbaum, H., & Tanila, H. (2005). Age-associated alterations of hippocampal place cells are subregion specific. *The Journal of Neuroscience*, *25*(29), 6877–6886.

Wilson, I.A., Ikonen, S., Gureviciene, I., McMahan, R.W., Gallagher, M., Eichenbaum, H., & Tanila, H. (2004). Cognitive aging and the hippocampus: How old rats represent new environments. *The Journal of Neuroscience*, *24*(15), 3870–3878.

Wilson, I.A., Ikonen, S., Gurevicius, K., McMahan, R.W., Gallagher, M., Eichenbaum, H., & Tanila, H. (2005). Place cells of aged rats in two visually identical compartments. *Neurobiology of Aging*, *26*(7), 1099–1106.

Wilson, I. A., Ikonen, S., McMahan, R.W., Gallagher, M., Eichenbaum, H., & Tanila, H. (2003). Place cell rigidity correlates with impaired spatial learning in aged rats. *Neurobiology of Aging*, *24*(2), 297–305.

Winocur, G., & Gagnon, S. (1998). Glucose treatment attenuates spatial learning and memory deficits of aged rats on tests of hippocampal function. *Neurobiology of Aging*, *19*, 233–241.

Wixted, J.T., Mickes, L., & Squire, L.R. (2010). Measuring recollection and familiarity in the medial temporal lobe. *Hippocampus*, *20*, 1195–1205.

Wong, G., Dolcos, S., Denkova, E., Morey, R., Wang, L., McCarthy, G., & Dolcos, F. (2012). Brain Imaging Investigation of the Impairing Effect of Emotion on Cognition. *Journal of Visualized Experiments*, *60*, e2434.

Yassa, M.A., Lacy, J.W., Stark, S.M., Albert, M.S., Gallagher, M., & Stark, C.E.L. (2010). Pattern separation deficits associated with increased hippocampal CA3 and dentate gyrus activity in nondemented older adults. *Hippocampus*, *21(9)*, 968–979.

Yassa, M.A., Mattfeld, A.T., Stark, S.M., & Stark, C.E.L. (2011). Age-related memory deficits linked to circuit-specific disruptions in the hippocampus. *PNAS*, *108*(21), 8873–8878.

Yassa, M.A., & Stark, C.E.L. (2011). Pattern separation in the hippocampus. *Trends in Neurosciences*, *34*(10), 515–525.

Yassa, M. A., Stark, S.M., Bakker, A., Albert, M.S., Gallagher, M., & Stark, C.E.L. (2010). High-resolution structural and functional MRI of hippocampal CA3 and dentate gyrus in patients with amnestic Mild Cognitive Impairment. *NeuroImage*, *51*(3), 1242–1252.

Yonelinas, A.P. (2002). The nature of recollection and familiarity: A review of 30 years of research. *Journal of Memory and Language*, *46*, 441–517.

Yonelinas, A.P., Aly, M., Wang, W.-C., & Koen, J.D. (2010). Recollection and familiarity: Examining controversial assumptions and new directions. *Hippocampus*, *20*(11), 1178–1194.

Zacks, R. T., Hasher, L., & Li, K. Z. H. (2000). Human memory. In F. I. M. Craik & T. A. Salthouse (Eds.), *The handbook of aging and cognition* (2nd edition, pp. 293–357). Mahwah, NJ: LEA.

Zhang, H., Lin, S.-C., & Nicolelis, M.A.L. (2010). Spatiotemporal coupling between hippocampal acetylcholine release and theta oscillations in vivo. *The Journal of Neuroscience*, *30*, 13431–13440.

3

RECOGNITION MEMORY

Tina Chen, Caren M. Rotello and Paul Verhaeghen

3.1   Introduction

Recognition memory plays an important role in everyday life, from meeting new people to remembering what you did on your last birthday. Sometimes, successful recognition comes with associated details, like remembering that a woman at a party is your friend's sister. Associated context details are frequently absent, though, like when you forget with whom you celebrated your birthday. Remembering these kinds of associations becomes more difficult as we grow older (see Old & Naveh-Benjamin, 2008a, for a meta-analysis). Understanding the nature of this normal age-related decline in memory can help direct useful strategies or interventions to improve memory.

3.2   Age-related episodic memory decline

Not all types of memory decline with age. For example, semantic memory – general knowledge that might be tapped for crossword puzzles or playing Jeopardy – remains relatively consistent and can even increase with age (e.g., Kausler & Puckett, 1980). In contrast, episodic memory – memory for specific events – declines with age, and this decline is especially noticeable for associative episodic memory – or memory for associations of an event (Old & Naveh-Benjamin, 2008a). This relatively greater decline for associative information is known as the age-related associative memory deficit (Naveh-Benjamin, 2000) and includes deficits in memory for context, like where you left your keys (see Spencer & Raz, 1995, for a meta-analysis), and source information, like who told you about an upcoming concert (e.g., Hashtroudi, Johnson, & Chrosniak, 1989).

   A common way to test the age-related associative deficit in the laboratory involves presenting younger and older adults with study lists of unrelated pairs of stimuli, like the word pairs "balloon-coffee" and "dolphin-flower" (e.g., Naveh-Benjamin,

2000). The participants are then tested for their memory of the individual items, e.g., "flower". They are also tested for their memory of the specific pairings: for this associative memory test, a target is an *intact* pair in which both items were studied as part of the same pair (e.g., "balloon-coffee"), whereas a lure is a *recombined* pair in which both words were studied, but not together (e.g., "dolphin-coffee"). These recombined pairs serve to test the memory of the specific binding of the pair; accurate responding requires that the particular combination of items be remembered as having occurred together. Familiarity for the individual items is not sufficient to perform accurately for this test. For example, remembering that "dolphin" was presented at study does not help the participant realize that "dolphin-coffee" is novel.

These methods are used to examine both the nature and cause of the associative memory deficit, and researchers propose models of the processes in recognition memory to understand what is happening. One particularly prominent model of recognition memory, the dual-process signal detection model (Yonelinas, 1994), has been used to explain the associative memory deficit. This model proposes that the process of remembering associated details is distinct from remembering in the absence of associated details. An account of the model follows.

3.3 Dual-process vs. single-process models of recognition memory

For many years, there has been a debate over whether recognition memory is most accurately modeled as a single signal detection process, or as a dual-process in which another component may play a role in addition to the single signal detection process (e.g., Mandler, 1980; Parks & Yonelinas, 2007; Reder et al., 2000; Wixted, 2007; Yonelinas, 1994; Yonelinas, 2002).

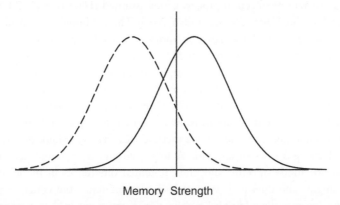

Memory Strength

FIGURE 3.1 A simple single-process signal detection model of recognition memory. The target distribution is represented with a solid line and the lure distribution is represented with a dotted line; these distributions differ in memory strength along the x-axis. A vertical line shows a decision criterion.

The single-process model (Figure 3.1) proposes that memories for episodes or items vary in strength continuously along a familiarity axis (e.g., Banks, 1970; Macmillan & Creelman, 2005). An item in a test list is recognized as old (i.e., previously studied) if its familiarity exceeds some decision criterion. On the other hand, the dual-process model posits that this familiarity process is sometimes supplemented with a recollection process in which one remembers the context of the item or its associated details.

A large body of literature has come from this debate (for reviews, see Diana, Reder, Arndt, & Park, 2006; Wixted, 2007; Yonelinas, 2001), but our focus is the application of these models to understanding age-related memory change. A prominent hypothesis for differences at retrieval is that older adults have problems recollecting the context of associations, though their familiarity-based responding remains intact (Light, Prull, LaVoie, & Healy, 2000; see Benjamin, 2010, for an alternative hypothesis). According to this dual-process explanation, recognition in the standard associative memory task requires some form of a recollective process, and the age-related decline in memory performance is driven by failures of recollection, not of familiarity. For example, a recall-to-reject process in which a studied pair ("dolphin-flower") is recalled and used to facilitate rejection of a test lure ("dolphin-coffee"; Rotello & Heit, 2000; Rotello, Macmillan, & Van Tassel, 2000) may be impaired for older adults, leading to higher false alarms in the associative memory task (Cohn, Emrich, & Moscovitch, 2008; Healy, Light, & Chung, 2005).

The data from these associative memory tasks appear to compel a dual-process interpretation in which older adults are selectively impaired on memory tasks that require recollection. However, a single-process model might be sufficient to explain the data. For example, Hautus, Macmillan, and Rotello (2008) proposed a model in which item memory and source information are represented on different dimensions of memory strength, but the same basic decision strategy applies. In this model, a separate recollection process is not assumed (Hautus et al., 2008; Starns, Pazzaglia, Rotello, Hautus, & Macmillan, 2013). Thus, although dominant explanations for the age-related associative memory deficit rely on dual-process theories, these conclusions may not be warranted.

Moreover, although much of the empirical support for the dual-process explanations comes in the form of interactions of task and age on performance measures, Newell and Dunn (2008; Bamber, 1979; Dunn & Kirsner, 1988) have shown that it is possible for some interactions to be accounted for by a single-process model. They described *state-trace analysis* as a method that may shed light on the number of underlying processes in any task. A major advantage of state-trace analysis is that it is not model-specific, and, thus, potential differences in model flexibility for the single- and dual-process models cannot influence the conclusion. This is important because the additional recollection component in dual-process models allows for greater flexibility in fitting data than in single-process models (Jang, Wixted, & Huber, 2009), meaning that even if data were generated by a single process, a dual-process model could artificially fit the data better.

3.4 State-trace analysis

The logic of state-trace analysis is that if two dependent variables rely upon a single underlying psychological resource, a *state-trace plot*—a scatterplot of their co-variation—should lie on one monotonic curve (Bamber, 1979; Dunn & Kirsner, 1988; Newell & Dunn, 2008). As Newell and Dunn (2008) say, these two variables "operate in a common 'currency' or metric" (pg. 287).

Thus, the values of the two performance measures both reflect the single underlying process (Figure 3.2A is an example of what this could look like for the current tasks). Interactions may still be observed when a single psychological process drives performance on both tasks to different degrees.

For example, if the function that maps familiarity to item recognition task performance is relatively flat over the range seen in the experiment, then item recognition will not differ much across conditions, as for the black and white dots in Figure 3.3A. A different mapping function for the associative recognition task might produce a more dramatic effect empirically, leading to a significant interaction and the appearance of selective influence. Figure 3.3B shows the corresponding state-trace plot, which is a monotonic function.

In contrast, if the two tasks rely on separate underlying psychological resources (as in Figure 3.2B and Figure 3.3C), then a scatterplot of their co-variation would *not* be likely to fall on a single monotonic function as seen in Figure 3.3D. The state-trace could show two curves because there would not be a single variable relating to the dependent variables.

State-trace analysis is especially important because the holy grail of the double dissociation falls apart when one considers the underlying logic of dissociations (Newell & Dunn, 2008). A dissociation requires that one effect is seen in the absence of another, but the lack of an effect is unverifiable, i.e., there may still be an effect on an unobservable latent process, but that effect has not reached a

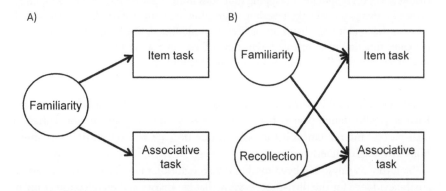

FIGURE 3.2 Single- and dual-process models in a typical age-related associative memory experiment. Model A shows a single process, here called familiarity, affecting item and associative task performance. Model B shows two distinct processes, familiarity and recollection, affecting both item and associative task performance.

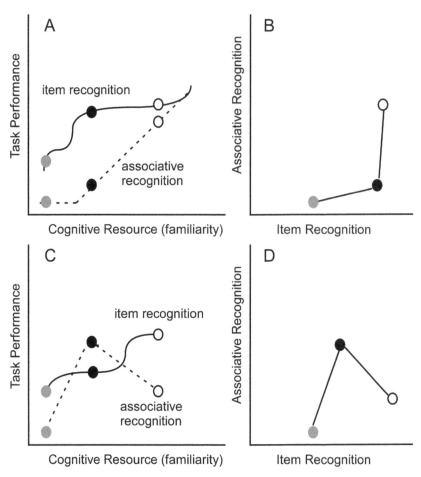

FIGURE 3.3 A) Hypothetical mapping functions from cognitive resource to task performance for two potential tasks, revealing interaction of resource and task. B) Corresponding state-trace plot that shows a single monotonic function. C) Another hypothetical mapping function that reveals interaction of resource and task. D) Corresponding state-trace plot that shows a non-monotonic function.

threshold that would manifest its presence in the dependent variable. Dunn and Kirsner (1988) demonstrated that even cross-over interactions do not demand a dual-process interpretation if the tasks in question are affected in opposite directions by a single underlying process.

State-trace analysis has been used in the recognition memory literature to evaluate the evidence for the dual-process view that familiarity and recollection contribute to judgments. Several major classes of data have been garnered in favor of the dual-process view, namely data collected in the remember-know paradigm (Tulving, 1985), in neuroimaging studies that reveal greater activity in hippocampus and perirhinal cortex for recollected items (e.g., Eichenbaum, Yonelinas, & Ranganath,

2007), and in event-related potential experiments that reveal differential signatures of familiarity (the FN400) and recollection (the LPC, late positive component, e.g., Curran, 1999; 2004; Rugg et al.,1998; Rugg & Curran, 2007; Rugg & Yonelinas, 2003). In each case, state-trace analysis has challenged the dual-process interpretation of the data, suggesting that a single process is sufficient to account for the data (Dunn, 2008; de Zubicaray, McMahon, Dennis, & Dunn, 2011; Freeman, Dennis, & Dunn, 2010). State-trace analyses have also been used for cognitive aging data, revealing that, for certain processes previously thought to be affected by age, aging deficits are actually reduced or non-existent (Verhaeghen, 2014; Verhaeghen & De Meersman, 1998; Verhaeghen, Steitz, Sliwinski, & Cerella, 2003).

Here, we use a state-trace analysis in conjunction with meta-analysis to examine the underlying psychological processes contributing to the age-related associative memory deficit. If there are two underlying psychological processes, familiarity and recollection, then we would expect both young and older adults to use familiarity in both the item and associative recognition tasks. Young adults are also expected to use recollection in both tasks, whereas the literature suggests that older adults' recollective process is especially impaired in the associative task. If older adults have impaired recollection, particularly for associative information, the data gathered across different experiments will not fall on a single, monotonic function; item recognition will depend on two processes and associative recognition on only (or mostly) just one. In the absence of that finding, a single-process account will be a more parsimonious explanation; there will be no strong evidence in favor of two separate processes in aging associative memory.

3.4.1 Concordance plots

Another way to examine the data with state-trace analysis is to look at *concordance plots*. Concordance plots examine the differences in scores between two levels of an experimental factor to assess whether those differences are consistent or inconsistent with a monotonic function (see, e.g., Dunn, 2008). For example, in a set of experiments that manipulated study time over two levels, one would expect longer exposure durations to lead to higher hit rates, i.e., correctly identifying an old item as old; the difference in the hit rates across conditions (longer minus shorter exposure) should be non-negative in each experiment. Non-negative differences are *concordant* with the predicted outcome, and negative differences are *discordant*. Points in the upper right (or lower left) quadrant indicate data consistent with the monotonic function (concordant points); the others are discordant.

For the purpose of examining the data another way in addition to the state-trace plots, we reviewed all of the studies of associative and item recognition that fit the inclusion criteria in our meta-analysis and used concordance plots to examine the differences between younger and older adults' performance. If item and associative memory are positively and monotonically related, then any manipulation that increases performance on one task cannot produce a decrease in performance on the other task. So, item memory performance differences across experimental conditions should have the same sign as associative memory performance differences (i.e., concordance). For example, younger adults may perform better than older adults on item tasks, but this performance advantage would also appear in associative tasks because younger adults have more of that underlying resource available in both item and associative tasks than older adults. Any point that does not reflect this pattern is discordant. If there are a large number of discordant points that are not due to measurement noise, item and associative memory performance may depend on different underlying processes.

3.4.2 Method

Sample of Studies

Articles published before mid-2006 were compiled from the Old and Naveh-Benjamin (2008a) meta-analysis. Articles published after mid-2006 were found via the PsycInfo database, searching for terms including: assoc*, aging, memory, context, source, and binding. The search was completed in June 2012.

The following criteria were necessary for inclusion in the meta-analysis: participation of both younger adults and older adults without known dementia or memory problems, and use of hits, i.e., responding "old" to targets; false alarms, i.e., responding "old" responses to lures; or d', i.e., in signal-detection terms, the "distance" between the target and the lure distributions, as the summary measure for both item and associative memory performance. Articles were also included in the d' analyses if d' could be calculated from the published statistics.

We found 19 articles with a total of 34 experiments that fulfilled the first criteria (see Appendix). All but two of the articles concluded there was an age-related deficit in associative memory compared to item memory. Of the remaining two articles, one found no age effects on memory for facial expression (D'Argembeau & Van der Linden, 2004), perhaps because the study face and facial expression were bound together in a unitized fashion, which may reduce the associative memory deficit (Bastin et al., 2013). The second article reported that older adults performed slightly better than younger adults at remembering whether a word was externally or internally generated (Gregory, Mergler, Durso, & Zandi, 1988). However, participants were unaware that there would be a memory test, and incidental encoding can reduce the associative memory deficit (Old & Naveh-Benjamin, 2008a).

Thirty experiments were used for analysis of hits, 25 for false alarms, and 20 for d'.

3.4.3 Results

The state-trace plots for hits, false alarms, and d' can be found in Figure 3.4.

No obvious non-monotonicity was observed. Younger adults had higher hit rates and lower false alarm rates than older adults for both item and associative tests. These hit and false alarm rate differences led to the overall finding that younger

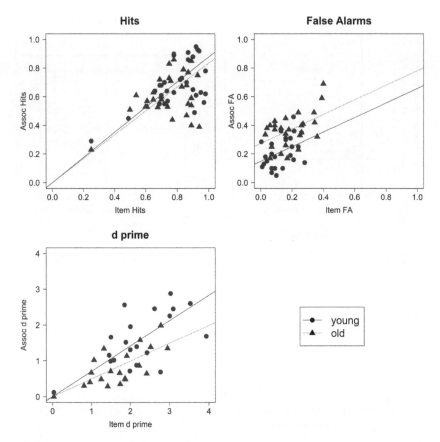

FIGURE 3.4 State-trace plots for hits, false alarms, and d' with final hierarchical linear model lines.

adults had higher d' scores than older adults on both tasks, reflecting better overall memory performance. No obvious duality of processes was seen, but since the data were noisy, we also looked at concordance plots.

The concordant plots for hits, false alarms, and d' are shown in Figure 3.5. The points on this plot are the difference scores between younger adults' performance and older adults' performance (younger minus older). Because d' scores were calculated from the overall experiments' hits and false alarms rather than from individual participants' hits and false alarms, standard errors for each d' score could not be calculated.

The hit rates show overwhelming concordance in the age effects for item and associative tests; performance on these tasks is monotonically related. The difference between younger and older adults' hit rates increased for item tests as it increased for associative tests. Only one of these three points appears to be significantly discordant (larger than the estimated standard error). This discordant point is from

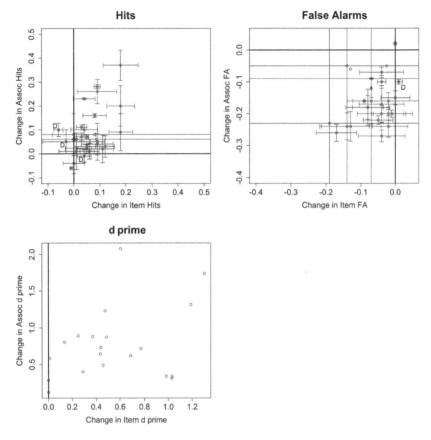

FIGURE 3.5 Concordance plots for hits, false alarms, and d'. Each point represents older adults' performance subtracted from younger adults' performance for a single experiment. Discordant points are labelled D. Standard errors for the differences were calculated assuming a correlation of r = 0.1 (correlations as large as 0.9 did not much influence the estimated error bars).

Kim and Giovanello (2011), which provides the only between-subjects comparison in the meta-analysis. All other points were concordant or could be easily made concordant.

The concordance plot for the false alarm rates shows a similar pattern: the difference between younger and older adults' false alarm rates decreased for item tests as it decreased for associative tests.[1] Only one point was discordant, and that may be due to measurement noise: the size of the effect is not larger than the estimated standard error. The discordant point in the false alarms analysis (Kim & Giovanello, 2011) was due to older adults having atypically higher false alarm rates for items compared to younger adults (0.18 v. 0.01).

The d' concordance plot shows that there is a highly variable but positive trend for the difference scores. Most notably, there were no discordant points, so according to the concordance analysis and consistent with our visual conclusion for the state-trace plots, there is no strong evidence for multiple underlying processes.

3.4.4 Statistical analysis

Despite its usefulness, mere visual inspection of the data is not sufficient to reach strong conclusions, and statistical analysis is required. The inferential statistics for state-trace analysis are not yet clear and widely accepted, since the possible shapes of the functions relating performance on the two tasks are both undefined and unknown (Newell & Dunn, 2008). There are recent efforts to develop tests for departures from monotonicity for fully within-subject designs (e.g., Prince, Brown, & Heathcote, 2012). However, for between-subjects designs, a hierarchical linear modeling approach is currently the best option (e.g., Sliwinski & Hall, 1998).

The item and associative recognition tasks were varied within-subjects, so we nested the data points within studies. We used an empty model to test the necessity of an explanatory variable: $A = \beta_0$, where A is associative performance and β_0 is the intercept. Also, there was a simple linear model including item task performance as an explanatory variable: $A = \beta_0 + \beta_1 I$, where β_1 is the slope relating item performance to associative performance, and I is item performance.[2] Finally, we fit the full model including item task performance, categorical age, and item by age interaction variables:

$$A = \beta_0 + \beta_1 I + \beta_2 C + \beta_3 I \times C \tag{1}$$

where C is the categorical age of younger adult or older adult. If the slopes for age or the item by age interaction are significant, then younger and older adults' performance fall on different state-trace functions and cannot be explained by the same single process.

Applying these statistical methods to the data led to a different conclusion than simple visual interpretation of the state-trace and concordance plots. For the hit rates, false alarm rates, and d' data, fit separately, the predictions of the best fitting model are shown superimposed on the data in Figure 3.4. In all cases, different linear functions are needed for each age group, consistent with their use of different processes.

For the hit rates, the significant model parameters were $\beta_0 = 0.88$ (SE = 0.32) and $\beta_3 = -0.044$ (SE = 0.022), indicating a significant interaction of item and categorical age, and no main effects for item recognition performance or age. Compared to the young adults, older adults' associative hit rates did not increase as steeply with item recognition hit rates, though the interaction effect was small. For the false alarm rates, the significant model parameters were $\beta_0 = 0.15$ (SE = 0.03), $\beta_1 = 0.51$ (SE = 0.15), and $\beta_2 = 0.12$ (SE = 0.02), indicating a significant intercept, effect of item recognition performance, and effect of age, but no interaction of age with item recognition. Older adults' had uniformly higher associative recognition false alarm rates than younger adults. For d', the significant model parameters were

$\beta_1 = 0.71$ (SE = 0.06) and $\beta_3 = -0.21$ (SE = 0.04), indicating a significant effect of item performance and interaction with categorical age: compared to young adults, older adults' associative d' scores did not increase as quickly with their item recognition scores. In each of the measures, younger adults and older adults' data separated, revealing that a single monotonic function was not sufficient to capture both younger and older adults' performance.

Thus, the two interpretive approaches yielded different conclusions. The visual state-trace and, especially, the concordance plot analysis showed no strong evidence that two processes underlie the age-related associative memory deficit. On the other hand, hierarchical linear modeling suggested that two distinct processes are involved in the age-related relative decline in associative memory performance.

3.4.5 Discussion

A state-trace analysis of 34 experiments on the age-related associative memory deficit reveals some evidence for a dual-process account. The dual-process signal detection model assumptions mean that state-trace analysis should yield dissociable representations of the underlying psychological processes if one, but not the other, of those processes is impaired. The state-trace analysis yielded distinct functions for the young and older adults' data, reflecting different contributions of the underlying psychological processes that influence hit rates, false alarm rates, and d' scores. While the visual analysis of the concordance plots showed all but one point was consistent with a single monotonic curve, hierarchical linear modeling revealed that younger and older adults' associative memory performance could not be explained by a single monotonic function. Younger and older adults' task performance did not rely on the same unique process.

It is worth noting that the analysis is atheoretical: the state-trace analysis cannot infer which processes occur, merely that more than one process is necessary to explain the data. Aging therefore affects associative episodic memory by impacting at least one psychological process, where at least two processes are operating. Though it is unknown what the affected process may be, current dual-process explanations of aging recognition memory suggest it is a recall-like process. Our analysis also showed a dissociation in the hits.

There are two main limitations of the current meta-analysis. First is the number of excluded studies. Only 34 experiments, from 19 separate articles, were included in the analysis: a small fraction of the literature. Indeed, over 100 articles were considered but ultimately excluded because of incomplete data reporting.

A second limitation of our analysis is that the data in these studies were very noisy, which likely accounts for the conflicting conclusions in our analyses. The state-trace plot of within-subjects factors is generally cleaner (e.g., Dunn, 2008, Newell, Dunn, & Kalish, 2010), as any between-subjects or across studies comparison will necessarily have more variability. Standardization of the data can help with between-study comparisons but requires the assumption that the slope of each condition is the same (Dunn, 2008), a point violated in our data.

3.5   Conclusions and looking ahead

The results of our meta-analysis indicate potential avenues for improving memory in older adults. Because these results are consistent with dual-process signal detection theories and these theories are prominent, it may be fruitful to attempt to improve the component processes proposed by the theories.

One approach is to improve recollection, perhaps by targeting its strategic use. Older adults are less likely to spontaneously use strategies to remember information than younger adults, though using associative strategies can improve their memory (Naveh-Benjamin, Brav, & Levy, 2007). Naveh-Benjamin and colleagues (2007) presented younger and older adults with unrelated word pairs and either gave no specific instruction or asked them to create sentences with the words during study and to retrieve those sentences at test. This strategy greatly improved older adults' associative memory, whereas younger adults benefitted less.

Another approach is to improve the familiarity process in older adults, specifically by *unitization*, or the grouping of items into a single cohesive whole. In experiments by Bastin et al. (2013), participants were asked to unitize word-color associations by imagining the object in the color of the background of the screen. In comparison to a condition in which the associations were not made familiar via unitization, older adults exhibited a reduced associative deficit. Other empirical examples of unitization include associating the features of a face into a single whole (Yonelinas, Kroll, Dobbins, & Soltani, 1999) or creating interactive imagery (Rhodes & Donaldson, 2008). While defining unitization *a priori* can be difficult (Harlow, Mackenzie, & Donaldson, 2010; Mayes et al., 2004), it does seem clear that the extent to which information can be made more cohesive and less disparate will improve associative memory, potentially because this may reduce the reliance on recollection.

Though state-trace analysis is agnostic as to whether recollection is specifically affected by aging, our results suggest that the age-related associative memory deficit is due to impairment of at least one memory process. A single-process signal detection theory of memory is, therefore, not sufficient to explain the effects of aging on associative memory, and the prevalent dual-process explanations of recognition memory suggesting that aging specifically affects a recall process may provide a better theoretical framework to understanding age-related changes in associative memory.

APPENDIX A

Studies	n		Stimuli		Hits			
					Young		Old	
	Young	Old	Item	Associative	Item	Associative	Item	Associative
Chua, Chen, & Park (2006)	26	26	statements	statements and speaker	0.98	0.62	0.94	0.39
	26	28	statements	statements and speaker	0.97	0.56	0.89	0.40
Cohn, Emrich, & Moscovitch (2008)	24	24	words	word pairs	0.82	0.72	0.76	0.71
D'argembeau &Van der Linden (2004)	32	32	faces	faces and expressions	0.74	0.64	0.65	0.58
Dennis, Hayes, Prince, Madden, Huettel, & Cabeza (2008)	14	14	faces	face–scene pairs	0.49	0.45	0.50	0.51
			faces	face–scene pairs	0.25	0.29	0.25	0.23
Gopie, Craik, & Hasher (2010)	20	20	faces	facts and faces	0.83	0.73	0.86	0.68
	20	20	faces	facts and faces	0.98	0.78	0.93	0.75
Gregory, Mergler, Durso, & Zandi (1988)	20	20	words	words and source (imagined or perceived)	0.69	0.55	0.68	0.53
Kersten & Earles (2010)	16	16	actions	action–person pairs	0.90	0.65	0.89	0.59
	24	24	actions	action–person pairs	0.95	0.63	0.87	0.55
Kilb & Naveh-Benjamin (2011)	24	24	faces, scenes	face–scene pairs	0.70	0.68	0.70	0.60
	26	25	faces, scenes	face–scene pairs	0.66	0.64	0.65	0.63
Kim & Giovanello (2011)	12	12	words	word pairs	0.78	0.89	0.84	0.79
Naveh–Benjamin & Craik (1995)	25	25	words	words and fonts	0.70	0.61	0.61	0.57
			words	words and fonts	0.78	0.63	0.74	0.53
	25		words	words and voice	0.72	0.55	0.61	0.53
			words	words and voice	0.74	0.57	0.70	0.58

Studies	n		Stimuli					
	Young	Old	Item	Associative				
	35	35	words	words and voice	0.91	0.49	0.86	0.47
			words	words and voice	0.92	0.61	0.89	0.54
Naveh–Benjamin, Guez, & Shulman (2004)	22	22	words	word pairs	0.78	0.90	0.60	0.53
Naveh–Benjamin, Hussain, Guez, & Bar-On (2003)	18	18	objects	object pairs	0.93	0.93	0.75	0.73
	30	30	objects	object pairs	0.86	0.70	0.77	0.44
			objects	object pairs	0.87	0.86	0.75	0.83
Naveh–Benjamin, Shing, Kilb, Werkle–Bergner, Lindenberger, & Li (2009)	24	23	names	name face pairs	0.69	0.68	0.69	0.72
Old & Naveh–Benjamin (2008b)	42	42	names	name face pairs	0.72	0.70	0.54	0.61
	28	28	actions	action-person pairs	0.87	0.91	0.78	0.86
Wang, Dew, & Giovanello (2010)	60	56	words	word pairs	0.94	0.92	0.89	0.85
			words	word pairs	0.90	0.88	0.87	0.77
Wegesin, Friedman, Varughese, & Stern (2002)	14	14	words	words and list	0.92	0.95	0.83	0.67

False Alarms

Studies	n		Stimuli		Young		Old	
	Young	Old	Item	Associative	Item	Associative	Item	Associative
Cohn, Emrich, & Moscovitch (2008)	24	24	words	word pairs	0.28	0.14	0.36	0.32
			words	word pairs	0.10	0.05	0.17	0.17
Cyr & Anderson (2012)	33	31	words	words and context	0.01	0.29	0.03	0.34

(Continued)

Studies	n		Stimuli		False Alarms			
					Young		Old	
	Young	Old	Item	Associative	Item	Associative	Item	Associative
Dennis, Hayes, Prince, Madden, Huettel, & Cabeza (2008)	14	14	faces	face-scene pairs	0.07	0.10	0.16	0.26
			faces	face-scene pairs	0.24	0.25	0.24	0.23
Dywan, Segalowitz, & Arsenault (2002)	13	13	words	words and list	0.09	0.18	0.13	0.38
Gopie, Craik, & Hasher (2010)	20	20	faces	facts and faces	0.07	0.27	0.09	0.43
	20	20	faces	facts and faces	0.03	0.18	0.07	0.25
Kersten & Earles (2010)	16	16	actions	action-person pairs	0.19	0.31	0.26	0.40
	24	24	actions	action-person pairs	0.13	0.36	0.27	0.41
			actions	action-person pairs	0.21	0.46	0.40	0.69
Kilb & Naveh-Benjamin (2011)	24	24	faces, scenes	face-scene pairs	0.07	0.20	0.09	0.40
	26	25	faces, scenes	face-scene pairs	0.04	0.15	0.09	0.37
Kim & Giovanello (2011)	12	12	words	word pairs	0.01	0.11	0.18	0.37
Memon, Bartlett, Rose, & Gray (2003)	84	88	faces	faces and list	0.26	0.35	0.39	0.59
			faces	faces and list	0.20	0.25	0.34	0.49
Naveh-Benjamin, Guez, & Shulman (2004)	22	22	words	word pairs	0.14	0.10	0.16	0.34
Naveh-Benjamin, Hussain, Guez, & Bar-On (2003)	18	18	objects	object pairs	0.02	0.13	0.06	0.40
	30	30	objects	object pairs	0.21	0.16	0.25	0.33
			objects	object pairs	0.19	0.19	0.26	0.35

Studies	n		Stimuli		d'			
					Young		Old	
	Young	Old	Item	Associative	Item	Associative	Item	Associative
Naveh–Benjamin, Shing, Kilb, Werkle-Bergner, Lindenberger, & Li (2009)	24	23	names	name face pairs	0.16	0.30	0.16	0.45
Old & Naveh–Benjamin (2008b)	42	42	names	name face pairs	0.16	0.31	0.24	0.49
	28	28	actions	action-person pairs	0.03	0.18	0.04	0.38
Wang, Dew, & Giovanello (2010)	60	56	words	word pairs	0.07	0.07	0.06	0.17
			words	word pairs	0.09	0.10	0.13	0.20
Cohn, Emrich, & Moscovitch (2008)	24	24	words	word pairs	1.50	1.66	1.06	1.02
D'argembeau & Van der Linden (2004)	32	32	faces	faces and expressions	1.99	0.72	0.96	0.40
Dennis, Hayes, Prince, Madden, Huettel, & Cabeza (2008)	14	14	faces	face-scene pairs	1.45	1.16	0.99	0.67
			faces	face-scene pairs	0.03	0.12	0.03	0.00
Gopie, Craik, & Hasher (2010)	20	20	faces	facts and faces	2.43	1.23	2.42	0.64
	20	20	faces	facts and faces	3.93	1.69	2.95	1.35
Kersten & Earles (2010)	16	16	actions	action-person pairs	2.16	0.88	1.87	0.48
	24	24	actions	action-person pairs	2.77	0.69	1.74	0.35
Kilb & Naveh–Benjamin (2011)	24	24	faces, scenes	face-scene pairs	2.00	1.31	1.87	0.51
	26	25	faces, scenes	face-scene pairs	2.16	1.39	1.73	0.66
Kim & Giovanello (2011)	12	12	words	word pairs	3.10	2.45	1.91	1.14
Naveh-Benjamin, Guez, & Shulman (2004)	22	22	words	word pairs	1.85	2.56	1.25	0.49
Naveh-Benjamin, Hussain, Guez, & Bar-On (2003)	18	18	objects	object pairs	3.53	2.60	2.23	0.87

(Continued)

APPENDIX A Continued

Studies	n		Stimuli		d'			
					Young		Old	
	Young	Old	Item	Associative	Item	Associative	Item	Associative
	30	30	objects	object pairs	1.89	1.52	1.41	0.29
			objects	object pairs	2.00	1.96	1.32	1.34
Naveh-Benjamin, Shing, Kilb, Werkle-Bergner, Lindenberger, & Li (2009)	24	23	names	name face pairs	1.49	0.99	1.49	0.71
	42	42	names	name face pairs	1.58	1.02	0.81	0.30
Old & Naveh-Benjamin (2008b)	28	28	actions	action-person pairs	3.01	2.26	2.52	1.39
Wang, Dew, & Giovanello (2010)	60	56	words	word pairs	3.03	2.88	2.78	1.99
			words	word pairs	2.62	2.46	2.25	1.58

Acknowledgements

This research was supported in part by grant AG16201 from the National Institute on Aging to P.V.

Notes

1 A few points have associated error bars that are an order of magnitude larger than those for other experiments with similar sample sizes. We suspect that those reflect reporting errors in the original articles, such as reported standard deviations being mislabeled as standard errors.
2 Introducing curvilinearity to the model did not improve any fits.

References

★ = study included in meta-analysis

Bamber, D. (1979). State-trace analysis: A method of testing simple theories of causation. *Journal of Mathematical Psychology, 19*, 137–181. doi:10.1016/0022-2496(79)90016-6

Banks, W.P. (1970). Signal detection theory and human memory. *Psychological Bulletin, 74*, 81–99.

Bastin, C., Diana, R.A., Simon, J., Collette, F., Yonelinas, A.P., & Salmon, E. (2013). Associative memory in aging: The effect of unitization on source memory. *Psychology and Aging, 28*, 275–283. doi:10.1037/a0031566

Benjamin, A.S. (2010). Representational explanations of "process" dissociations in recognition: The DRYAD theory of aging and memory judgments. *Psychological Review, 117*, 1055–1079. doi:10.1037/a0020810

★Chua, H.F., Chen, W., & Park, D. C. (2006). Source memory, aging and culture. *Gerontology, 52*(5), 306–313. doi:10.1159/000094612

★Cohn, M., Emrich, S.M., & Moscovitch, M. (2008). Age-related deficits in associative memory: The influence of impaired strategic retrieval. *Psychology and Aging, 23*, 93–103. doi:10.1037/0882-7974.23.1.93

Curran, T. (2004). Effects of attention and confidence on the hypothesized ERP correlates of recollection and familiarity. *Neuropsychologia, 42*(8), 1088–1106. doi:10.1016/j.neuropsychologia.2003.12.011

Curran, T. (1999). The electrophysiology of incidental and intentional retrieval: ERP old/new effects in lexical decision and recognition memory. *Neuropsychologia, 35*, 1035–1049.

★Cyr, A.-A., & Anderson, N.D. (2012). Trial-and-error learning improves source memory among young and older adults. *Psychology and Aging, 27*, 429–439. doi:10.1037/a0025115

★D'Argembeau, A., & Van der Linden, M. (2004). Identity but not expression memory for unfamiliar faces is affected by ageing. *Memory, 12*, 644–654. doi:10.1080/09658210344000198

de Zubicaray, G.I., McMahon, K.L., Dennis, S., & Dunn, J.C. (2011). Memory strength effects in fMRI studies: A matter of confidence. *Journal of Cognitive Neuroscience, 23*, 2324–2335. doi:10.1162/jocn.2010.21601

★Dennis, N.A., Hayes, S.M., Prince, S.E., Madden, D.J., Huettel, S.A., & Cabeza, R. (2008). Effects of aging on the neural correlates of successful item and source memory encoding. *Journal of Experimental Psychology: Learning, Memory, and Cognition, 34*, 791–808. doi:10.1037/0278-7393.34.4.791

Diana, R. A., Reder, L.M., Arndt, J., & Park, H. (2006). Models of recognition: A review of arguments in favor of a dual-process account. *Psychonomic Bulletin & Review, 13*, 1–21. doi:10.3758/BF03193807

Dodson, C.S., Bawa, S., & Slotnick, S.D. (2007). Aging, source memory, and misrecollections. *Journal of Experimental Psychology. Learning, Memory, and Cognition, 33*, 169–181. doi:10.1037/0278-7393.33.1.169

Dunn, J.C., & Kirsner, K. (1988). Discovering functionally independent mental processes: The principle of reversed association. *Psychological Review, 95*, 91–101.

Dunn, J.C. (2008). The dimensionality of the remember-know task: A state-trace analysis. *Psychological Review, 115*(2), 426–46. doi:10.1037/0033-295X.115.2.426

★Dywan, J., Segalowitz, S., & Arsenault, A. (2002). Electrophysiological response during source memory decisions in older and younger adults. *Brain and Cognition, 49*, 322–340. doi:10.1006/brcg.2001.1503

Eichenbaum, H., Yonelinas, A.P., & Ranganath, C. (2007). The medial temporal lobe and recognition memory. *Annual Review of Neuroscience, 30*, 123–152. doi:10.1146/annurev. neuro.30.051606.094328

Freeman, E., Dennis, S., & Dunn, J.C. (2010). An examination of the ERP correlates of recognition memory using state-trace analysis. In S. Ohlsson & R. Catrambone (Eds.), *Proceedings of the 32nd Annual Conference of the Cognitive Science Society* (pp. 97–102). Austin, TX: Cognitive Science Society.

Gallo, D.A., Cotel, S.C., Moore, C.D., & Schacter, D.L. (2007). Aging can spare recollection-based retrieval monitoring: The importance of event distinctiveness. *Psychology and Aging, 22*, 209–213. doi:10.1037/0882-7974.22.1.209

Glisky, E.L., Rubin, S.R., & Davidson, P.S.R. (2001). Source memory in older adults: An encoding or retrieval problem? *Journal of Experimental Psychology: Learning, Memory, and Cognition, 27*, 1131–1146. doi:10.1037//0278-7393.27.5.1131

★Gopie, N., Craik, F.I.M., & Hasher, L. (2010). Destination memory impairment in older people. *Psychology and Aging, 25*, 922–928. doi:10.1037/a0019703

★Gregory, M., Mergler, N., Durso, F., & Zandi, T. (1988). Cognitive reality monitoring in adulthood. *Educational Gerontology, 14*(1), 1–13.

Harlow, I.M., Mackenzie, G., & Donaldson, D.I. (2010). Familiarity for associations? A test of the domain dichotomy theory. *Journal of Experimental Psychology. Learning, Memory, and Cognition, 36*(6), 1381–1388. doi:10.1037/a0020610

Hashtroudi, S., Johnson, M.K., & Chrosniak, L.D. (1989). Aging and source monitoring. *Psychology and Aging, 4*, 106–112.

Hautus, M.J., Macmillan, N.A., & Rotello, C.M. (2008). Toward a complete decision model of item and source recognition. *Psychonomic Bulletin & Review, 15*, 889–905. doi:10.3758/ PBR.15.5.889

Healy, M.R., Light, L.L., & Chung, C. (2005). Dual-process models of associative recognition in young and older adults: Evidence from receiver operating characteristics. *Journal of Experimental Psychology. Learning, Memory, and Cognition, 31*, 768–788. doi:10.1037/0278-7393.31.4.768

Jang, Y., Wixted, J.T., & Huber, D.E. (2009). Testing signal-detection models of yes/no and two-alternative forced-choice recognition memory. *Journal of Experimental Psychology: General, 138*, 291–306. doi:10.1037/a0015525

Kausler, D.H., & Puckett, J.M. (1980). Adult age differences in recognition memory for a nonsemantic attribute. *Experimental Aging Research, 6*, 349–355.

Kelley, R., & Wixted, J.T. (2001). On the nature of associative information in recognition memory. *Journal of Experimental Psychology: Learning, Memory, and Cognition, 27*, 701–722. doi:10.1037//0278-7393.27.3.701

★Kersten, A.W., & Earles, J.L. (2010). Effects of aging, distraction, and response pressure on the binding of actors and actions. *Psychology and Aging, 25*, 620–630. doi:10.1037/a0019131

★Kilb, A., & Naveh-Benjamin, M. (2011). The effects of pure pair repetition on younger and older adults' associative memory. *Journal of Experimental Psychology: Learning, Memory, and Cognition, 37,* 706–719. doi:10.1037/a0022525

★Kim, S.-Y., & Giovanello, K.S. (2011). The effects of attention on age-related relational memory deficits: Evidence from a novel attentional manipulation. *Psychology and Aging, 26,* 678–688. doi:10.1037/a0022326

Light, L.L., Prull, M.W., La Voie, D.J., & Healy, M.R. (2000). Dual process theories of memory in old age. In T.J. Perfect & E.A. Maylor (Eds.), *Models of cognitive aging* (pp. 239–300). Oxford: Oxford University Press.

Macho, S. (2004). Modeling associative recognition: A comparison of two-high-threshold, two-high-threshold signal detection, and mixture distribution models. *Journal of Experimental Psychology: Learning, Memory, and Cognition, 30,* 83–97. doi:10.1037/0278-7393.30.1.83

Macmillan, N.A., & Creelman, C.D. (2005). *Detection Theory: A User's Guide.* Mahwah, New Jersey: Lawrence Erlbaum Associates, Inc.

Mandler, G. (1980). Recognizing: The judgment of previous occurrence. *Psychological Review, 87*(3), 252–271.

Mayes, A.R., Holdstock, J.S., Isaac, C.L., Montaldi, D., Grigor, J., Gummer, A., . . . Norman, K.A. (2004). Associative recognition in a patient with selective hippocampal lesions and relatively normal item recognition. *Hippocampus, 14*(6), 763–784. doi:10.1002/hipo.10211

★Memon, A., Bartlett, J., Rose, R., & Gray, C. (2003). The aging eyewitness: Effects of age on face, delay, and source-memory ability. *The Journals of Gerontology, 58,* P338–345.

Mickes, L., Wais, P.E., & Wixted, J.T. (2009). Recollection is a continuous process: Implications for dual-process theories of recognition memory. *Psychological Science, 20,* 509–515. doi:10.1111/j.1467-9280.2009.02324.x

Naveh-Benjamin, M. (2000). Adult age differences in memory performance: Tests of an associative deficit hypothesis. *Journal of Experimental Psychology: Learning, Memory, and Cognition, 26,* 1170–1187. doi:10.1037//0278-7393.26.5.1170

★Naveh-Benjamin, M., Brav, T.K., & Levy, O. (2007). The associative memory deficit of older adults: The role of strategy utilization. *Psychology and Aging, 22,* 202–208. doi:10.1037/0882-7974.22.1.202

★Naveh-Benjamin, M., & Craik, F.I. (1995). Memory for context and its use in item memory: Comparisons of younger and older persons. *Psychology and Aging, 10,* 284–293.

Naveh-Benjamin, M., Craik, F.I.M., Guez, J., & Kreuger, S. (2005). Divided attention in younger and older adults: Effects of strategy and relatedness on memory performance and secondary task costs. *Journal of Experimental Psychology: Learning, Memory, and Cognition, 31,* 520–537. doi:10.1037/0278-7393.31.3.520

★Naveh-Benjamin, M., Guez, J., & Shulman, S. (2004). Older adults' associative deficit in episodic memory: Assessing the role of decline in attentional resources. *Psychonomic Bulletin & Review, 11,* 1067–1073.

★Naveh-Benjamin, M., Hussain, Z., Guez, J., & Bar-On, M. (2003). Adult age differences in episodic memory: Further support for an associative-deficit hypothesis. *Journal of Experimental Psychology: Learning, Memory, and Cognition, 29,* 826–837. doi:10.1037/0278-7393.29.5.826

Naveh-Benjamin, M., Shing, Y. L., Kilb, A., Werkle-Bergner, M., Lindenberger, U., & Li, S. C. (2009). Adult age differences in memory for name–face associations: The effects of intentional and incidental learning. *Memory, 17*(2), 220-232.

Newell, B.R., & Dunn, J.C. (2008). Dimensions in data: Testing psychological models using state-trace analysis. *Trends in Cognitive Sciences, 12,* 285–290. doi:10.1016/j.tics.2008.04.009

Newell, B. R., Dunn, J. C., & Kalish, M. (2010). The dimensionality of perceptual category learning: A state-trace analysis. *Memory & Cognition, 38*(5), 563–581.

Old, S.R., & Naveh-Benjamin, M. (2008a). Differential effects of age on item and associative measures of memory: A meta-analysis. *Psychology and Aging, 23*, 104–118. doi:10.1037/0882-7974.23.1.104

*Old, S.R., & Naveh-Benjamin, M. (2008b). Memory for people and their actions: Further evidence for an age-related associative deficit. *Psychology and Aging, 23*, 467–472. doi:10.1037/0882-7974.23.2.467

Parks, C.M., & Yonelinas, A.P. (2007). Moving beyond pure signal-detection models: Comment on Wixted (2007). *Psychological Review, 114*, 188–202. doi:10.1037/0033-295X.114.1.188

Pazzaglia, A. M., Dube, C., & Rotello, C.M. (2013). A critical comparison of discrete-state and continuous models of recognition memory: Implications for recognition and beyond. *Psychological Bulletin, 139*(6), 1173–1203. doi:10.1037/a0033044

Prince, M., Brown, S., & Heathcote, A. (2012). The design and analysis of state-trace experiments. *Psychological Methods, 17*(1), 78–99. doi:10.1037/a0025809

Reder, L.M., Nhouyvanisvong, A., Schunn, C.D., Ayers, M.S., Angstadt, P., & Hiraki, K. (2000). A mechanistic account of the mirror effect for word frequency: A computational model of remember-know judgments in a continuous recognition paradigm. *Journal of Experimental Psychology: Learning, Memory, and Cognition, 26*, 294–320. doi:10.1037//0278-7393.26.2.294

Rhodes, S.M., & Donaldson, D.I. (2008). Electrophysiological evidence for the effect of interactive imagery on episodic memory: Encouraging familiarity for non-unitized stimuli during associative recognition. *NeuroImage, 39*(2), 873–884. doi:10.1016/j.neuroimage.2007.08.041

Rotello, C.M., & Heit, E. (2000). Associative recognition: A case of recall-to-reject processing. *Memory and Cognition, 28*, 907–922.

Rotello, C.M., Macmillan, N.A., & Van Tassel, G. (2000). Recall-to-reject in recognition: Evidence from ROC curves. *Journal of Memory and Language, 43*, 67–88.

Rugg, M.D., & Curran, T. (2007). Event-related potentials and recognition memory. *Trends in Cognitive Sciences, 11*(6), 251–257. doi:10.1016/j.tics.2007.04.004

Rugg, M.D., Fletcher, P.C., Allan, K., Frith, C.D., Frackowiak, R.S., & Dolan, R.J. (1998). Neural correlates of memory retrieval during recognition memory and cued recall. *NeuroImage, 8*(3), 262–273. doi:10.1006/nimg.1998.0363

Rugg, M.D., & Yonelinas, A.P. (2003). Human recognition memory: A cognitive neuroscience perspective. *Trends in Cognitive Sciences, 7*(7), 313–319. doi:10.1016/S1364-6613(03)00131–1

Sliwinski, M., & Hall, C.B. (1998). Constraints on general slowing: A meta-analysis using hierarchical linear models with random coefficients. *Psychology and Aging, 13*, 164–175.

Spencer, W.D., & Raz, N. (1995). Differential effects of aging on memory for content and context: A meta-analysis. *Psychology and Aging, 10*, 527–539.

Starns, J.J., Pazzaglia, A. M., Rotello, C.M., Hautus, M.J., & Macmillan, N.A. (2013). Unequal-strength source zROC slopes reflect criteria placement and not (necessarily) memory processes. *Journal of Experimental Psychology: Learning, Memory, and Cognition, 39*, 1377–1392

Tulving, E. (1985). Memory and consciousness. *Canadian Psychology/Psychologie Canadienne, 26*, 1–12. doi:10.1037/h0080017

Verhaeghen, P. (2014). *The elements of cognitive aging: Meta-analyses of age-related differences in processing speed and their consequences.* New York, NY: Oxford University Press.

Verhaeghen, P., & De Meersman, L. (1998). Aging and the negative priming effect: A meta-analysis. *Psychology and Aging, 13*, 435–444.

Verhaeghen, P., Steitz, D.W., Sliwinski, M.J., & Cerella, J. (2003). Aging and dual-task performance: A meta-analysis. *Psychology and Aging, 18*, 443–460. doi:10.1037/0882-7974.18.3.443

★Wang, W.-C., Dew, I.T.Z., & Giovanello, K.S. (2010). Effects of aging and prospective memory on recognition of item and associative information. *Psychology and Aging, 25*, 486–491. doi:10.1037/a0017264

★Wegesin, D.J., Friedman, D., Varughese, N., & Stern, Y. (2002). Age-related changes in source memory retrieval: An ERP replication and extension. *Brain Research, 13*, 323–338. Retrieved from http://www.ncbi.nlm.nih.gov/pubmed/11918998

Wixted, J.T. (2007). Dual-process theory and signal-detection theory of recognition memory. *Psychological Review, 114*, 152–176. doi:10.1037/0033-295X.114.1.152

Yonelinas, A.P. (1994). Receiver-operating characteristics in recognition memory: Evidence for a dual-process model. *Journal of Experimental Psychology: Learning, Memory, and Cognition, 20*(6), 1341–1354.

Yonelinas, A.P. (1997). Recognition memory ROCs for item and associative information: The contribution of recollection and familiarity. *Memory & Cognition, 25*, 747–763.

Yonelinas, A.P. (2001). Consciousness, control, and confidence: The 3 Cs of recognition memory. *Journal of Experimental Psychology: General, 130*, 361–379. doi:10.1037/0096-3445.130.3.361

Yonelinas, A.P. (2002). The nature of recollection and familiarity: A review of 30 years of research. *Journal of Memory and Language, 46*, 441–517. doi:10.1006/jmla.2002.2864

Yonelinas, A.P., Kroll, N.E.A., Dobbins, I.G., & Soltani, M. (1999). Recognition memory for faces: When familiarity supports associative recognition judgments. *Psychonomic Bulletin & Review, 6*(4), 654–661.

4

REMEMBERING THE SOURCE

Directions for intervention in ageing

Noeleen M. Brady and Richard A. P. Roche

4.1 Source memory

Our ability to remember the origin of a piece of information or the contextual details of an event – *who* told us something, *where* we were when it happened, *when* it took place – is an aspect of memory that is crucial for our ability to function independently in the world. The scientific study of this capacity – termed *source memory* – dates back to the early 1990s when a number of studies suggested that humans often have difficulty in differentiating between something we *remember* and something that we *know* or that seems *familiar* (see also Chapter 3 for a similar dichotomy, i.e., recollection and familiarity). For example, your daily commute to work represents a very familiar activity, but you probably do not remember the specific journey to work, say, two days ago.

Evidence to support this distinction came from a variety of studies showing, among other things, that people sometimes had issues telling apart real from imagined actions (Hashtroudi, Johnson, & Crosniak, 1990) or events (Cohen & Faulkner, 1989), famous from non-famous faces (Bartlett, Strater, & Fulton, 1991; Dywan & Jacoby, 1990), male from female voices (Senkfor & Van Petten, 1998), and memories for spoken words from memory for words rehearsed sub-vocally (Hashtroudi, Johnson, & Crosniak, 1989).

Originally, source memory was defined as the recollection of the *context* in which an event happened (Schmitter-Edgecombe, Woo, & Greeley, 2009), *how* an item was encoded (Schacter, Osowiecki, Kaszniak, Kihlstrom, & Valdiserri, 1994) or *when* and *where* facts were acquired (Jacoby, Shimizu, Daniels, & Rhodes, 2005). When a specific episode took place, source memory was considered as the ability to recall that particular episode's source, i.e., the origin of the memory (Schacter, Kaszniak, Kihlstrom, & Valdiserri, 1991). However, according to Glisky and Kong (2008), this definition is too narrow, and the term source memory has since been extended to include any and all specific aspects of the associated context in which an event occurred or an item was acquired (Glisky & Kong, 2008; Glisky, Rubin, & Davidson, 2001). As source memory is responsible for allowing us to identify the origin of information, it gives us our ability to exercise control over our own opinions, beliefs and knowledge (Johnson, Hashtroudi, & Lindsay, 1993), as it allows one to distinguish between internal and external events (Dennis et al., 2008; Johnson & Raye, 1981).

Source memory is not considered an entirely separate function from episodic memory. Episodic memory refers to the entire content of a specific event, while source memory refers to the *context* of the information alone and the *process* of forming a memory (Brickman & Stern, 2009). Although they are not considered as entirely separate functions, it is clear that memory for content and memory for context may rely on different processes (Siedlecki, Salthouse, & Berish, 2005; Wilding, Doyle, & Rugg, 1995; Wilding & Rugg, 1996). For example, individuals can recall specific items of information but may have more difficulty recollecting the origin of this information. Therefore, there may be a distinction between the mechanisms involved in the retrieval of factual content as opposed to the source of this information. It is theorised that source memory is dependent on recollection, while content memory relies on the recognition of, or familiarity with, the item in the absence of the contextual information (Dobbins, Foley, Schacter, & Wagner, 2002; Siedlecki et al., 2005; Yonelinas, 2002; see Chapter 3).

In a typical test of source memory, one is required to recall specific details or features of a memory peripheral to the memory itself (Dennis et al., 2008). The Encoding Specificity Principle states that if the learning context remains stable between encoding and retrieval of a memory (that is, the learning environment matches the test environment), recollection will be facilitated and aspects that were attended to can be more easily recalled (Tulving, 1974; Tulving & Thomson, 1973). This implies that if item and source are bound together at the time of encoding, memory performance will be enhanced. If binding occurs, the contextual elements that are bound to the item can act as cues, allowing for easier access to the information (Smith, 1979; Tulving, 1974; Tulving & Thomson, 1973). Therefore, when different aspects of context combine to form a source, this allows individuals to more readily identify the information, which in turn allows for better recollection of an event (Mammarella & Fairfield, 2008).

4.2   Source memory and ageing

It has been suggested that source memory is one of the first types of cognition to decline in the ageing process (Jennings & Jacoby, 1997). A particular difficulty with this capacity was identified among older adults in tasks involving famous names (Dywan, Segalowitz, & Williamson, 1994) and later with word-list stimuli (Jennings & Jacoby, 1997). Importantly, however, Multhaup (1995) demonstrated that with proper instruction, this deficit in the elderly could be overcome. One explanation for this decline may be seen in the age-related reduction of function (and neuronal integrity) in brain regions such as the pre-frontal cortex (PFC) and the medial temporal lobes (MTL; Friedman, 2000; Morcom, Good, Frackowiak, & Rugg, 2003; Rajah & D'Esposito, 2005; Reuter-Lorenz, 2002), which have been closely linked to source memory ability (Eichenbaum, Yonelinas, & Ranganath, 2007; Leshikar & Duarte, 2012; Mitchell & Johnson, 2009). The literature indicates a large decrement in source compared to content memory with increasing age, typically from approximately 55 years and onwards (Siedlecki et al., 2005; Spencer & Raz, 1994).

This source memory decline in ageing has been identified across different cultures (Chua, Chen, & Park, 2006), and across various cognitive domains. For example, Schacter and colleagues (1991) have shown that older adults have more difficulty in identifying *who* provided the source of the information in laboratory tasks than younger controls. In this study, different speakers read statements aloud and, when tested later, older adults performed more poorly than young in identifying the *specific* source, i.e., in pairing the statement to the original speaker. Furthermore, this performance difference has been shown to extend to a *partial* source whereby older adults struggled more than younger controls when attempting to identify the correct gender of the source (Simons, Dodson, Bell, & Schacter, 2004). Therefore, not only is there evidence of a relative decline in source memory but this decline can sometimes be extremely pronounced, extending to an inability to distinguish the source as a male or female speaker. Even when external factors such as excessive information or distraction are accounted for, this age-related difference in accuracy remains apparent and substantial (Schacter et al., 1994). By manipulating attentional resources in two separate experiments, Schacter and colleagues (1994) found evidence in support for source memory decline being independent of external conditions but associated with the progression of age. Further evidence indicates that an age-related reduction in source recall remains despite achieving accurate recollection of the content of a memory (Brickman & Stern, 2009). This further cements the concept that source memory and content memory are separate processes and that source memory displays a downward trajectory in ageing before such impairments are evident in item memory.

Various studies have provided evidence for an underlying age-related decline in the ability to bind contextual and content information together (Glisky & Kong, 2008; Henkel, Johnson, & De Leonardis, 1998; Kessels, Hobbel, & Postma, 2007). Older adults have been shown to display poorer performance than younger controls on target/item memory, contextual memory and a combination of the two (Kessels et al., 2007). Particularly, older adults showed more errors when required to bind target and context. Dennis et al. (2008) have additionally shown an age-related deficit in source memory when asking older adults to bind face-scene pairs, although this deficit is not so pronounced when faces and scenes are encoded separately (i.e., item memory). Glisky and Kong (2008) have stated that a decline in source memory may become prominent when greater demands are set on older adults to bind items to contextual information, while Henkel and colleagues (1998) suggest that source memory in older adults will be poorer if the items are similar. Therefore, additional resources in the binding process need to be deployed in order to compensate for this decline in source memory in such cases of similarity and context.

Taken together, the above studies all seem to suggest that older adults' recall may suffer due to an underlying problem in binding contextual and item information in memory (Dennis et al., 2008; Kessels et al., 2007).

4.3   Theories of source memory decline

The main theories explaining this source memory decline in ageing posit a problem in the formation of associations or binding of information in memory. These theories include the *Associative Deficit Hypothesis*, the *Source Monitoring Framework* and the *Misrecollection Hypothesis*. Naveh-Benjamin's (2000) Associative Deficit Hypothesis suggests that individual units of information are linked or joined together in a network of connections, and that these collections or combinations of units form what we experience as episodes or memories. This model postulates that a breakdown in creating and retrieving these links is caused by the ageing process, resulting in poorer memory recall in older adults (Naveh-Benjamin, Hussain, Guez, & Bar-On, 2003). The Associative Deficit Hypothesis further suggests that older adults have particular difficulty with the binding aspect of the process, and if the units appear to be unrelated, this becomes especially problematic (Naveh-Benjamin, Guez, & Shulman, 2004).

The Source Monitoring Framework (Johnson et al., 1993) states that features, which can be perceptual, spatial, temporal, semantic and/or emotional, are bound together to create the entire context of an event or memory (Johnson, 2006; Johnson et al., 1993; Johnson & Raye, 1981; Mitchell & Johnson, 2009). This framework suggests that the entire context of an episode is recalled by directly accessing these features or cues; as such, the binding of such features is critical for source memory recall (Mammarella & Fairfield, 2008). Therefore, if there is a deficit in monitoring (i.e., a lapse of attention), this results in a decrement in source memory performance (Johnson et al., 1993). Johnson and colleagues (1993) have suggested that the ageing process causes a separation of the features; as a result, when one feature is identified through source monitoring, it no longer reactivates the remaining features, as the cues have become distinct items in memory (Johnson et al., 1993), leading to a recollection failure.

The Misrecollection Hypothesis states that older adults incorrectly bind the context of an episode within memory, and that this faulty binding accounts for the source memory deficit that can be seen in ageing (Dodson, Bawa, & Slotnick, 2007). This incorrect binding procedure results in false recollections of events but produces a highly convincing misrecollection, leading to high confidence in the source of the information despite this source being erroneous (Dodson, Bawa, & Krueger, 2007; Dodson & Krueger, 2006). Older adults have been shown to report higher confidence in the source of information compared to young adults, although this high level of confidence was accompanied by poorer accuracy (Bryce & Dodson, 2013; Dodson, Bawa, & Krueger, 2007; Dodson & Krueger, 2006).

The main theories on source memory decline in ageing, and the literature, all indicate a discrepancy in the process of binding contextual information in memory, either in the form of insufficient or misdirected binding. Therefore, the best way to compensate for this impairment appears to lie in enhancing the binding process. This can be achieved by promoting semantic processing as part of the memory trace.

4.4   The preservation of source memory in ageing

A sedentary lifestyle or reduced practise of mental skills may lead to a decline in neural systems, which can in turn result in serious consequences on mental capabilities (Hultsch, Hertzog, Small, & Dixon, 1999). Therefore, identifying novel means by which cognitive function can be enhanced in older adults is an important task, and compelling evidence suggests that mental activities can protect against the deterioration of cognitive performance (Greiner, Snowdon, & Schmitt, 1996; Riley, Snowdon, Desrosiers, & Markesbery, 2005; see also Chapter 10). We have argued above that the age-related memory decline observed is predominantly associated to a loss of source memory ability. As such, it is important to investigate whether interventions can ameliorate the age-related decline in source memory.

A number of techniques have been successfully demonstrated to enhance memory. Previous research has shown how the use of mnemonic strategies (i.e., techniques that aid retrieval of information) significantly improved recall in the aged (Saczynski, Rebok, Whitfield, & Plude, 2007; Verhaeghen, Marcoen, & Goossens, 1992). Additionally, Dornburg and McDaniel (2006) have shown amelioration of memory decline in older adults with the use of a Cognitive Interview, wherein instructions before beginning the interview emphasised the reinstatement of context and reliance on numerous cues and sensory stimuli to facilitate recall (Dornburg & McDaniel, 2006; Geiselman, Fisher, MacKinnon, & Holland, 1985). However, one of the most effective techniques involves promoting an emphasis on the meaning, inference and implications of item memory at the encoding phase, leading to a deeper level of processing and better recall/a slower rate of information loss. This approach is known as the Levels of Processing Framework (Craik, 2002; Craik & Lockhart, 1972), and has been shown to be effective at easing the memory impairment seen in older adults (Froger, Taconnat, Landré, Beigneux, & Isingrini, 2008; Jacoby, Shimizu, Velanova, & Rhodes, 2005; see also Chapter 8).

The Levels of Processing approach suggests that the depth at which an item is encoded is inherently linked to the strength of a memory trace, so an item that is processed at a deeper level (e.g., thinking about the *meaning* of a word) will have a longer-lasting memory trace than one processed at a shallow level (e.g., attending to the font in which the word is presented; Craik & Tulving, 1975; Craik & Lockhart, 1972; Moscovitch & Craik, 1976). This suggests that if one engages with deep processing at the time of learning, information will be retained for a longer period of time. Furthermore, if the information is lost, it will be lost at a much slower rate than information that was processed at a shallow level (Craik & Lockhart, 1972; Craik & Tulving, 1975; Moscovitch & Craik, 1976). Moscovitch and Craik (1976) have further suggested that it is very probable that the process of encoding regulates the storage of memory. However, since testing recall or recognition is the only way that the presence of memory can be inferred, enhanced recollection following deeper processing results in the somewhat circular conclusion that such measures have enhanced the encoding process (Moscovitch & Craik, 1976). This is unavoidable in the absence of an objective measure of encoding depth.

Craik and Tulving (1975) were among the first to demonstrate that deeper processing can enhance memory retention. They suggested that people do not necessarily learn best when they are merely told to learn in the absence of any instruction on *how* to do so (Craik & Tulving, 1975); therefore, by instructing people on how to learn, memory performance can be enhanced. Moscovitch and Craik (1976) provided evidence in favour of deep processing facilitating item memory, and they further proposed that the level of recall is a direct result of the quality of the trace. In this experiment, the authors asked participants a variety of questions about the items being presented during a study block. When the participants were tested at a later stage, it was found that deeper encoding took longer to achieve, but subsequently led to an increase in the retention of the information (Moscovitch & Craik, 1976). Memory performance can be improved via deep processing, as it requires semantic binding of the item information, thus allowing for easier identification and better overall recall (Craik & Tulving, 1975). It therefore follows that deeper processing should be advantageous for the source memory deficit in ageing.

Jacoby, Shimizu, Daniels and Rhodes (2005) indicated that deep processing could lead to an increase in source memory for foil (new) words compared to item (old) words. Initially, participants were required to make pleasantness ratings of visually presented words (deep processing) or make vowel judgements (shallow processing). When tested on recognition memory, those words that were deeply processed were more readily identified. To extend the effect to source memory, the authors then presented participants with words either visually or aurally, manipulating the mode of presentation, and participants were required to rate how pleasant they found the visually presented words, i.e., deep processing, while no further processing was required for aurally presented words, i.e., shallow processing (Jacoby, Shimizu, Daniels et al., 2005). The participants were tested under one of three conditions, either respond "yes" to all previously presented words, visual and aural; respond "yes" to only pleasantness rated words; or respond "yes" to only heard words. Participants also completed a standard recognition test. Superior memory performance was obtained for those words that were presented visually under pleasantness ratings compared to both standard recognition and aurally presented words, and the authors concluded that this was due to the level of semantic processing involved in the pleasantness ratings of the words. In a different study, Jacoby, Shimizu, Velanova and Rhodes (2005) suggested that deeper processing can not only enhance source memory in general, but that it can further reduce source memory impairments in older adults. Participants were required to rate the pleasantness of visually presented words (deep encoding) or to make vowel judgements on the words (shallow encoding). The authors found that deeper processing resulted in better recognition for target words for a group of older adults, thus concluding that deeper processing could help alleviate the source memory impairments that are commonly seen in ageing (Jacoby, Shimizu, Velanova et al., 2005). Further research has shown that deeper processing approaches can elicit increased brain activity in studies using imaging techniques such as MEG (e.g., Walla et al., 2001) and fMRI (e.g., Dennis et al., 2008). This may be attributed to the recruitment of additional neural resources during processing, thus allowing the information to be retained for longer periods of time with easier access (Walla et al., 2001). As deeper processing had been shown to improve both item and source memory in older adults, the use of a depth of processing intervention may be applicable to one of the most commonly used tasks in source memory research, the Opposition task (Jennings & Jacoby, 1993; 1997).

The Opposition task is a variation on the classic Old/New memory paradigm developed by Egan (1958, as cited in Banks, 1970, p. 81) in which a study list of items is learned and followed by a test list of the study items and new distractors for identification as 'old' or 'new'. In the Opposition paradigm, source memory is taxed by manipulating the stage of the task (i.e., study or test block) at which items are acquired, thereby placing memory and familiarity in opposition to each other (Jennings & Jacoby, 1993; 1997). The design utilises a lag procedure allowing both source and item recollection to be investigated – participants must judge whether a previously encountered stimulus was first presented as part of the study block or merely earlier within the test block (Jennings & Jacoby, 1997). Studies have indicated that ageing severely affects retention in the Opposition task and that older adults display more errors on repeated items compared to young, even when the repetition is at a very short interval, i.e., the lag between first and second presentations is very short (Jennings & Jacoby, 1997). The original version of the task repeated new items only; however, in order to further test the effects of repetition on source memory, the task was modified to include repetitions of both new (Distractor) and old (Target) words. Drawing on the common failure of repeating oneself, in the test phase, both new and old words are presented at three different intervals: lag 0 (i.e., no words between the first and second presentation), lag 4 (four words between the first and second presentation) and lag 16 (i.e., 16 words between the first and second repetitions). Participants must rely on conscious memory to avoid repetition errors. The longer the lag between repetitions, the more likely one is to incorrectly identify the second presentation of a Distractor (new) word as being a Target word (old).

In a study by Brady and Roche (unpublished data), three groups of adults completed this modified Opposition task: young controls (18–30 years, mean = 25.5 years, n = 20), older controls (55+ years, mean = 64.52, n = 20) and an older group using an intervention (55+, mean = 63.55, n = 20). Both control groups completed the task without the use of any intervention. However, the older intervention group used a technique employing deep processing whereby they were required during encoding to put each of the presented words into a sentence that provided a clear meaning of that word, thus engaging with the information on a semantic level. The young group were used as controls, as it was believed that they would perform at ceiling source memory performance. As semantic elaboration represents the deepest level of processing (Craik & Lockhart, 1972; Craik & Tulving, 1975), this method was predicted to be potentially most beneficial, as one must understand and comprehend the meaning of the word in order to create a sentence around it. Thus, it was anticipated that this strategy could potentially lead to an advantage with recollection at a later stage.

The groups were approximately equal on estimates of IQ and self-reports of cognitive failures (i.e., everyday lapses of memory or attention, such as walking into a room and forgetting why you went there). Figure 4.1 (below) shows the total accuracy represented as a percentage for each of the conditions. A one-way between groups ANOVA indicated that there was a statistically significant difference on total accuracy across the three groups, $F (2, 57) = 25.92, p < 0.001$, with *post hoc* tests revealing that these differences lay between the young and older group, $p < 0.01$, the young and intervention group, $p < 0.01$, and the older and intervention group, $p < 0.001$, with the highest percentage accuracy in the intervention group, followed by the young and finally the older control groups.

It is apparent from the results that the older control group was more affected by source memory errors than the young control group and the older group using an intervention. By contrast, the older intervention group appeared to show few source memory failures, as their performance was superior to both the older and young control groups, the latter of which was expected to be performing at ceiling. These results may indicate that a deep processing strategy at encoding (in this case, semantic elaboration) can lead to better source recall. The repetition of Distractor

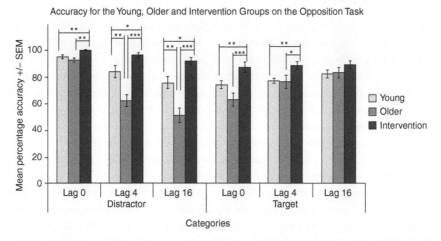

FIGURE 4.1 Mean percentage accuracy scores +/- SEM between the young, older and intervention groups at lags 0, 4 and 16 for Distractor and Target words on the Opposition task.

(* p < 0.05, ** p < 0.01, *** p < 0.001)

(new) words in the Opposition task is known to be a sensitive index of source memory processing, and results for these stimuli indicate that the older control adults showed a decrement in recall that was not apparent for young adults, with this impairment particularly evident for longer lag length (i.e., lags 4 and 16). These results indicate that older adults were more likely to misidentify items as being previously encountered when they were not, as these conditions consisted of the longest time delay between the presentations of items. Furthermore, these results offer support for the idea that older adults have more difficulty with identifying the correct time of the occurrence of an event (Jennings & Jacoby, 1993; 1997), in this case, the study or test block.

However, when older adults were given an intervention involving depth of processing, they performed with a level of accuracy superior to both older and young control groups in all but one condition. This would suggest that the older adults engaged in a deeper level of processing by utilising the semantic meaning of the to-be-learned words, which led to a greater level of retention. This finding is supported by previous studies suggesting that using semantic-based depth of processing can increase memory performance (Eysenck & Eysenck, 1980; Jacoby, Shimizu, Daniels et al., 2005; Moscovitch & Craik, 1976), while others have reported similar enhancing effects in the elderly (Froger et al., 2008; Jacoby, Shimizu, Velanova et al., 2005). Such a semantically based depth of processing approach to to-be-learned material at the time of encoding may therefore represent an easily applicable and potentially effective strategy for reducing source memory impairments in older adults.

4.5   Conclusion

The ability to bind together the individual elements or contextual details that combine to form our memory of an event or a fact is a vital function that allows us to distinguish real from imagined events and actual memories from familiar-seeming scenarios. Research has confirmed that this capacity appears to be subject to deterioration with increasing age, as source memory deficits appear to emerge long before impairments of item memory are detected in old age. These deficits are likely the result of deteriorating tissue integrity in key memory regions of the ageing brain, including the prefrontal cortices and medial temporal lobes. Prominent theories of the age-related decline in source memory emphasise the importance of the binding process, positing either insufficient or erroneous binding as causal in this decrement in memory performance. Some successful attempts to reduce or even reverse this impairment focus on conditions at the time of memory encoding, employing strategies that promote the development of a more elaborate memory trace by means of increasing the depth of processing engaged at study. Studies have demonstrated that such approaches can restore memory accuracy of older groups to levels comparable – or, in some cases, superior – to young and older controls, and may therefore represent a fruitful avenue of research to pursue in the search for effective and low-cost approaches to memory remediation.

References

Banks, W.P. (1970). Signal detection theory and human memory. *Psychological Bulletin, 74*(2), 81–99.

Bartlett, J.C., Strater, L., & Fulton, A. (1991). False recency and false fame of faces young adulthood and old age. *Memory and Cognition, 19*(2), 177–188.

Brickman, A. M., & Stern, Y. (2009). Aging and memory in humans. *Encyclopedia of Neuroscience, 1*, 175–180.

Bryce, M.S., & Dodson, C.S. (2013). Cross-age effect in recognition performance and memory monitoring for faces. *Psychology and Aging, 28*(1), 87–98.

Chua, H.F., Chen, W., & Park, D. C. (2006). Source memory, aging and culture. *Gerontology, 52*, 306–313.

Cohen, C., & Faulkner, D. (1989). Age differences in source forgetting: Effects of reality monitoring on eyewitness testimony. *Psychology and Aging, 4*(1), 10–17.

Craik, F.I.M. (2002). Levels of processing: Past present . . . and future? *Memory, 10*(5/6), 305–318.

Craik, F.I.M., & Lockhart, R. (1972). Levels of processing: A framework for memory research. *Journal of Verbal Learning and Verbal Behavior, 11*, 671–684.

Craik, F.I.M., & Tulving, E. (1975). Depth of processing and the retention of words in episodic memory. *Journal of Experimental Psychology: General, 104*(3), 268–294.

Dennis, N.A., Hayes, S.M., Prince, S.E., Madden, D.J., Huettel, S.A., & Cabeza, R. (2008). Effects of aging on the neural correlates of successful item and source memory encoding. *Journal of Experimental Psychology. Learning, Memory, and Cognition, 34*(4), 791–808.

Dobbins, I.G., Foley, H., Schacter, D.L., & Wagner, A. D. (2002). Executive control during episodic retrieval: Multiple prefrontal processes subserve source memory. *Neuron, 35*, 989–996.

Dodson, C.S., Bawa, S., & Krueger, L.E. (2007). Aging, metamemory, and high-confidence errors: A misrecollection account. *Psychology and Aging, 22*(1), 122–133.

Dodson, C.S., Bawa, S., & Slotnick, S.D. (2007). Aging, Source Memory, and Misrecollections. *Journal of Experimental Psychology: Learning, Memory, and Cognition, 33*(1), 169–181.

Dodson, C.S., & Krueger, L.E. (2006). I misremember it well: Why older adults are unreliable eyewitnesses. *Psychonomic Bulletin & Review, 13*(5), 770–775.

Dornburg, C.C., & McDaniel, M.A. (2006). The Cognitive Interview enhances long-term free recall of older adults. *Psychology and Aging, 21*(1), 196–200.

Dywan, J., & Jacoby, L.L. (1990). Effects of aging on source monitoring: Differences in susceptibility to false fame. *Psychology and Aging, 5*(3), 379–387.

Dywan, J., Segalowitz, S.J., & Williamson, L. (1994). Source monitoring during name recognition in older adults: Psychometric and electrophysiological correlates. *Psychology and Aging, 9*(4), 568–577.

Eichenbaum, H., Yonelinas, A.R., & Ranganath, C. (2007). The medial temporal lobe and recognition memory. *Annual Review of Neuroscience, 30*, 123–152.

Eysenck, M.W., & Eysenck, M.C. (1980). Effects of processing depth, distinctivness, and word frequency on retention. *British Journal of Psychologfy, 71*, 263–274.

Friedman, D. (2000). Event-related brain potential investigations of memory and aging. *Biological Psychology, 54*, 175–206.

Froger, C., Taconnat, L., Landré, L., Beigneux, K., & Isingrini, M. (2008). Effects of level of processing at encoding and types of retrieval task in mild cognitive impairment and normal aging. *Journal of Clinical and Experimental Neuropsychology, 31*(3), 312–321.

Geiselman, R.E., Fisher, R.P., MacKinnon, D.P., & Holland, H.L. (1985). Eyewitness memory enhancement in the police interview: Cognitive retrieval mnemonics versus hypnosis. *Journal of Applied Psychology, 70*(2), 401–412.

Glisky, E.L., & Kong, L.L. (2008). Do young and older adults rely on different processes in source memory tasks? A neuropsychological study. *Cognition, 34*(4), 809–822.

Glisky, E.L., Rubin, S.R., & Davidson, P.S.R. (2001). Source memory in older adults: An encoding or retrieval problem? *Journal of Experimental Psychology: Learning, Memory, and Cognition, 27*(5), 1131–1146.

Greiner, P.A., Snowdon, D.A., & Schmitt, F.A. (1996). The loss of independence in activities of daily living: The role of low normal cognitive function in elderly nuns. *American Journal of Public Health, 86*(1), 62–66.

Hashtroudi, S., Johnson, M.K., & Crosniak, L.D. (1989). Aging and source monitoring. *Psychology and Aging, 4*(1), 106–112.

Hashtroudi, S., Johnson, M.K., & Chrosniak, L.D. (1990). Aging and qualitative characteristics of memories for perceived and imagine complex events. *Psychology and Aging, 5*(1), 119–126.

Henkel, L.A., Johnson, M.K., & De Leonardis, D.M. (1998). Aging and source monitoring: Cognitive processes and neuropsychological correlates. *Journal of Experimental Psychology. General, 127*(3), 251–268.

Hultsch, D.F., Hertzog, C., Small, B.J., & Dixon, R.A. (1999). Use it or lose it: Engaged lifestyle as a buffer of cognitive decline in aging? *Psychology and Aging, 14*(2), 245–263.

Jacoby, L.L., Shimizu, Y., Daniels, K.A., & Rhodes, M.G. (2005). Modes of cognitive control in recognition and source memory: Depth of retrieval. *Psychonomic Bulletin & Review, 12*(5), 852–857.

Jacoby, L.L., Shimizu, Y., Velanova, K., & Rhodes, M.G. (2005). Age differences in depth of retrieval: Memory for foils. *Journal of Memory and Language, 52*, 493–504.

Jennings, J.M., & Jacoby, L.L. (1993). Automatic versus intentional uses of memory: Aging, attention, and control. *Psychology and Aging, 8*(2), 283–293.

Jennings, J.M., & Jacoby, L.L. (1997). An opposition procedure for detecting age-related deficits in recollection: Telling effects of repetition. *Psychology and Aging, 12*(2), 352–361.

Johnson, M.K. (2006). Memory and reality. *The American Psychologist, 61*(8), 760–771.

Johnson, M.K., Hashtroudi, S., & Lindsay, D. (1993). Source monitoring. *Psychological Bulletin, 114*(1), 3–28.

Johnson, M.K., & Raye, C.L. (1981). Reality monitoring. *Psychological Review, 88*(1), 67–85.

Kessels, R.P.C., Hobbel, D., & Postma, A. (2007). Aging, context memory and binding: A comparison of "what, where and when" in young and older adults. *International Journal of Neuroscience, 117*, 795–810.

Leshikar, E.D., & Duarte, A. (2012). Medial prefrontal cortex supports source memory accuracy for self-referenced items. *Society for Neuroscience, 7*(2), 126–145.

Mammarella, N., & Fairfield, B. (2008). Source monitoring: The importance of feature binding at encoding. *European Journal of Cognitive Psychology, 20*(1), 91–122.

Mitchell, K.J., & Johnson, M.K. (2009). Source monitoring 15 years later: What have we learned from fMRI abou the neural mechanisms of source memory? *Psychological Bulletin, 135*(4), 638–677.

Morcom, A. M., Good, C.D., Frackowiak, R.S.J., & Rugg, M.D. (2003). Age effects on the neural correlates of successful memory encoding. *Brain, 126*(1), 213–229.

Moscovitch, M., & Craik, F.I.M. (1976). Depth of processing, retrieval cues, and uniqueness of encoding as factors in recall. *Journal of Verbal Learning and Verbal Behavior, 15*, 447–458.

Multhaup, K.S. (1995). Aging, source, and decision criteria: When false fame errors do and do not occur. *Psychology and Aging, 10*(3), 492–497.

Naveh-Benjamin, M. (2000). Adult age differences in memory performance: Tests of an associative deficit hypothesis. *Journal of Experimental Psychology: Learning, Memory, and Cognition, 26*(5), 1170–1187.

Naveh-Benjamin, M., Guez, J., & Shulman, S. (2004). Older adults' associative deficit in episodic memory: Assessing the role of decline in attentional resources. *Psychonomic Bulletin & Review, 11*(6), 1067–1073.

Naveh-Benjamin, M., Hussain, Z., Guez, J., & Bar-On, M. (2003). Adult age differences in episodic memory: Further support for an associative-deficit hypothesis. *Journal of Experimental Psychology: Learning, Memory, and Cognition, 29*(5), 826–837.

Rajah, M.N., & D'Esposito, M. (2005). Region-specific changes in prefrontal function with age: A review of PET and fMRI studies on working and episodic memory. *Brain, 128,* 1964–1983.

Reuter-Lorenz, P.A. (2002). New visions of the aging mind and brain. *Trends in Cognitive Sciences, 6*(9), 394–400.

Riley, K.P., Snowdon, D.A., Desrosiers, M.F., & Markesbery, W.R. (2005). Early life linguistic ability, late life cognitive function, and neuropathology: Findings from the Nun Study. *Neurobiology of Aging, 26*(3), 341–347.

Saczynski, J.S., Rebok, G.W., Whitfield, K.E., & Plude, D.L. (2007). Spontaneous production and use of mnemonic strategies in older adults. *Experimental Aging Research, 33,* 273–294.

Schacter, D.L., Kaszniak, A.W., Kihlstrom, J.F., & Valdiserri, M. (1991). The relation between source memory and aging. *Psychology and Aging, 6*(4), 559–568.

Schacter, D.L., Osowiecki, D., Kaszniak, A.W., Kihlstrom, J.F., & Valdiserri, M. (1994). Source memory: Extending the boundaries of age-related deficits. *Psychology and Aging, 9*(1), 81–89.

Schmitter-Edgecombe, M., Woo, E., & Greeley, D.R. (2009). Characterizing multiple memory deficits and their relation to everyday functioning in individuals with mild cognitive impairment. *Neuropsychology, 23*(2), 168–177.

Senkfor, A.J., & Van Petten, C. (1998). Who said what? An event-related potential investigation of source and item memory. *Journal of Experimental Psychology: Learning, Memory, and Cognition, 24*(4), 1005–1025.

Siedlecki, K.L., Salthouse, T.A., & Berish, D.E. (2005). Is there anything special about the aging of source memory? *Psychology and Aging, 20*(1), 19–32.

Simons, J.S., Dodson, C.S., Bell, D., & Schacter, D.L. (2004). Specific- and partial-source memory: Effects of aging. *Psychology and Aging, 19*(4), 689–694.

Smith, S.M. (1979). Remembering in and out of context. *Journal of Experimental Psychology: Human Learning & Memory, 5*(5), 460–471.

Spencer, W.D., & Raz, N. (1994). Memory for facts, source, and context: Can frontal lobe dysfunction explain age-related differences? *Psychology and Aging, 9*(1), 149–159.

Tulving, E. (1974). Cue dependent forgetting. *American Scientist, 62*(1), 74–82.

Tulving, E., & Thomson, D.M. (1973). Encoding specificity and retrieval processes in episodic memory. *Psychological Review, 80*(5), 352–373.

Verhaeghen, P., Marcoen, A., & Goossens, L. (1992). Improving memory performance in the aged through mnemonic training: A meta-analytic study. *Psychology and Aging, 7*(2), 242–251.

Walla, P., Hufnagl, B., Lindinger, G., Imhof, H., Deecke, L., & Lang, W. (2001). Left temporal and temporoparietal brain activity depends on depth of word encoding: A magnetoencephalographic study in healthy young subjects. *NeuroImage, 13,* 402–409.

Wilding, E.L., Doyle, M.C., & Rugg, M.D. (1995). Recognition memory with and without retrieval of context: An event-related potential study. *Neuropsychologia, 33*(6), 743–767.

Wilding, E.L., & Rugg, M.D. (1996). An event-related potential study of recognition memory with and without retrieval of source. *Brain, 119,* 889–905.

Yonelinas, A.P. (2002). The nature of recollection and familiarity: A review of 30 years of research. *Journal of Memory and Language, 46*(3), 441–517.

PART II

Assessment and prediction

5

FROM CLICK TO COGNITION

Detecting cognitive decline through daily computer use

Gemma Stringer, Peter Sawyer, Alistair Sutcliffe and Iracema Leroi

5.1 Introduction

Dementia is a rapidly growing worldwide concern. The Alzheimer's Society reports that there are currently over 35 million people with dementia in the world and this is expected to double every 20 years, resulting in increased health risks and a potentially negative economic and social impact. Currently, the total estimated cost of dementia worldwide is $604 billion (£380 billion). Detection of dementia in the early stages is infrequent and as many as 28 million people living with dementia worldwide do not have a diagnosis and access to care.

In the UK, over 800,000 people are living with some form of dementia and it is estimated that this figure will rise to one million by 2021. The financial cost of dementia to the UK is currently £23 billion per year. Formal diagnoses of dementia is often very late, and at present, more than 50% of people with dementia have yet to receive one. A diagnosis and earlier intervention might increase the chances of delaying the onset of dementia. If the onset can be delayed by five years, the number of deaths directly attributable to dementia would be reduced by 30,000 per year (Alzheimer's Society, 2013).

Several countries now have national dementia strategies in which national policy is urging the earlier identification of cognitive impairment, when still in the mild cognitive stages (Arai, Arai, & Mizuno, 2010; Banerjee, 2010; Brodaty & Cumming, 2010; Nakanishi & Nakashima, 2014; Robert, 2010; Todd, Wilson, McGuinness, Craig, & Passmore, 2010). Countries without national dementia strategies are being advised to develop them in order to provide a quicker response to the most problematic issues in dementia care, such as the need for a timely diagnosis (Alzheimer's Society of Canada, 2010; Mateos, Franco, & Sanchez, 2010). The ability to monitor the progression of dementia from the early 'prodromal' stage, which is commonly referred to as 'mild cognitive impairment' (MCI), is increasingly important due to developments in disease modifying therapies for clinical use in Alzheimer's disease (AD). For such interventions to be effective, therapy must be initiated before extensive tissue damage has occurred, such as when the disease reaches the 'dementia' stage. Early detection also provides the opportunity for those affected to make future plans at a time when symptoms are mild and it is still possible to make informed decisions, undertake self-management of the condition and intervene to slow disease progression through life-style modification (Saxton et al., 2009).

The conventional approach to detecting and diagnosing cognitive impairment involves the clinic-based administration of neuropsychological tests of various cognitive domains. Such cognitive assessments are usually performed only in response to patient or family concerns about possible cognitive dysfunction. These screening tests, such as the Mini-Mental State Exam (Folstein, Folstein, & McHugh, 1975), the Montreal Cognitive Assessment (Smith, Gildeh, & Holmes, 2007) and the Addenbrooke's Cognitive Examination – III (Hsieh, Schubert, Hoon, Mioshi, & Hodges, 2013), have several drawbacks. For example, they often rely on trained clinical staff for their administration, they capture only a cross-sectional point-in-time and they are generally unable to detect the more subtle decline in functional ability that signals the onset of cognitive impairment. The limitations of these methods have been noted by clinicians, patients and caregivers alike, and the 'clinical meaningfulness' of changes in such tests over time have also been called into question (Mitnitski, Hoffman, Rockwood, & Richard, 2012; Rockwood, Fay, Gorman, Carver, & Graham, 2007).

In recent years, in order to address some of the concerns about conventional clinic-based cognitive test methods, several neuropsychological assessments have been designed for use with a standard personal computer (Saxton et al., 2009). However, most of these tests still have to be administered and scored by a clinician, and are therefore subject to the same limitations as equivalent pen and paper methods. In contrast, self-administered online tests do not require a professional input, at the same time maintaining the sensitivity and specificity to detect cognitive impairment (Saxton et al., 2009). One issue with these tests, however, is that they are dependent upon the individuals' desire and motivation to access the testing materials and complete the tests. One way to overcome these limitations is through continuous unobtrusive or semi-passive monitoring of daily computer use. Computer use is a complex task that relies on both cognitive and functional abilities. Being able to detect changes in daily computer use may provide an opportunity for older computer users to detect and self-manage cognitive decline at an earlier stage rather than relying on conventional means of detection and diagnosis.

New methods in unobtrusive or semi-passive computerised observation of cognitive performance in a home environment also offer the possibility of detecting trends and changes in cognitive performance in a natural setting over time. This reduces the delay and expense associated with current established cognitive assessment methods used in clinical practice and increases the ecological validity of the findings. The use of frequent, unobtrusive measures would also reduce the need to rely on population norms that can be confounded by cultural and language differences because measurement would be based on within-individual changes, using individual elders as their own control. Such methods could have profound economic and social implications, especially in view of the upcoming challenges due to a rapidly growing demographic of elders and escalating health care costs, particularly within ethnic minority communities (Pavel et al., 2008).

Monitoring of cognition in peoples' own homes has the added advantage of enabling people to take ownership of their health and well-being by having a heightened awareness of their cognitive abilities on an ongoing basis. This may in turn enable people to maintain independence for longer as they devise strategies to compensate for the onset of deficits. Moreover, continuous information about cognitive performance can also help to track the effectiveness of therapies and other interventions, and reveal acute problems such as physical illness or medication side effects earlier. Finally, the assessment of cognitive and functional changes related to ageing, as detected by continuous computer use monitoring, will further enhance the understanding of such systems in healthy elderly computer users (Pavel et al., 2008). This chapter provides an overview of this approach as well as outlining alternative uses of the computer in the assessment and management of cognitive impairment, including using motor function as a marker of cognitive decline, the use of computer-based language assessments and the application of *serious games* (SG).

5.2 Older adults and computer technology

Older adults now make up the fastest growing group of Internet users (Hart, Chaparro, & Halcomb, 2008). In April 2012, the Pew Research Center found for the first time that more than half of older adults (defined as those aged 65 or older) were Internet users (Pew Research Center, 2014). According to the Office of National Statistics, 71% of adults aged between 64 and 75, and 37% aged over 75, have used the Internet – in the over 75 years age group, this figure has increased by 13% since 2011.

The next generation of older adults will be even more dependent on technology than the present generation. Of people between the ages of 55–64, 88% use the Internet and this figure increases to 96% for the 35–54 years age group, suggesting that unobtrusive computer-based assessments in relation to health and well-being will be even more relevant in coming years (Office for National Statistics, 2014).

The most popular online services for older adults include e-mail, general information searching and e-banking (Vuori & Holmlund-Rytkönen, 2005). The main purpose for using the computer is word processing, keeping in touch with others, and generally increasing the experience and ability on a computer. Older adults' computer use mainly takes place at home and, if support is needed, it most often comes from immediate family members and close relations (Selwyn, 2004). Increased use of information technology by older adults thus provides a rich opportunity for detecting cognitive change over time. The amount of data that can be captured from a person's use of a computer is vast and complex, ranging from measures and error detection that need to be systematically organised in order to provide clinically useful information about a person's level of cognitive functioning.

5.3 Computer actions as proxy measures of cognitive function

Computer use is a complex task requiring the activation of multiple cognitive domains (e.g., attention, working memory, episodic memory and executive function) and is therefore likely to be *highly sensitive to cognitive change* (Kaye et al., 2014). For example, computer use errors such as incomplete requests and repetitive or idiosyncratic computer use behaviour patterns might be early indicators of cognitive pathology, while text mining could identify expressions of memory loss and frustration in user-generated content, or early deficits in language function. Using a computer is also a highly *interactive activity* that presents special challenges to older adults ranging from increased difficulty in psychomotor ability in using the computer mouse, to sensory and cognitive abilities such as speed of searching for icons, to issues with learning, memory and executive function, all of which may be compromised with age (Tun & Lachman, 2010). In this manner, computer use can be used as a proxy measure of distinct cognitive functions through the deconstruction of computer actions of varying complexity. This fertile source of information can be used to develop a profile that enables people to become more aware of changes in their cognitive functioning and to seek further clinical assessment as appropriate.

One method for analysing computer use data is to apply a structure of hierarchical 'layers' ranging from simpler functions, such as routine typing and mouse interactions, which provide information on motor speed and sensorimotor information, through to the more complex analysis of the content of naturalistic typing in e-mail and word documents, which can inform aspects of linguistic complexity. At the highest level, computer games, or SG, can be used to provide evidence about a wide range of cognitive functions. For example, word finding or memory games can provide information about verbal and semantic fluency, and memory functioning, respectively.

We have conceptualised the hierarchical layers of data capture complexity in five levels. Layer I is dedicated to detecting keyboard and mouse movements; Layer II to monitoring the user's navigation of the operating system; Layer III serves to detect e-mail and Internet searching strategies; Layer IV focuses on analysing text language in e-mails and word documents; and Layer V analyses semi-active tasks such as a weekly diary and various cognitive games such as a card game or quiz. This model allows translation of each computer use parameter from each layer into possible 'clinical indicators' on both an individual and cohort level. These indicators will then be examined by a clinical consensus team able to interpret them and assess whether clinical change, however subtle, has taken place over time.

The specific form of the clinical indicator will depend on the type of computer specification. For example, a dissection of the components of mouse movements could be indicated graphically in a dashboard style (e.g., short direct moves, long curved moves, etc.), or by spatial maps of screen traces.

Clinically, the most relevant cognitive domains underpinning the high level functions required in computer use include executive function, visual attention and memory. Impaired executive function is common in some forms of MCI or early dementia and refers to the ability to respond to novel situations in an adaptive manner. It includes aspects of volition, planning, anticipation and effective performance (Lezak, Howieson, Bigler, & Tranel, 2012). Impaired executive function can manifest clinically through personality changes, a reduction in impulse control, lack of cognitive flexibility and impaired insight. In the context of computer use, users with executive dysfunction may make inappropriate decisions and sequencing errors. Visual attention and scanning is a process that selects visual stimuli based on their spatial location. Such a complex form of attention is critical for computer screen navigation and, if impaired, could result in 'drag and drop' operation errors, incorrect highlighting of screen icons or failure to detect an icon. Impaired visual attention is a frequent early feature of dementia although is not specific to any single diagnostic sub-type of dementia. Episodic memory includes the registration, acquisition and encoding of information. Everyday computer-based tests of episodic memory are, for example, remembering log-in details and passwords. Procedural memory refers to the ability to use a learned skill in an unconscious automatic way, such as using a mouse and keyboard correctly or navigating tiers of folders. Short term memory refers to the temporarily retaining of a limited amount of information in a very accessible state. This translates to computer functioning as the ability to successfully undertake games such as online card games, memory games or managing multiple simultaneously open folders.

No single computer use indicator will be sufficient to predict clinically significant cognitive dysfunction accurately, so the opportunity to secure data from a variety of sources is an enormous advantage. However, development work is needed to establish the optimal thresholds for signalling clinically significant changes in cognition. Furthermore, several of the clinical indicators for MCI or dementia are not necessarily a part of regular computer use functions, and may therefore not be detected through passive and unobtrusive means. Consequently, it will be necessary to incentivise users to perform specific tasks that provide data with clear links to the cognitive processes that go awry in MCI or early dementia. For example, the computer user might have to be prompted to undertake card games or regular diary entries from which to derive data on memory or language functions. This active form of data collection can then be combined with the more natural and unobtrusive passive detection of computer use to provide a range of relevant data. Below, we will detail methods of analysis of the hierarchical layers of computer functions for potential conversion into clinical indicators. An example of a planned system that follows these guidelines is SAMS, described in Box 5.1.

5.3.1   Layer I: motor function

At this fundamental layer, the use of the keyboard and mouse can provide information about motor functioning. Ageing is associated with functional decline in motor performance, as has already been established through assessments of changes in gait in elderly people. A decline in gait speed is positively associated with declines in global cognition and executive and visuo-spatial function, and may be an early marker of non-Alzheimer dementias, including Parkinson's disease dementia, vascular dementia and dementia with Lewy bodies (Mielke et al., 2013). However, with more relevance to computer use, finer motor control, as manifested in handwriting or computer mouse and keyboard movements, may be more discriminating, and may manifest in MCI and AD as well (Yan, Rountree, Massman, Doody, & Li, 2008). Movement kinematics' investigations have revealed that slower, less smooth, less coordinated and less consistent handwriting is associated with cognitive impairment, even in the MCI stage. These changes become even more evident as dementia, even of the AD type, emerges (Yan et al., 2008).

5.3.2   Layer II and III: higher cognitive functions

These layers include various, more complex, computer functions such as switching between windows (Layer II), and reading and deleting e-mails (Layer III), which could be analysed as proxy measures of higher cognitive functions. For example, resizing a window is underpinned by the cognitive domains of attention, perception and procedural memory. Likewise, cutting and pasting within a Word document is underpinned by procedural memory, attention and executive scheduling.

5.3.3   Layer IV: language

With the onset of dementia, deterioration of various aspects of language functioning manifests primarily as language repetition, a decline in vocabulary word specificity, use of the passive voice, grammatical complexity and idea density. The large amount of text and language produced via the computer enables the clinician to infer subtle and early changes in cognitive function. The potential for detecting MCI with online questionnaires (Brehmer, McGrenere, Tang, & Jacova, 2012) and text analysis of diaries and novels has already been demonstrated (Le, Lancashire, Hirst, & Jokel, 2011), and it has also been shown that topic density measures correlate with MCI (Snowdon et al., 1996).

5.3.4   Layer V: cognition and games

Computer games represent the 'highest level' (i.e., Layer V) of computer activity detection for analysis. Such games have already been demonstrated to be a feasible means of measuring a computer user's cognitive performance, even in older computer users. In particular, such exploration can characterise normal variations in user performance and task learning in order to detect sustained trends in cognitive performance. Moreover, measures of cognitive performance and task difficulty can be used to adapt the user interface and future computer interactions (Jimison, Jessey,

McKanna, Zitzelberger, & Kaye, 2006; Jimison, Pavel, Bissell, & McKanna, 2007; Jimison, Pavel, McKanna, & Pavel, 2004).

SG are one type of digital application specially adapted for purposes other than entertaining, including rehabilitation, training and education. There are a number of benefits to the use of SG in the assessments and monitoring of people with cognitive decline. SG allow for game interfaces to be created that adapt to the user's capacities and interests, and because of their playful character, SG can enhance motivation and improve the mood of the users. Observing and quantifying a person's behaviour when participating in a SG may provide information that is even more reliable than information acquired with traditional performance assessments because the person engaged in a gaming task is less focused on *being tested*, which may often cause stress (Cassady & Johnson, 2002). SG have the flexibility to be used for home-based skill practice and self-assessment, are safe to use and allow for the analysis of performance in real time (Robert et al., 2014).

Recently, there has been an increase of interest in the use of SG targeting patients with AD and other related disorders. There is evidence that SG can be successfully employed to train physical and cognitive abilities in elderly people, and recently, some studies have started to investigate the impact SG can have in improving performance in people with AD, MCI and related disorders. In a review of the literature of experiments conducted to date on the use of SG in neurodegenerative disorders, McCallum and Boletsis (2013) found that physical games can positively affect health areas such as balance and gait, cognitive games can improve cognitive functions such as attention, memory and visuo-spatial abilities, and the combination of physical and cognitive games can improve mood and increase positive affect and sociability. However, despite the positive results, a number of the studies have found that elderly people and people with AD and related disorders have problems using and accessing SG (Robert et al., 2014). SG specifically targeting older adults with cognitive decline are starting to emerge; however, products and research in this area is relatively sparse (Robert et al., 2014). Research that has been done suggests that assessments using Information and Communication Technology (ICT) are generally well-tolerated and they provide useful information regarding motor, cognitive and behavioural dimensions of diseases like dementia (Romdhane et al., 2012).

5.4 The challenges

One of the challenges of analysing daily computer use to detect cognitive change is determining a hierarchy for the data that establishes its clinical relevance. There is no gold standard diagnostic model of cognitive function and dementia progression, and the amount of data that can be collected from daily computer use is vast; therefore, it is essential to refine the data so that what is analysed is clinically meaningful. Furthermore, any change in performance should ideally be assessed both within the individual and across a range of computer users. This approach confers the advantage of obviating the need to rely on population norms, which may only approximate an individual's background and capabilities prior to decline. Collecting computer data longitudinally can also enable comparisons with the individual's capabilities prior to decline based on a 'within-subject' experimental design. However, matching the clinical indicators for dementia with the interaction data collected using computers will require detailed clinical expertise, which in turn will depend upon a process of gaining expert input from clinical and academic neuropsychology and neuropsychiatry to determine the association between the computer data and the clinical indicators, as well as to determine which of the derived clinical indicators will have the most clinical relevance.

BOX 5.1: OVERVIEW OF THE SAMS STUDY

The SAMS study: Software Architecture for Mental Health Self-Management

SAMS is computer software being developed to detect changes in daily computer use due to cognitive and functional decline. The overarching aim of the SAMS project is to determine whether personalised passive, directed and semi-directed monitoring data from computer use in elderly people is sensitive enough to detect clinically significant changes in cognition and function.

The pilot stage of SAMS will determine whether a profile of computer-generated output by people with mild cognitive impairment (MCI) and mild Alzheimer's disease (mild AD) has a significantly different pattern to people with no cognitive impairment.

The pilot proof-of-concept reliability study will aim to enrol a total of 30 participants with MCI/mild AD and 30 cognitively healthy age-matched controls and collect data on their computer use by means of the SAMS software. The profile of computer-generated output will be compared in the two groups of participants in order to detect significant differences. Information gained from this pilot study will be used to inform a subsequent 12 month follow-up study with 60 elderly computer users, aged 65 and over, who meet criteria for 'age associated memory impairment' (AAMI). With SAMS installed on their home computers, several computer use parameters will be captured and analysed on a continuous basis in order to provide information about cognitive change.

Finally, a further challenge in regard to ethics involves establishing how best to inform computer users of a possible decline in their cognitive functioning. The aim of using computer data in this way would not be to diagnose, but rather to encourage the computer user to act on signs of cognitive decline by taking a recognised online test or consulting their health care provider. Throughout the process of collecting computer use data, it is ethically imperative that people are aware they are being monitored and the system must be designed to remind people of their involvement and provide an option to opt out. However, when communicating signs of cognitive decline, if not presented in an appropriate manner, the information provided by the system has the potential to cause uncertainty and anxiety in the user, and do more harm than good. Careful consideration needs to be given to the design of a persuasive user interface based on user choice and models of patient stereotypes in order to develop the optimal combination of motivators and triggers for different types of individuals.

5.5 Conclusions

Monitoring daily computer use to detect cognitive change has the potential to improve the early diagnosis of dementia, as well as providing meaningful and continuous information about longitudinal change. The information gained could then be used to alert the individual, or their health professionals, about the observed changes in order to undergo more specific diagnostic tests or plan appropriate interventions. The most significant challenges in doing this include interpreting the data collected in a way that is consistent with the clinical knowledge and also encouraging users to (a) adopt the software and (b) act on any warnings.

References

Alzheimer's Society. (2013, July). Demography. Retrieved from http://www.alzheimers.org. uk/site/scripts/documents_info.php?documentID=412

Alzheimer's Society of Canada. (2010). Rising Tide: The Impact of Dementia on Canadian Society. Retrieved from http://www.alzheimer.ca/~/media/Files/national/Advocacy/ASC_Rising_Tide_Full_Report_e.pdf

Arai, Y., Arai, A., & Mizuno, Y. (2010). The national dementia strategy in Japan. *International Journal of Geriatric Psychiatry, 25*(9), 896–899.

Banerjee, S. (2010). Living well with dementia—development of the national dementia strategy for England. *International Journal of Geriatric Psychiatry, 25*(9), 917–922.

Brehmer, M., McGrenere, J., Tang, C., & Jacova, C. (2012). *Investigating interruptions in the context of computerised cognitive testing for older adults.* Paper presented at the Proceedings of the SIGCHI Conference on Human Factors in Computing Systems, Austin, Texas, USA.

Brodaty, H., & Cumming, A. (2010). Dementia services in Australia. *International Journal of Geriatric Psychiatry, 25*(9), 887–995.

Cassady, J.C., & Johnson, R.E. (2002). Cognitive Test anxiety and academic performance. *Contemporary Educational Psychology, 27*(2), 270–295. doi: http://dx.doi.org/10.1006/ceps.2001.1094

Folstein, M.F., Folstein, S.E., & McHugh, P.R. (1975). "Mini-mental state": A practical method for grading the cognitive state of patients for the clinician. *Journal of Psychiatric Research, 12*(3), 189–198.

Hart, T.A., Chaparro, B.S., & Halcomb, C.G. (2008). Evaluating websites for older adults: Adherence to 'senior-friendly' guidelines and end-user performance. *Behaviour & Information Technology, 27*(3), 191–199. doi:10.1080/01449290600802031

Hsieh, S., Schubert, S., Hoon, C., Mioshi, E., & Hodges, J.R. (2013).Validation of the Adden-brooke's Cognitive Examination III in frontotemporal dementia and Alzheimer's disease. *Dementia and Geriatric Cognitive Disorders, 36*(3–4), 242–250.

Jimison, H., Jessey, N., McKanna, J., Zitzelberger, T., & Kaye, J. (2006). *Monitoring Computer Interactions to Detect Early Cognitive Impairment in Elders.* Paper presented at the 1st Trans-disciplinary Conference on Distributed Diagnosis and Home Healthcare, April 2–4.

Jimison, H., Pavel, M., McKanna, J., & Pavel, J. (2004). Unobtrusive monitoring of computer interactions to detect cognitive status in elders. *IEEE Transactions in Information Technology and Biomedicine, 8*(3), 248–252.

Jimison, H.B., Pavel, M., Bissell, P., & McKanna, J. (2007). A framework for cognitive moni-toring using computer game interactions. *Studies in Health Technology and Informatics, 129*(Pt 2), 1073–1077.

Kaye, J., Mattek, N., Dodge, H.H., Campbell, I., Hayes, T., Austin, D., . . . Pavel, M. (2014). Unobtrusive measurement of daily computer use to detect mild cognitive impairment. *Alzheimer's & Dementia, 10*(1), 10–17. doi: http://dx.doi.org/10.1016/j.jalz.2013.01.011

Le, X., Lancashire, I., Hirst, G., & Jokel, R. (2011). Longitudinal detection of dementia through lexical and syntactic changes in writing: A case study of three British novelists. *Literary and Linguistic Computing, 26*(4), 435–461. doi:10.1093/llc/fqr013

Lezak, M.D., Howieson, D.B., Bigler, E.D., & Tranel, D. (2012). *Neuropsychological Assessment* (5th edition). Oxford: Oxford University Press.

Mateos, R., Franco, M., & Sanchez, M. (2010). Care for dementia in Spain: The need for a nationwide strategy. *International Journal of Geriatic Psychiatry, 25*(9), 881–884.

McCallum, S., & Boletsis, C. (2013). Dementia Games: A Literature Review of Dementia-Related Serious Games. In M. Ma, M. Oliveira, S. Petersen, & J. Hauge (Eds.), *Serious Games Development and Applications* (Vol. 8101, pp. 15–27): Springer Berlin Heidelberg.

Mielke, M. M., Roberts, R. O., Savica, R., Cha, R., Drubach, D. I., Christianson, T., . . . Petersen, R. C. (2013). Assessing the temporal relationship between cognition and gait: Slow gait predicts cognitive decline in the Mayo Clinic Study of Aging. *The Journals of Gerontology Series A: Biological Sciences and Medical Sciences, 68*(8), 929–937.

Mitnitski, A., Hoffman, D., Rockwood, K., & Richard, M. (2012). Assessing the ability of ADAS-Cog to capture all clinically meaningful changes in symptoms over time. *Al-zheimer's & Dementia: The Journal of the Alzheimer's Association, 8*(4), P127. doi:10.1016/j.jalz.2012.05.334

Nakanishi, M., & Nakashima, T. (2014). Features of the Japanese national dementia strat-egy in comparison with international dementia policies: How should a national demen-tia policy interact with the public health- and social-care systems? [Research Support, Non-U S Gov't]. *Alzheimer's & Dementia, 10*(4), 468–476.

Office for National Statistics. (2014). Internet access quarterly update, Q1 2014. London: Office for National Statistics.

Pavel, M., Jimison, H., Hayes, T., Kaye, J., Dishman, E., Wild, K., & Williams, D. (2008). *Con-tinuous, Unobtrusive Monitoring for the Assessment of Cognitive function. Handbook of Cognitive Aging: Interdisciplinary Perspectives.* Thousand Oaks, CA: SAGE Publications, Inc.

Pew Research Center. (2014). Older Adults and Technology Use: Adoption is increasing, but many seniors remain isolated from digital life. Retrieved from http://www.pewinternet.org/2014/04/03/older-adults-and-technology-use/

Robert, P.H. (2010). The French National Alzheimer disease plan 2008–2012. *International Journal of Geriatric Psychiatry, 25*(9), 900–901.

Robert, P.H., Konig, A., Amieva, H., Andrieu, S., Bremond, F., Bullock, R., . . . Manera, V. (2014). Recommendations for the use of Serious Games in people with Alzheimer's Dis-ease, related disorders and frailty. *Frontiers in Aging Neuroscience, 6*(54).

Rockwood, K., Fay, S., Gorman, M., Carver, D., & Graham, J.E. (2007). The clinical meaningfulness of ADAS-Cog changes in Alzheimer's disease patients treated with donepezil in an open-label trial. *BMC Neurology, 7,* 26.

Romdhane, R., Mulin, E., Derreumeaux, A., Zouba, N., Piano, J., Lee, L., . . . Robert, P.H. (2012). Automatic video monitoring system for assessment of Alzheimer's disease symptoms. *Journal of Nutrition Health and Aging, 16*(3), 213–218.

Saxton, J., Morrow, L., Eschman, A., Archer, G., Luther, J., & Zuccolotto, A. (2009). Computer assessment of mild cognitive impairment. *Postgraduate Medicine, 121*(2), 177–185.

Selwyn, N. (2004). The information aged: A qualitative study of older adults' use of information and communications technology. *Journal of Aging Studies, 18*(4), 369–384.

Smith, T., Gildeh, N., & Holmes, C. (2007). The Montreal Cognitive Assessment: Validity and utility in a memory clinic setting. [Comparative Study]. *Canada Journal of Psychiatry, 52*(5), 329–332.

Snowdon, D.A., Kemper, S.J., Mortimer, J.A., Greiner, L.H., Wekstein, D.R., & Markesbery, W.R. (1996). Linguistic ability in early life and cognitive function and Alzheimer's disease in late life. Findings from the Nun Study. *JAMA, 275*(7), 528–532.

Todd, S., Wilson, D., McGuinness, B., Craig, D., & Passmore, A.P. (2010). Northern Ireland dementia strategy. *International Journal of Geriatric Psychiatry, 25*(9), 902–904.

Tun, P.A., & Lachman, M.E. (2010). The association between computer use and cognition across adulthood: Use it so you won't lose it? *Psychology and Aging, 25*(3), 560–568.

Vuori, S., & Holmlund-Rytkönen, M. (2005). 55+ people as internet users. *Marketing Intelligence & Planning, 23*(1), 58–76. doi:10.1108/02634500510577474

Yan, J.H., Rountree, S., Massman, P., Doody, R.S., & Li, H. (2008). Alzheimer's disease and mild cognitive impairment deteriorate fine movement control. *Journal of Psychiatric Research, 42*(14), 1203–1212.

6

THE MEMORY EDUCATION AND RESEARCH INITIATIVE

A model for community-based clinical research

Chelsea Reichert, John J. Sidtis and Nunzio Pomara

6.1 The MERI program

The Memory Education and Research Initiative, or "MERI program", was established as a platform for bringing current research in aging and Alzheimer's disease (AD) to the world of clinical practice while providing a community mental health service at no cost to the participants. The initial funding for this program was provided in part by Rockland County, New York, which has had a strong commitment to the health of its residents. The MERI program enables the collection of an array of data from a diverse adult population, facilitating the exploration of relationships among the participant's presenting complaints, clinical status, demographic characteristics, the results of behavioral and medical assessments, and genetic and other biomarkers. Our particular areas of interest have been the evaluation of potential biomarkers for pathological aging, including genetic risk factors, phenotypic patterns, and the role of late-life depression.

MERI participants receive a neuropsychiatric evaluation at no cost to them. A report provides neuropsychological test results with age-appropriate normalized scores to provide a gauge of a participant's level of performance. The MERI reports are clinically valuable, and community physicians have become a major referral source. Many participants are self-referred as well, or brought in by a concerned spouse in response to advertisements or word-of-mouth recommendation.

The MERI program has become increasingly popular with the growing awareness and acceptance of AD within general culture, and the prevalence of advertisements for pharmaceuticals that target AD. Further, individuals who have had experience with AD through a family member or friend can have an increased concern about their own status, often triggered by otherwise normal cognitive failures.

As suggested earlier, an important aspect of the MERI program is that it is a clinical research study and not a diagnostic machine. Responsible diagnoses are beyond the scope and resources of this program and are appropriately the province of the participant's treating physician. Rather, we can comment through written reports to the participants, and if they consent, to their physicians. If a diagnosis of AD or other dementia has already been made, the compatibility of the MERI results with the diagnosis will be commented on. If no diagnosis exists and the results warrant one, a recommendation to seek a neurological evaluation is made. If a medical or psychiatric condition or current medications raise concerns, a recommendation for further evaluation of the suspected problem is made, or a review of medications is suggested. Most often, the participants are reassured that the results are within normal limits.

The MERI evaluation consists of both clinical and neuropsychological examinations. It is typically completed in three to four hours. The structure of the evaluation enables the examination to be repeated every 12 to 18 months and allows comparisons of the results over time. Whether it is a one-time check-up or a yearly occurrence, the results can assist a participant's primary medical provider in routine care. Likewise, this evaluation is designed to identify a pattern of symptoms and behaviors that may suggest the development or presence of Alzheimer's disease, while distinguishing other possible causes of subjective complaints or abnormal test results.

The structured framework of the MERI evaluation is similar to a routine clinical trial visit: review of medical history and medications, basic physical evaluation, neuropsychological testing, and clinical assessment. The clinical trial structure of the evaluation facilitates the identification of potential participants for other clinical trials and exposes participants to what is involved in such studies. The medical information and neuropsychological results decreases the chance that an individual will be inappropriately introduced to a treatment trial only to be disappointed by failing a screening evaluation. Our experience with the participants in the MERI also increases the chance of finding the best-fitting study for each individual.

6.2 The "MERI program" protocol

The MERI protocol defines three identifiable parts of each visit: the intake, the neuropsychological testing, and the investigator interview. The intake portion of the visit includes reviews of medical history, prescribed medications, and current medical state. The neuropsychological testing assesses the areas of performance that are affected in a memory-related disorder such as Alzheimer's disease, including general intellectual functioning, verbal memory, confrontation naming, verbal fluency, visual-spatial problem solving, and psychomotor functioning. The neuropsychological evaluation is not modeled after traditional longer neuropsychological test batteries, but rather evolved from experience in the Brain Tumor Cooperative Group and the Neuro-AIDS Study Group, which employed shorter, time-limited, objective tests. The aim is to efficiently assess the cardinal features of intellectual function much like a neurological examination assesses systems. In an older adult population, like most other populations, additional hours of neuropsychological testing do not ensure a proportionate amount of useful information. Nevertheless, the MERI test battery allows the investigators to assess the likelihood that the participant's presentation suggests AD or some other neurologic or psychiatric problem. The final part of the visit is the investigator interview, which is composed of inquiry about general lifestyle (e.g., sleep and appetite), possible psychiatric factors (e.g., depression and anxiety), recent reductions in functional ability, and any recent stressors (e.g., death of a family member, loss of a job, serious medical event) that might produce subject complaints of cognitive decline.

6.2.1   The intake

The intake is comparable to a first visit with a primary care doctor. The staff performs a comprehensive review of the participant's medical history, medications, and psychiatric and medical status. This review enables the staff to assess any medical-based problems that could account for memory complaints, such as medication interactions, which may be otherwise overlooked in participants seeing multiple physicians. The intake records demographic information, medical history, family history, lifestyle, vital signs, psychiatry status scales, and subjective memory complaints. A blood sample is taken for genetic testing and proteomics if consent is provided.

An important part of the intake is the determination of the reason for participation. This involves questions about perceived or experienced cognitive problems. It is important to establish the time of onset of the cognitive problem, the nature of the onset (i.e., whether the problem started abruptly or more gradually), the rate or absence of progression of the cognitive problem, the stability of the problem, the functional impact of the problem, and whether the severity of the problem is influenced by specific factors (e.g., worse at certain times of the day). The history of the cognitive problem is generally more informative than the family history, which can contribute to unnecessary anxiety in participants.

A Mini Mental State Exam (MMSE; Folstein, Folstein, & McHugh, 1975; Mitchell, 2009; Tombaugh & McIntyre, 1992) test is also performed. The MMSE provides a general cognitive status assessment, and it is widely used to categorize the mental status of participants in clinical trials and research studies. The MMSE consist of 30 questions and takes approximately 10 minutes to administer. This test touches on several domains of cognitive functioning: orientation, memory, registration, arithmetic, and the ability to follow commands. The severity of depressive and anxiety symptoms that a patient is currently experiencing are assessed using the Hamilton Depression (HAM-D; Hamilton, 1960) and Anxiety rating scales (HAM-A; Hamilton, 1959). The complete intake typically lasts approximately 45 minutes for a new participant and 30 minutes for a returning one. Information captured during intake is ideally verified through medical records provided by the patient or from the primary care physician or neurologist.

6.2.2   The neuropsychological exam

The neuropsychological assessment is a critical part of the MERI evaluation and it provides quantitative estimates of the participant's level of performance in several areas. This is useful in interpreting the participant's complaints (e.g., the presence or absence of a significant memory problem) and assessing whether the pattern of performance is consistent with some stage of AD, some other condition, or normal function. This portion lasts approximately one hour for cognitively intact participants and up to one and a half hours for cognitively impaired participants. The neuropsychological evaluation examines several broad areas of functioning using standardized measures: intellectual functioning, verbal memory, word-finding and fluency, visual-spatial problem solving, and psychomotor functioning. These areas of assessment represent the general cognitive domains that can be affected in Alzheimer's disease or related brain disorders. Moreover, because the cognitive presentation of a cognitive disorder like AD varies from person to person, with the potential to affect any cognitive domain in addition to memory, it is important that the neuropsychological evaluation extends beyond simply testing memory (Whitehouse, Lerner, & Hedera, 1993).

The use of standardized measures enables comparison of assessments across cognitive domains as well as across time. It is important that the individual administering the neuropsychological tests is properly trained, both to ensure standard administration of the assessments and to have the sensitivity to optimize the testing experience with the range of participants who exhibit diverse abilities. It is also essential for the neuropsychological examiner to be attuned to the behavior of the participants as well as the quality and nature of their communication. Incidental observations of a participant's behavior, like the history, can provide valuable information about possible etiologies, which can guide the clinical recommendations.

6.2.3 The assessments

Performance is categorized as average, above or below average, or significantly above or below average. Terms like "impaired" are avoided, as they communicate clinical judgments that extend beyond the scope of our program. When a result or a pattern of results raise a concern in our case review, the participant is advised to seek further work-up with his or her private physician.

Descriptions of the tests, where they can be obtained, and collections of normative values for different populations can be found in various sources (Lezak, Howieson, & Loring, 2004; Mitrushina, Boone, Razani, & D'Elia, 2005; Spreen & Strauss, 1998). Some commercial tests are frequently updated, but the selection of which edition to use is more often dictated by the desire to maintain consistency over time than by a desire to acquire the latest test version. The skills assessed by these tests are not subject to rapid evolutionary pressures, so frequent updates are not deemed essential.

The tests and their order of administration are as follows:

1   *Orientation* – The orientation test from the Wechsler Memory Scale consists of 14 open-ended questions about awareness of self, time, and location at the time of testing.

2   *Mental Control* – The mental control test, also from the Wechsler Memory Scale, consists of four questions that measure highly learned material, such as reciting the alphabet and counting. Poor performance on this test will influence the decision to administer the Trail Making tests described later.

3   *Rey Auditory Verbal Learning Test* – This test assesses the learning and retention of verbal material. It consists of three parts: the learning phase, immediate memory test, and delayed memory and recognition tests. The learning phase consists of five consecutive trials in which 15 words are read to the participant followed by immediate recall. An interference word list is presented and recall is requested. The participant is then asked to recall the original word list. The next series of tests in the evaluation do not involve material that might interfere with the word list and fill a 20–25 minute period, after which delayed recall is tested.

4   *Grooved Pegboard* – This is a timed test in which the participant places grooved pegs in a five by five array of holes in which notches matching the grooves on the pegs occur in varied orientation. The task is described as fitting a key in a lock and is performed as quickly as possible. Each hand is tested separately. This evaluates psychomotor speed, manual dexterity, and coordination, and is only administered to patients with full use of their hands (e.g., without carpal tunnel or severe arthritis).

5   *Trail Making A & B* – Test A consists of circles numbered 1 to 25 randomly placed on a page. Test B consists of circles that contain either numbers (1–13) or letters (A–L). Subjects are asked to connect circles in order as quickly as possible. It can be described to participants as a "connect the dots" test. Part A requires connecting circles in numerical order and part B involves alternating in order between numbers and letters. Both tests assess visual processing, attention, working memory, manual control, and executive functioning.

6   *Digit Symbol Substitution* – from the Wechsler Adult Intelligence Scale, is a coding test that requires participants to transcribe as many symbols as possible to a number series using a template. A fixed period of time (90 or 120 seconds, depending on the version) is allowed. This test is complementary to the Trail Making B test.

7   *Finger Tapping* – This test, administered to each hand, consists of tapping a key with the index finger as quickly as possible for 10 seconds. Five trials are obtained. This is a test of motor speed and fatigue.

8   *Delayed Recall (Rey Auditory Verbal Learning)* – Delayed recall is assessed 20–25 minutes after the completion of the learning trials. This assesses longer term recall of the originally learned words from the 15 item list.

9   *Delayed Recognition* – After the delayed recall, a two alternative forced choice procedure is used to assess recognition. Recognition is a well preserved ability and poor performance in an otherwise relatively intact participant raises the possibility of poor compliance or a psychogenic problem interfering with performance.

10   *Vocabulary* – The vocabulary test from the Wechsler Adult Intelligence Scale is administered only at the first visit. It provides a good estimate of intellectual attainment, similar to years of education.

11 *Confrontation Naming* – The Boston Naming test is administered in abridged versions consisting of 30 line drawings (the 60 item test is divided into two alternative versions). The participant is asked to name each picture. If the participant has difficulty naming the picture, a stimulus cue is provided. If that fails, a phonetic cue is provided.

12 *Verbal Fluency* – The test is often referred to as FAS but is formally named the Controlled Oral Word Association Test (COWAT). Participants are asked to name as many words as possible in 60 seconds. Three trials are given, each with a different letter (e.g., F, A, and S).

13 *Visual-spatial Problem Solving* – The Block Design test from the Wechsler Adult Intelligence Scale consists of nine blocks, each of which has two sides that are red, two sides that are white, and two sides that are half red and half right. The subject is asked to recreate a series of designs that range in difficulty from very easy to complex. This is one of the most difficult tests and is often the most frustrating.

14 *Mood* – The Profile of Mood States (POMs) is a questionnaire that assesses mood states (McNair, Lorr, & Droppleman, 1971). It consists of 65 different mood-related adjectives and participants are requested to report how each mood-related adjective applies to them in a given time frame.

15 *Subjective Memory Ability* – The MACs, or the Memory Assessment Complaint Questionnaire, is a survey that measures participant's concerns and beliefs about current memory status (Crook, Feher, & Larrabee, 1992). The survey consists of 33 questions. The first set of questions address how participants perceive their memory as compared with other people their age. The second set of questions address how participants perceive themselves compared with 10 years prior. The third set of questions address how often the subject recalls committing a number of memory-related mistakes. The final three questions ask the participants to provide an overall judgment of their memory, the speed with which they remember, and their concerns regarding their memory problems.

6.2.4 Additional assessments

It is highly recommended that participants come to the evaluation accompanied by another individual, whether it is a family member or a close friend, who is able to act as a reliable informant. If willing, the informant is asked to complete a 30 minute assessment with a member of the staff to evaluate the severity of possible dementia. This assessment is called the Clinical Dementia Rating Scale (CDR; Morris, 1993). The CDR is a structured interview that is conducted first with the informant and then completed with the participant. It is administered by a certified rater. This assessment covers a number of domains that are affected in people with dementia, including memory, orientation, judgment and problem solving, community affairs, home and hobbies, and personal care (Morris, 1993). After completing the CDR, the rater scores the assessment, based both on the informant's objective report and the subject's performance, and receives a score of 0.0 (not demented) to 3.0 (severely demented).

6.2.5 Psychiatric evaluation

The psychiatric evaluation is a semi-structured interview that is conducted by a geriatric psychiatrist. The interview is administered to the participant as well as the informant. The objective of the interview is to evaluate potential factors that could contribute to either real or perceived decline in memory. The result of the psychiatric evaluation is an evaluation of likelihood of the appropriateness of a diagnosis of a memory disorder like AD, a psychiatric condition like late-life major depression, or normal cognition. This assessment is further considered in the context of the neuropsychological test results. Quite frequently, subjective memory complaints reported during this visit are not supported by the neuropsychological testing. In such instances, one should consider the possibility that the perceived memory problems may be the result of stress, anxiety, depression, or other factors unrelated to neuropathological changes associated with AD or related brain disorders.

6.2.6 MERI report

On a weekly basis, the results of the MERI evaluations are reviewed by a team consisting of a psychiatrist, neuropsychologist, evaluator, and study coordinator. The purpose of the case conference is to review the results and determine the best clinical recommendations for each participant. There are a number of meaningful elements that are considered when reviewing each case, including the presenting complaint, medical history, overall test performance, and possible causes of the complaint and test abnormalities. The presenting complaint (i.e., perceived decline in short-term memory, difficulty remembering words or names, or general forgetfulness) is considered in comparison with the subject's test performance. Second, the medical history is reviewed for possible psychiatric or medical conditions, or possible use of medications with central anticholinergic effects or benzodiazepines, which are known to be associated with adverse cognitive effects. Carriers of the APOE-ε4 allele, an established risk factor for AD, have an elevated risk of adverse cognitive effects from such medications (Pomara, Belzer, Hernando, De La Pena, & Sidtis, 2008; Pomara et al., 2015; Pomara, Willoughby, Wesnes, Greenblatt, & Sidtis, 2005; Pomara, Willoughby, Wesnes, & Sidtis, 2004). Finally, the complaint and performance are evaluated in terms of the possible cause. Organic causes, such as AD or late-life major depression, result in recommendations for neurological work-ups or evaluation by a psychiatrist, whereas unsubstantiated cognitive complaints are explained in terms of illness, or the stress of an event such as moving or loss of a job, and typically result in recommendations for stress reduction.

The MERI report is a one-page summary of the neuropsychological testing, an interpretation of the testing and other information gathered, as well as recommendations. This report is the main benefit that patients receive when they come for the MERI evaluation. While all of the information gathered is used to interpret the testing, only select information is included on the report, specifically the neuropsychological testing. The raw score of each neuropsychological assessment is converted to a standardized score. This conversion allows for comparison with measures that assess similar cognitive domains (i.e., intellectual function); this also allows for ease of interpretation for the patient because each standardized score has a classification (i.e., average, above average, below average, etc.).

6.3   Who participates in the MERI?

The participants in the MERI program represent a diverse population of individuals from Rockland County, New York. To date, nearly 1,000 people have completed at least one MERI evaluation, over 12 years. The average MERI participant has completed approximately three years of college. There have been slightly more female participants (57%), and Figure 6.1 shows that the majority of these participants fall in the age range of 70–79 years, with an average age of 71.3 years.

In general, 95% of the participants who completed the initial MERI evaluation reported that they came because of a personal concern about memory. Participants described these concerns as forgetfulness, short-term memory loss, and difficulty producing words. The remaining 5% of subjects initially participated in the MERI program because of a family history of dementia, to accompany a spouse that they were concerned about, or because they wanted to serve as a research volunteer even though they had no memory complaint. Less than half of the individuals who completed an initial visit returned for a follow-up visit (Figure 6.2). The participants who typically responded to invitations for a follow-up evaluation were those who were cognitively normal, having benign subjective memory complaints that can occur with increasing age. Participants with objective cognitive impairments who come for the evaluation with a pre-existing AD diagnosis make up approximately 15% of the MERI population. Conversely, a considerable number of participants who come for an evaluation without a pre-existing diagnosis of dementia exhibit

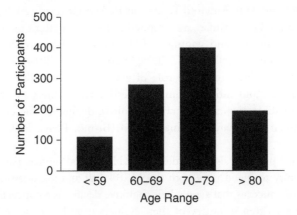

FIGURE 6.1   The numbers of participants by age group who have completed the baseline MERI visit.

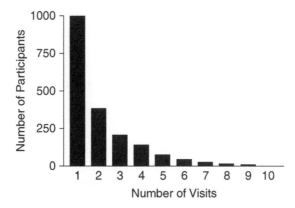

FIGURE 6.2   The number of participants who have had one or more MERI evaluations. Some participants have been remarkably stable over several years. Other participants have exhibited fluctuations in performance that would earn them a classification of mild cognitive impairment (MCI) at one visit but not the next.

significantly poor neuropsychological performance across multiple testing domains. For these participants, a neurological evaluation is recommended.

6.4   The value of the MERI program

For various administrative reasons, the program was named the Memory Education and Research Initiative. This has turned out to be an appropriate name. As noted previously, the MERI has been a valuable resource for research, both by providing a recruitment tool and by educating participants to what it is like to participate in clinical studies. The program has facilitated participation in federally funded studies, such as the Alzheimer's Disease Neuroimaging Initiative (the ADNI study) and Anti-Amyloid Treatment in Asymptomatic Alzheimer's study (the "A4" study). These studies are designed to develop better biological markers to aid in the diagnosis and staging of AD and to explore preventive pharmacological strategies (Mueller et al., 2005; Sperling et al., 2014). The MERI has also enabled us to investigate the role of genetics, medical illnesses, cardiovascular risk factors, and sub-syndromal depressive and anxiety symptoms in the emergence of subjective and objective cognitive decline in the elderly (Bruno, Brown, Kapucu, Marmar, & Pomara, 2014; Bruno, Reiss, Petkova, Sidtis, & Pomara, 2013).

The MERI program also provides a valuable clinical service. Participants have the opportunity to spend time with the MERI staff and ask questions about the wide range of concerns that arise when cognitive decline is a concern. Participants also receive a written summary of their evaluation with a contact number of a senior member with significant clinical experience in the evaluation of individuals with neurological disorders. This has led to numerous conversations that usually alleviate concerns. At other times, these conversations try to prepare a participant or spouse for what is likely to occur in the future. While the MERI staff educate the participants, the participants also continue to educate the staff. The MERI provides a good model for a mutually beneficial relationship between the community and clinical research.

References

Bruno, D., Brown, A. D., Kapucu, A., Marmar, C.R., & Pomara, N. (2014). Cognitive reserve and emotional stimuli in older individuals: Level of education moderates the age-related positivity effect. *Experimental Aging Research, 40*(2), 208–223.

Bruno, D., Reiss, P.T., Petkova, E., Sidtis, J.J., & Pomara, N. (2013). Decreased recall of primacy words predicts cognitive decline. *Archives of Clinical Neuropsychology, 28*(2), 95–103.

Crook, T.H., Feher, E.P., & Larrabee, G.J. (1992). Assessment of memory complaint in age-associated memory impairment: The MAC-Q. *International Psychogeriatrics, 4*(2), 165–176.

Folstein, M.F., Folstein, S.E., & McHugh, P.R. (1975). "Mini-Mental State". *Journal of Psychiatric Research, 12,* 189–198.

Hamilton M. (1959). The assessment of anxiety states by rating. *British Journal of Medical Psychology, 32,* 50–55.

Hamilton, M. (1960). A rating scale for depression. *Journal of Neurology Neurosurgery Psychiatry, 23,* 56–62.

Lezak, M.D., Howieson, D.B., & Loring, D.W. (2004). *Neuropsychological Assessment.* New York, Oxford University Press.

McNair, D.M., Lorr, M., & Droppleman, L.F. (1971). *Manual: Profile of mood states.* San Diego: Educational and Industrial Testing Service.

Mitchell, A.J. (2009). A meta-analysis of the accuracy of the mini-mental state examination in the detection of dementia and mild cognitive impairment. *Journal of Psychiatric Research, 43,* 411–431.

Mitrushina, M., Boone, K.B., Razani, J., & D'Elia, L.F. (2005). *Handbook of Normative Data for Neuropsychological Assessment.* New York, Oxford University Press.

Morris, J.C. (1993). The Clinical Dementia Rating (CDR): Current version and scoring rules. *Neurology, 43*(11), 2412–2414.

Mueller, S.G., Weiner, M.W., Thal, L.J., Petersen, R.C., Jack, C.R., Jagust, W., . . . Beckett, L. (2005). Ways toward an early diagnosis in Alzheimer's disease: The Alzheimer's Disease Neuroimaging Initiative (ADNI). *Alzheimer's & Dementia, 1*(1), 55–66.

Pomara, N., Belzer, K., Hernando, R., De La Pena, C., & Sidtis, J.J. (2008). Increased mental slowing associated with the APOE epsilon4 allele after trihexyphenidyl oral anticholinergic challenge in healthy elderly. *American Journal of Geriatric Psychiatry, 16*(2),116–124.

Pomara, N., Lee, S.H., Bruno, D., Silber, T., Greenblatt, D.J., Petkova, E., & Sidtis, J.J. (2015). Adverse performance effects of acute lorazepam administration in elderly long-term users: Pharmacokinetic and clinical predictors. *Progress in Neuropsychopharmacology & Biological Psychiatry, 56,* 129–135.

Pomara, N., Willoughby, L., Wesnes, K., Greenblatt, D.J., & Sidtis, J.J. (2005). Apolipoprotein E epsilon4 allele and lorazepam effects on memory in high-functioning older adults. *Archives of General Psychiatry, 62*(2), 209–216.

Pomara, N., Willoughby, L.M., Wesnes, K., & Sidtis, J.J. (2004). Increased anticholinergic challenge-induced memory impairment associated with the APOE-epsilon4 allele in the elderly: A controlled pilot study. *Neuropsychopharmacology, 29*(2), 403–409.

Sperling, R.A., Rentz, D.M., Johnson, K.A., Karlawish, J., Donohue, M., Salmon, D.P., & Aisen, P. (2014). The A4 study: Stopping AD before symptoms begin? *Science Translational Medicine, 6*(228), 228fs13.

Spreen, O., & Strauss, E. (1998). *A Compendium of Neuropsychological Tests.* New York, Oxford University Press.

Tombaugh, T.N., & McIntyre, N.J. (1992). The Mini-Mental State Examination: A comprehensive review. *Journal of the American Geriatric Society, 40,* 922–935.

Whitehouse, P.J., Lerner, A., & Hedera, P. (1993). *Dementia.* In K. M. Heilman & E. Valenstein (Eds.), *Clinical Neuropsychology.* New York: Oxford University Press.

PART III

From the laboratory to the home

Practical applications for ageing populations

7

USING THE BACKGROUND TO REMEMBER THE FOREGROUND

The role of contextual information in memory

Gerasimos Markopoulos

7.1 Introduction

Environmental context-dependent memory is a ubiquitous memory phenomenon that is intuitive and easy to relate to everyday experience. It is also at the core of most cognitive theories attempting to explain human memory function. No memory theory would be complete without postulating a role for the processing of contextual information (see also Chapter 4) and a mechanism through which the reinstatement of encoded contextual information at retrieval contributes to item memory. Considering how important context is for memory function, it is perhaps not surprising that there is much debate about its role and the nature of its contribution. Understanding the role of context in memory function as fully as possible is crucial for many theoretical and practical reasons; among these, the need to understand the effects of age-related and neurodegenerative changes on memory function, and how this knowledge may contribute to the development of techniques and strategies for helping people with memory preservation.

7.2 The nature of environmental context-dependent memory

Environmental context (EC) refers to information that is peripheral to the memory target. The term peripheral does not necessarily refer solely to the spatial properties of the information but also to its relationship with the target; EC is incidental in the sense that it does not affect the interpretation of the target (cf. semantic context; Light & Carter-Sobell, 1970) and participants are not explicitly instructed to meaningfully associate the target with the context (cf. Eich, 1985). EC will be the focus of this chapter, although other types of context information will be considered.

Most would be familiar with the influence of EC on memory in everyday life. One example would be realising you need a specific item located in another room in the house. Once you reach that other room, you have forgotten what it was you needed. Importantly, you remember again when you return to the original room. Presumably, the item needed is remembered because memory is aided by the environmental cues that were present when the thought of needing the item was initially formed. Another example would be returning to a former place of residence after a long time of absence. Such an experience is often accompanied by the apparent re-emergence of memories associated with the place, possibly of events that might have been considered forgotten otherwise.

In addition to anecdotal evidence, EC-dependent memory has a long research history. Many of the early studies suggest the influence of associationism and the principle of contiguity, which purports that items contiguous in space and/or time are likely to become mentally linked. On the basis of this principle, it is inevitable to hypothesise that encoding information in a specific physical or mental environment will create a link between the information and the environment such that, when the environment is reinstated, the retrieval of the information is facilitated. Early in the history of psychology, Carr (1913) conducted a series of experiments to test the effects of several environmental manipulations on the learning of a maze by a rat (e.g., illumination, cleanliness of the maze). He concluded that "an experience can be recalled most readily in those environmental situations with which it has the most direct, the strongest and the most numerous associations" (Carr, 1925, p. 250). Since then, many studies have been conducted demonstrating the effects of EC on memory employing a variety of different experimental designs. A classic and very frequently cited study was conducted by Godden and Baddeley (1975) employing the reinstatement paradigm. In the reinstatement paradigm, encoding takes place in one EC and, at retrieval, the encoding EC is reinstated or changed. An EC effect is observed if retrieval is superior when the encoding EC is reinstated. In Experiment 1, Godden and Baddeley employed divers as participants. They encoded a list of words aurally either on land or while diving underwater. Subsequently, participants retrieved the words using written free recall either in the same EC as the one at encoding or in the different EC. Participants retrieving in the encoding EC recalled significantly more items than the participants who switched, regardless of what the testing environment was (i.e., on land or underwater).

Since the Godden and Baddeley (1975) study, others have employed a variety of less extreme environmental manipulations to demonstrate the EC reinstatement effect. One of the most common EC manipulations involves rooms. Smith, Glenberg and Bjork (1978, Experiment 3) instructed participants to sort words into categories in one of two different rooms. At encoding, participants were not aware that another room was involved in the study or that their memory would be tested later. Therefore, the significance of the environment did not become apparent until retrieval, if at all. A day later, participants returned to the same room where encoding had occurred or to the other room, and their memory was tested via free recall. As anticipated, retrieval was superior when it occurred in the original encoding EC. Other studies employing the EC reinstatement paradigm have included background and font colour manipulations (e.g., Markopoulos, Rutherford, Cairns, &

Green, 2010), testing in person or via telephone (Canas & Nelson, 1986) and more (see Smith & Vela, 2001, for a review).

Interestingly, Smith (1985) employed music as EC in two experiments. A crucial difference with previous EC reinstatement experiments is that the music manipulation allowed for a condition where the encoding EC was not reinstated but was not changed either. Using music as EC allowed for a 'no context' condition, where participants were exposed to music at encoding and to quiet (as opposed to different music) at retrieval. The pattern of results confirmed that it is not the change in context between encoding and retrieval that reduces performance per se, but rather it is the reinstatement of the encoding context at retrieval that has a beneficial effect probably through a cuing effect.

Such experimental findings are consistent with the Encoding Specificity Principle (ESP) as formulated by Tulving and Osler (1968) and Tulving and Thomson (1973). The ESP states that a retrieval cue will be effective in cueing the target item only to the extent that information in the cue was present and incorporated in the memory trace during encoding. An impressive demonstration of the principle was provided by Tulving and Thomson (1973). At Stage 1, target words were presented and encoded along with a weakly associated word (e.g., BLACK – train). At Stage 2, participants completed a filler task. The apparently unrelated filler task was to generate six associates to words that, unbeknownst to the participants, were strong associates of the target words from Stage 1 (e.g., WHITE). A large number of target words were produced in response (e.g., WHITE: black). At Stage 3, participants performed a recognition test on the associates they had produced and attempted to identify the ones they had seen at Stage 1 (e.g., BLACK). At the fourth and final stage, cued recall was tested where the cue provided was the weakly associated word paired with the target at encoding (e.g., train for the target BLACK). Participants performed better at cued recall at Stage 4 than at recognition at Stage 3, demonstrating that recognition is not always easier than recall. More critically, weakly related associates were shown to be more effective retrieval cues than strong associates, presumably because the weak associates were encoded along with the target. This result is consistent with the ESP and with EC-dependent memory, both of which place emphasis on the match between encoding and retrieval conditions. Specifically, the ESP and related theories such as Global Activation Models (e.g., Hintzman, 1988) would suggest that there is a direct and causal relationship between retrieval cue and memory trace match and retrievability.

The ESP, although both intuitive and supported by empirical evidence, has faced some criticism. Baddeley (1997) points out that the principle involves a circular argument. If a retrieval cue is effective, it is assumed that it is effective because it matches the memory trace formed at encoding. If a retrieval cue is not effective, the assumption made is that it does not match the memory trace sufficiently. Therefore, it is practically impossible to produce evidence against the principle (see an analogous circular argument in relationship to levels of processing in Chapter 4). A second criticism relating to the first is expressed by Nairne (2002), who argues that retrieval is not a function of the match between the cue and the memory trace, but that retrieval depends on the usefulness of the cue in distinguishing between the memory trace and competing or distracting items. According to Nairne, the relationship between cue-trace match and retrievability is correlational rather than causal. When the retrieval cue matches the memory trace, it is more likely to assist in differentiating between the target and competing items. This rather subtle point is illustrated very effectively by a thought experiment provided by Nairne (2002); at encoding, participants are asked to read aloud a list of homophones in a particular order (1: write, 2: right, 3: rite, etc.). At retrieval, half of the participants are asked to recall in writing the third word from the list (i.e., rite). The other half of the participants are provided with an additional retrieval cue and are told that the target word sounds like 'rayt'. According to the ESP, the second condition provides a relatively increased match between the retrieval cues and the memory trace. Therefore, the second group should demonstrate higher recall probability. However, in this particular instance, the increased cue-trace match does not help differentiate between the target (rite) and other competing items (write, right). An important point to be made is that Nairne's argument and the ESP itself refer to the functional match rather than the nominal match. In other words, they refer to the relationships formed in the participant's mind rather than to any objective relationship between the presented stimuli. This is the main reason Nairne has employed thought experiments to illustrate his point. Actual experimental manipulations can only indirectly explore functional relationships, making it difficult to eliminate alternative interpretations. However, there is empirical evidence that can be interpreted to support Nairne's position (e.g., Goh & Lu, 2012).

The criticisms aimed against the ESP also largely transfer to EC-dependent memory studies. With regard to Nairne's (2002) argument, it is very probable that not all EC manipulations will result in better retrieval performance when the encoding and retrieval ECs match due to the potentially poor diagnostic value of the cues provided. Indeed, EC reinstatement effects are typically not particularly strong (see Smith & Vela, 2001) and they are frequently not observed at all. The rather modest effect sizes of EC reinstatement studies are to be anticipated and they are actually desirable. Learning something in a specific EC and largely forgetting the information learnt, if required to retrieve it elsewhere, would not be a property of an effective memory system. Consistent with this idea, null effects in EC reinstatement studies have often been observed (e.g., Fernandez & Glenberg, 1985). EC reinstatement effects have also been elusive when recognition memory is tested as opposed to free recall (e.g., Godden & Baddeley, 1980; cf. Smith & Vela, 2001). Additionally, few studies have obtained reverse EC reinstatement effects, with retrieval performance being superior when the retrieval EC does not match the encoding EC (e.g., Markopoulos, 2005; McDaniel, Anderson, Einstein, & O'Halloran, 1988). Such unexpected results cannot be readily explained, but they do suggest that EC effects can vary dramatically and are sensitive to differences in instructions and tasks at encoding and retrieval.

In an attempt to extrapolate patterns and explain apparent inconsistencies in the EC-dependent memory literature, Smith and Vela (2001) conducted a review and meta-analysis. They included studies that manipulated incidental context as defined earlier in this section, employed human participants, and operationalised EC as global as opposed to local. The distinction between global and local EC is not very clear. Typically, global EC is operationalised through the use of rooms, while local EC is operationalised as the background colour of the screen on which the target stimuli are presented and/or the position and font colour of the stimuli (see Markopoulos et al., 2010). Although Smith and Vela only included global EC manipulations, it is not clear if the two types of EC produce different behavioural results or involve different mechanisms in how they operate (cf. Markopoulos, 2005). Some revealing patterns and conclusions were drawn from the meta-analysis. For one, mental reinstatement of the EC appears to be as effective in cuing the target stimuli as physical EC reinstatement. In other words, at retrieval, it is not essential that the encoding EC is physically present for EC reinstatement effects to occur as long as the participants are reminded of the encoding EC or spontaneously choose to mentally reinstate it as a retrieval strategy. Additionally, some evidence was found that EC effects are reduced when attention is drawn away from the EC at encoding (overshadowing) and/or at retrieval (outshining) through the provision of more effective or stronger cues. These findings are consistent with Nairne's (2002) position that effective cues are more diagnostic. EC cues will be more effective (and diagnostic) when other cues are not available. Smith and Vela's work is highly valuable and it generated several important conclusions and testable hypotheses. However, many questions still remain particularly with regard to reverse EC reinstatement effects, the relationship between global and local EC and their respective underlying mechanisms, and a full taxonomy of EC.

7.3   Context and the brain

In recent years, much progress has been made in terms of understanding how memory operates and how the underlying hypothesised mechanisms involved relate to specific brain areas and functions. This progress is largely attributable to neuroimaging technology, which has brought cognitive psychology and neurophysiological research closer together. Even before such technological advances, the role of the medial temporal lobe (MTL) and the hippocampus in particular in episodic memory was well-established, if not fully understood, through lesion studies and research in the amnestic syndrome (e.g., Scoville & Milner, 1957). Episodic memory involves the encoding and retrieval of specific episodes or events as opposed to general knowledge (see Tulving, 1983). What differentiates it from other types of memory is that the event (i.e., memory item) is accompanied by peripheral information such as when, where and under what circumstances the event took place (i.e., context information). Part of the contribution of recent neuroimaging literature is in attempting to determine the precise role of specific MTL regions and other brain areas in the processing of item and context information, and how these regions coordinate to result in the effective encoding and retrieval of episodic memories.

One particularly influential theory of how item and context information relate to specific brain regions has been the BIC (Binding of Item and Context) account as expressed by Diana, Yonelinas and Ranganath (2007). On the basis of a review of neuroimaging studies employing different methods and materials to distinguish between the processing of item and context information during encoding and retrieval, a model was formulated that identifies three main MTL regions as having distinct roles. The perirhinal cortex (PrC) processes item information, the parahippocampal cortex (PhC) processes context information (spatial and non-spatial), while the hippocampus processes item-context associations. An interesting prediction of the model is that although the hippocampus supports item-context associations and therefore associative retrieval, when the item and context are 'unitised' and processed as a single item, the PrC will be involved. This prediction has been supported by several studies. In an fMRI study, Haskins, Yonelinas, Quamme and Ranganath (2008) scanned participants during the encoding of unrelated word pairs. Word pairs were either presented within a sentence or they formed novel compound words (unitisation condition). At test, recognition memory was tested for intact or rearranged word pairs outside the scanner. In agreement with the BIC model prediction, PrC activation at encoding was higher for word pairs forming novel compound words than for pairs presented in a sentence. Both the BIC model and the unitisation prediction suggest that the manner in which contextual information is processed may have dramatic effects in which specific brain areas are involved. Despite this caveat, there is abundant evidence of the involvement of PhC in the processing of context information, and several theories concur with BIC although they differ in their theoretical assumptions and the interpretation of the evidence (e.g., Davachi, 2006; Montaldi & Mayes, 2010).

Models such as BIC (Diana et al., 2007) are based on neuroimaging studies that typically do not investigate the incidental influence of EC on memory as discussed in the previous section. Instead, they utilise experimental paradigms exploring associative memory or memory for context. Therefore, although the role of PhC in the intentional encoding and retrieval of context information has been demonstrated, it is not clear whether it has a role in EC reinstatement effects. It is impractical, if not impossible, to manipulate global EC in conjunction with fMRI measurements. However, Hayes, Nadel and Ryan (2007) explored this issue in an fMRI study testing object memory and manipulating local EC (Experiment 5). Everyday objects were presented at encoding either in a naturalistic scene or isolated in a white background. Encoding was incidental and participants were not given instructions regarding the background scenes. At retrieval, participants completed a recognition test for the objects. Three main conditions were employed: objects presented in a scene were tested in the same scene (scene-scene), objects presented on white background were tested on white background (object-object) and objects presented in a scene were tested on white background (scene-object). Recognition performance was superior in the same EC condition (scene-scene) than in the different EC condition (scene-object). Brain activity at encoding showed that PhC was associated with subsequent retrieval success in the scene-object and the scene-scene conditions but not in the object-object condition. At recognition, PhC activity was associated with retrieval success in the scene-object condition. Brain activity at recognition was contrasted between hits in the scene-object condition and hits in the object-object condition. This analysis revealed increased PhC activity in the scene-object condition, suggesting the possibility that the PhC is involved in the mental reinstatement of the encoding EC, which in turn facilitates correct item recognition. Overall, the neuroimaging evidence presented here strongly indicates the involvement of the MTL – if not specifically the PhC – in EC reinstatement effects.

7.4   The role of context in Alzheimer's disease

Alzheimer's disease (AD) is a type of dementia characterised by gradually progressive neurodegeneration, often preceded by mild cognitive impairment (MCI). MCI is defined as presenting signs of memory impairment and subjective memory complaints in the absence of additional cognitive impairments, which would be present in mild AD (see Albert et al., 2011, for MCI criteria, and McKhann et al., 2011, for AD criteria). Reflecting the progressive nature of AD, Braak and Braak (1991) have identified six stages of the disease on the basis of an extensive post-mortem study that allowed the specification of the brain damage involved at each stage. The earliest stages of AD involve damage of the entorhinal cortex (ErC), which is an MTL region and part of a pathway linking the hippocampus to neocortical areas. The damage eventually progresses to other MTL regions and later to neocortical areas. Consequently, the first cognitive impairment to manifest in AD is anterograde amnesia – which corresponds to a difficulty in acquiring new information.

It has been suggested that, in early AD, item memory is selectively impaired with context memory and/or context-bound memory being largely intact (Didic, Barbeau, Felician, Tramoni, & Guedj, 2011). This hypothesis is consistent with the initial damage of anterior sub-hippocampal structures, which include ErC and PrC. Additionally, it is consistent with BIC (Diana et al., 2007). Provided the posterior MTL including PhC remains intact, it is possible that context processing remains functional for considerably longer (i.e., including stages 1 and 2; Braak & Braak, 1991). However, more substantial experimental evidence is required to test this hypothesis further – this may not prove easy, since, as Didic et al. (2011) reasonably assume, context-rich memory impairment is more likely to result in an AD diagnosis.

Contrary to the hypothesis formulated by Didic et al. (2011), there is substantial evidence that context-based memory is impaired considerably early in AD, while item processing still remains relatively unimpaired. This pattern of pathology in AD is so widely accepted that tasks based on the ESP are employed for early diagnosis of AD on the basis that AD patients do not seem to fully benefit from the matching cues at encoding and retrieval (e.g., Adam et al., 2007). Della Barba (1997) employed the Remember-Know task (Tulving, 1985), which involves participants classifying recognition judgments on whether context details were also retrieved (Remember) or the retrieved item only felt familiar (Know). Della Barba (1997) found that AD patients produced fewer Remember responses than controls, but they did not differ in terms of Know responses, and they even produced more correct Know responses than controls in certain conditions. Irrespective of theoretical perspectives (see Yonelinas, 2002), it is widely agreed that Remember responses require context processing while Know responses reflect item memory. Also, according to the BIC model, Remember responses rely on the integrity of the hippocampus and the PhC, while Know responses rely on the integrity of the PrC. Similar findings have been obtained with other measures and paradigms, including source memory (i.e., memory for the context information present at encoding), with AD patients manifesting substantial misattribution errors (e.g., Mitchell, Sullivan, Schacter, & Budson, 2006). The Remember-Know task and source memory are both paradigms employed by studies reviewed by Diana et al. (2007), further suggesting the involvement of PhC and the hippocampus in memory for context.

Similar results to those obtained by Della Barba (1997) with AD patients have been obtained with MTL amnesic patients, with amnesic patients producing fewer Remember responses than controls but not differing in item-based Know responses (e.g., Aggleton et al., 2005). One of the early explanations for the amnesic syndrome that gathered much support was the Context Memory Deficit hypothesis (Mayes, 1988) which purported that MTL amnesic patients' memory problems originated from a failure to process contextual information. Since then, the hypothesis has evolved further, incorporating current theoretical perspectives, but the key role of context information processing remains (see Kopelman & Bright, 2012).

7.5 The use of context in rehabilitation

Haj and Kessels (2013) conducted a review of the literature on context memory in AD. Studies exploring EC reinstatement effects are conspicuously absent, while most reviewed studies focus on memory for context or employ semantic context in the form of word pairs. Haj and Kessels hypothesise that impaired context memory may be compensated for by the provision of cues from encoding on the basis of the ESP, although they do not mention EC reinstatement specifically. However, there is some indirect evidence that AD patients may benefit from EC reinstatement. Barak, Vakil and Levy (2013) tested traumatic brain injury (TBI) patients and controls using a variety of materials and different types of retrieval tests. TBI patients have different pathology to people with AD but their episodic memory impairment is rather similar at the early stages of AD. Barak et al. (2013) employed the EC reinstatement paradigm using rooms to manipulate encoding and retrieval EC match. EC reinstatement effects were obtained for both TBI patients and healthy controls. The effects were stronger for free recall than for cued recall, and no effects were obtained for recognition. These findings partially concur with Smith and Vela's (2001) meta-analysis suggesting an outshining effect with EC cues employed less at retrieval the more other cues are available. Interestingly, TBI patients benefitted more from EC reinstatement than controls. This finding demonstrates that episodic memory patients may benefit from EC reinstatement (see also Fernandez & Alonso, 2001, for similar findings with healthy elderly participants). Perhaps more importantly and quite counter-intuitively, it suggests that intact memory for context is not necessary for EC reinstatement effects to occur.

Considering the findings of Barak et al. (2013), the behavioural and neuroimaging literature presented in this chapter, and the key role of context in theories of episodic memory, a more exhaustive and systematic investigation of EC reinstatement effects in AD patients may prove to be critical for the development of rehabilitation techniques. Memory stimulation techniques for AD patients based on ESP have been explored to some degree with promising results (see Grandmaison & Simard, 2003). However, the evidence is scarce and based on non-longitudinal studies using semantic or category membership cues. Therefore, global and local EC reinstatement paradigm studies need to be conducted with AD patients at all stages of the disease, employing a variety of encoding and retrieval tasks, and different types of EC operationalization. On the basis of the evidence presented here, a reasonable hypothesis is that AD patients would manifest stronger EC reinstatement effects than healthy controls because of – rather than in spite of – their impairment in processing associative information. If the outshining and overshadowing principles are valid (Smith & Vela, 2001), it is possible that AD patients will benefit relatively more from the reinstatement of incidental EC information in the absence of stronger or more diagnostic cues, depending on the stage of the disease and the extent of the damage. Therefore, rehabilitation techniques could eventually incorporate EC reinstatement in terms of considering the learning and testing environments, their richness and distinctiveness, the attention directed to the environments at encoding and at retrieval, and the availability of alternative but perhaps less effective cues.

7.6 Conclusion

A clear pattern of memory impairment in AD has not yet been established. Contributing to the lack of consistency is the progressive nature of the disease but also possibly the large variability in the distribution of damage between patients (Braak & Braak, 1991). Another factor may be the focus of neuroimaging studies on MTL. Some fMRI studies have obtained hyperactivations in AD patients outside of MTL, possibly reflecting compensatory activity (see Dickerson & Sperling, 2009). The possibility of compensatory activity by intact brain areas may result in inconsistent findings across studies, but also suggests the development of proper rehabilitation techniques may contribute substantially to the alleviation of AD symptoms. Considering the role of context processing in the manifestation of AD symptoms, rehabilitation technique development must involve a more systematic investigation of EC reinstatement effects both in terms of under what circumstances they are observed and how they are operationalised.

References

Adam, S., Van Der Linden, M., Ivanoiu, A., Juillerat, A.-C., Bechet, S., & Salmon, E. (2007). Optimization of encoding specificity for the diagnosis of early AD: The RI-48 task. *Journal of Clinical and Experimental Neuropsychology, 29*, 477–487.

Aggleton, J. P., Vann, S. D., Denby, C., Dix, S., Mayes, A. R., Roberts, N., & Yonelinas, A. P. (2005). Sparing of the familiarity component of recognition memory in a patient with hippocampal pathology. *Neuropsychologia, 43*, 1810–1823.

Albert, M. S., DeKosky, S. T., Dickson, D., Dubois, B., Feldman, H. H., Fox, N. C., . . . Phelps, C. H. (2011). The diagnosis of mild cognitive impairment due to Alzheimer's disease: Recommendations from the National Institute on Aging-Alzheimer's Association workgroups on diagnostic guidelines for Alzheimer's disease. *Alzheimer's & Dementia, 7*, 270–279.

Baddeley, A. D. (1997). *Human memory: Theory and practice*. Hove: Psychology Press.

Barak, O., Vakil, E., & Levy, D. A. (2013). Environmental context effects on episodic memory are dependent on retrieval mode and modulated by neuropsychological status. *The Quarterly Journal of Experimental Psychology, 66*, 2008–2022.

Braak, H., & Braak, E. (1991). Neuropathological staging of Alzheimer-related changes. *Acta Neuropathologica, 82*, 239–259.

Canas, J. J., & Nelson, D. L. (1986). Recognition and environmental context: The effect of testing by phone. *Bulletin of the Psychonomic Society, 24*, 407–409.

Carr, H. A. (1913). Maze studies with the white rat. *Journal of Animal Behaviour, 7*, 259–306.

Carr, H. A. (1925). *Psychology: A study of mental activity*. New York: Longmans, Green & Co.

Davachi, L. (2006). Item, context and relational episodic encoding in humans. *Current Opinion in Neurobiology, 16*, 693–700.

Della Barba, G. (1997). Recognition memory and recollective experience in Alzheimer's disease. *Memory, 5*, 657–692.

Diana, R. A., Yonelinas, A. P., & Ranganath, C. (2007). Imaging recollection and familiarity in the medial temporal lobe: A three-component model. *Trends in Cognitive Sciences, 11*, 379–386.

Dickerson, B. C., & Sperling, R. A. (2009). Large-scale functional brain network abnormalities in Alzheimer's disease: Insights from functional neuroimaging. *Behavioural Neurology, 21*, 63–75.

Didic, M., Barbeau, E. J., Felician, O., Tramoni, E., & Guedj, E. (2011). Which memory system is impaired first in Alzheimer's disease? *Journal of Alzheimer's Disease, 27*, 11–22.

Eich, J. E. (1985). Context, memory and integrated item/context imagery. *Journal of Experimental Psychology: Learning, Memory, and Cognition, 11*, 764–770.

Fernandez, A., & Alonso, M. A. (2001). The relative value of environmental context reinstatement in free recall. *Psicologica, 22*, 253–266.

Fernandez, A., & Glenberg, A. M. (1985). Changing environmental context does not reliably affect memory. *Memory & Cognition, 13*, 333–345.

Godden, D. R., & Baddeley, A. D. (1975). Context-dependent memory in two natural environments: On land and underwater. *British Journal of Psychology, 66*, 325–331.

Godden, D. R., & Baddeley, A. D. (1980). When does context influence recognition memory? *British Journal of Psychology, 71*, 99–104.

Goh, W. D., & Lu, S. H. X. (2012). Testing the myth of the encoding-retrieval match. *Memory & Cognition, 40*, 28–39.

Grandmaison, E., & Simard, M. (2003). A critical review of memory stimulation programs in Alzheimer's Disease. *The Journal of Neuropsychiatry and Clinical Neurosciences, 15*, 130–144.

Haj, M. E., & Kessels, R. P. C. (2013). Context memory in Alzheimer's disease. *Dementia and Geriatric Cognitive Disorders, 3*, 342–350.

Haskins, A. L., Yonelinas, A. P., Quamme, J. R., & Ranganath, C. (2008). Perirhinal cortex supports encoding and familiarity-based recognition of novel associations. *Neuron, 59*, 554–560.

Hayes, S. M., Nadel, L., & Ryan, L. (2007). The effect of scene context on episodic object recognition: Parahippocampal cortex mediates memory encoding and retrieval success. *Hippocampus, 17*, 873–889.

Hintzman, D. L. (1988). Judgments of frequency and recognition memory in a multiple-trace memory model. *Psychological Review, 95*, 528–551.

Kopelman, M. D., & Bright, P. (2012). On remembering and forgetting our autobiographical past: Retrograde amnesia and Andrew Mayes's contribution to neuropsychological method. *Neuropsychologia, 50*, 2961–2972.

Light, L. L., & Carter-Sobell, L. (1970). Effects of changed semantic context on recognition memory. *Journal of Verbal Learning and Verbal Behavior, 9*, 1–11.

Markopoulos, G. (2005). *Comparisons of global and local environmental context reinstatement effects.* Unpublished Doctoral Dissertation, Keele University, UK.

Markopoulos, G., Rutherford, A., Cairns, C., & Green, J. (2010). Encoding instructions and stimulus presentation in local environmental context-dependent memory studies. *Memory, 18*, 610–624.

Mayes, A. R. (1988). *Human organic memory disorders.* Cambridge: Cambridge University Press.

McDaniel, M. A., Anderson, C. D., Einstein, G. O., & O'Halloran, C. M. (1988). Modulation of environmental reinstatement effects through encoding strategies. *American Journal of Psychology, 102*, 523–548.

McKhann, G. M., Knopman, D. S., Chertkow, H., Hyman, B. T., Jack, C. R., Kawas, C. H., . . . Phelps, C. H. (2011). The diagnosis of dementia due to Alzheimer's disease: Recommendations from the National Institute on Aging-Alzheimer's Association workgroups on diagnostic guidelines for Alzheimer's disease. *Alzheimer's Dementia, 7*, 263–269.

Mitchell, J. P., Sullivan, A. L., Schacter, D. L., & Budson, A. E. (2006). Misattribution errors in Alzheimer's disease: The illusory truth effect. *Neuropsychology, 20*, 185–192.

Montaldi, D., & Mayes, A. R. (2010). The role of recollection and familiarity in the functional differentiation of the medial temporal lobes. *Hippocampus, 20*, 1291–1314.

Nairne, J. S. (2002). The myth of the encoding-retrieval match. *Memory, 10*, 389–395.

Scoville, W. B., & Milner, B. (1957). Loss of recent memory after bilateral hippocampal lesions. *Journal of Neurology, Neurosurgery and Psychiatry, 20*, 11–21.

Smith, S. M. (1985). Background music and context-dependent memory. *American Journal of Psychology, 98*, 591–603.

Smith, S. M., Glenberg, A., & Bjork, R. A. (1978). Environmental context and human memory. *Memory & Cognition, 6*, 342–353.

Smith, S. M., & Vela, E. (2001). Environmental context-dependent memory: A review and meta-analysis. *Psychonomic Bulletin & Review, 8*, 203–220.

Tulving, E. (1983). *Elements of Episodic Memory.* New York: Oxford University Press.

Tulving, E. (1985). Memory and consciousness. *Canadian Psychology, 26*, 1–12.

Tulving, E., & Osler, S. (1968). Effectiveness of retrieval cues in memory for words. *Journal of Experimental Psychology, 77*, 593–601.

Tulving, E., & Thomson, D. M. (1973). Encoding specificity and retrieval processes in episodic memory. *Psychological Review, 80*, 352–373.

Yonelinas, A. P. (2002). The nature of recollection and familiarity: A review of 30 years of research. *Journal of Memory and Language, 46*, 441–517.

8

CAN SURVIVAL PROCESSING HELP TO PRESERVE OUR MEMORIES?

Daniel P. A. Clark

8.1   Introduction

One of the central questions in memory research is 'how can we improve memory performance?' Over the years, a number of encoding processes, essentially learning strategies, have been shown to improve the performance of our memory systems. These include manipulating depth of processing at encoding (Craik & Lockhart, 1972), retrieving information in the same environment it was encoded (Godden & Baddeley, 1975), testing retention immediately after encoding (Roediger & Karpicke, 2006) and the application of self-referential encoding (Symons & Johnson, 1997), to name just a few. In a recent study, Nairne, Thompson and Pandeirada (2007) demonstrated that processing items with regards to their relevance to survival produces superior recall when compared to a number of tried and tested memory encoding techniques. These results provided the foundation for a new avenue of research exploring the survival processing effect. This research has predominantly, but not exclusively, found further evidence for the effect and has demonstrated that the recall advantage is robust. Indeed, the mounting evidence supporting the effect has led to the claim that survival processing may be "the 'best of the best' of known encoding procedures" (Nairne, Pandeirada, & Thompson, 2008, p. 180). However, despite growing empirical success, there have been limited efforts to apply this 'superior encoding technique' to populations that may particularly benefit from its use, such as an aging population.

This chapter will explore the research surrounding the survival processing effect and will then consider potential applications of these findings to help facilitate the preservation of memory.

8.2   Survival processing

Nairne, Thompson and Pandeirada (2007) adopted a functional approach to the study of human memory, placing an emphasis away from exploring how our memory system works and instead focusing on why our memory functions the way it does. This approach is founded upon the principle that our memory systems have been moulded by the process of natural selection (Nairne, 2005; Nairne & Pandeirada, 2010) and have been subject to the pressures of evolution and subsequently survival (since survival would increase the likelihood that these memory characteristics would be inherited by future generations). This rationale led Nairne et al. (2007) to explore the idea that our memory systems have adapted to achieve specific functions, particularly those associated with our survival. Thus, Nairne et al. (2007) set out to test the hypothesis that human memory may be specifically tuned to process and retain information that is relevant to our survival. To formally test this hypothesis, Nairne et al. (2007) conducted four experiments where different scenarios were manipulated during the study phase. Experiment 1 had a between participants design and each participant was assigned to either a Survival, Moving or Pleasantness scenario. In the Survival condition, participants were asked to imagine that they were stranded in a foreign grassland without any basic survival materials, and were informed they would need to find food and water in addition to protecting themselves from predators. In the Moving condition, participants were asked to imagine they were moving to a new home in a foreign land, and that they would need to locate a new residence and later move their belongings to the new home. In the Pleasantness condition, participants were simply asked to consider how pleasant they perceived each word item to be (e.g., a flower may be perceived more pleasant than a stone). All participants were shown 30 concrete nouns in turn and were asked to rate each item from 1–5 regarding their relevance to each scenario. After providing the rating judgments, participants were asked to complete a short distracter task and were then asked to perform a free recall task. The results of this experiment revealed that significantly more items were recalled when survival processing had been employed than in either the moving or pleasantness conditions. This finding was particularly interesting, as previous evidence has shown that rating an item with regards to its perceived pleasantness or relevance to moving would produce higher levels of recall, as both are effective deep encoding tasks (Craik & Lockhart, 1972; Packman & Battig, 1978). Nairne et al. (2007) conducted a number of additional experiments to explore this initial finding and found further evidence of the survival processing effect in a within participants design (Experiment 2), in recognition memory (Experiment 3), and also higher levels of recall accuracy than self-referential encoding (Experiment 4). Collectively, the evidence presented by Nairne et al. (2007) suggested that processing items with regards to their survival properties is a particularly effective encoding mechanism that would benefit from further investigation.

Given the initial empirical success of survival processing, it is not surprising that there has been an influx of studies attempting to probe the effect further. Indeed, survival processing (also known as adaptive memory, given the functional hypothesis that memory adapted as a result of natural selection) has been shown to produce superior recall than a number of effective encoding mechanisms, such as imagery, intentional learning, generation and pleasantness (Bröder, Krüger, & Schütte, 2011; Burns, Burns, & Hwang, 2011; Howe & Otgaar, 2013; Kang, McDermott, & Cohen, 2008; Klein, 2012; Nairne & Pandeirada, 2010; Nairne, Pandeirada, Gregory, & Van

Arsdall, 2009; Nairne et al., 2008; Nairne et al., 2007; Nairne, VanArsdall, Pandeirada, & Blunt, 2012; Nouchi & Kawashima, 2012; Otgaar et al., 2011; Seamon et al., 2012). While the majority of studies exploring the survival processing effect have been shown to produce higher proportions of recall when retrieving lists of words (e.g., Kang et al., 2008; Nairne et al., 2008; Nairne et al., 2007), there is also evidence of the effect when the target objects are images (Otgaar, Smeets, & van Bergen, 2010), and when location memory performance is evaluated (Nairne et al., 2012).

A key issue that has been explored in the survival processing literature is the longevity of the effect. This is an important matter, as while the effect has been shown to consistently improve memory performance, the majority of studies have employed an immediate recall task, demonstrating improved performance only over a period of less than 10 minutes. While improved short term recall is an interesting starting point, if survival processing is to be considered an effective memory preservation tool, it would be beneficial if the initial advantage were maintained for a longer time frame than 10 minutes. While the longevity of the survival processing effect is an underrepresented area of research, there are two key studies that have explored this: Raymaekers, Otgaar and Smeets (2014) and Abel and Bäuml (2013). In both of these studies, participants were asked to rate concrete nouns using either the standard survival processing paradigm (the foreign grassland scenario) or an alternative deep encoding mechanism (either facilitating a move to a foreign land or pleasantness ratings, respectively). Raymaekers et al. (2014) then asked participants to complete a free recall and a recognition task either immediately after the ratings, or after a 24 hour or 48 hour delay. In contrast, Abel and Bäuml (2013) explored the role of sleep in the longevity of the survival processing effect. They asked one group of participants to complete a surprise recall task immediately after encoding, one group after a 12 hour delay with sleep and one group after 12 hours without sleep. Both studies demonstrated evidence of the survival processing effect at the immediate test of recall, supporting the findings of Nairne et al. (2007). Furthermore, despite a general reduction in recall accuracy across the delay period, both studies found significantly higher levels of recall when survival processing had been employed, as opposed to either the moving scenario or the pleasantness ratings. This evidence suggests that despite a general reduction in the number of words recalled across time, the survival processing benefit is maintained for a period of at least 48 hours after encoding.

In summary, there is consistent and strong evidence that survival processing yields superior recall when compared to other well-established encoding paradigms. However, a number of questions and exceptions have also emerged from the research data. For example, Nairne and Pandeirada (2010) conducted a study where their participants were asked to rate items according to their relevance for survival in either a foreign grassland or a modern city. Both of these survival conditions were compared to the moving city scenario. While there was clear evidence of the survival processing effect in the foreign grassland (ancestral) scenario, where more items were recalled than in the moving scenario, the results for the modern city were not so conclusive. In the first experiment reported, the modern city scenario did not show the survival processing effect, demonstrating comparable recall to that observed in the moving scenario. In the second experiment, the modern city scenario did show significantly higher recall than observed with a pleasantness condition, but more items were still recalled in the ancestral scenario compared to the modern city scenario. These results show that, while both the ancestral and modern scenarios paint a similar picture in terms of the survival issues (e.g., avoiding harm and finding sustenance), the modern scenario does not yield the same level of recall advantage that the ancestral scenario does (see also Weinstein, Bugg, & Roediger, 2008).

A number of potential explanations for this discrepancy have been proposed, including an evolutionary account and a consideration of the novelty of the encoding scenario (Nairne & Pandeirada, 2010). Nairne and Pandeirada (2010) have suggested that it is possible that the ancestral grassland scenario is more effective at triggering neural systems, as it has a greater synergy to the environment where our cognitive systems evolved. Thus, is it possible that if our memory systems adapted to help recall information in a hunter-gatherer context, recall would be more effective when considering a grassland context, where gathering food would serve a direct survival promoting function? Other scenarios, such as a modern city, would have lower overlap to our ancestral survival problems and subsequently produce lower levels of recall. This explanation seems unlikely, as other studies have shown evidence for the survival processing effect in contexts that cannot be explained by this evolutionary theory, such as survival in outer space or surviving while stranded at sea. Kostic, McFarlan and Cleary (2012) explored the survival processing effect in both of these contexts and found comparable levels of recall accuracy in both of these conditions when compared to the ancestral grassland scenario. If survival processing is particularly effective in the ancestral scenario because of its proximity to our ancestor's survival pressures, why were comparable levels of recall observed in an outer space scenario? Additionally, Soderstrom and MacCabe (2011) explored the survival processing scenario with either an ancestral threat (animals found in a foreign grassland) or a fictional threat (zombies). The results of this study demonstrated higher recall when the fictional zombies were introduced as a threat in the ancestral scenario as opposed to the evolutionary salient predators. Again, if the ancestral scenario's empirical success was simply the result of an evolutionary salient environment, we would expect to observe lower levels of recall when zombies were employed as a predator. This is not the case, which suggests that this overlapping context alone cannot explain the disparity in recall observed between the modern and ancestral survival scenarios.

Second, Nairne and Pandeirada (2010) suggested the survival processing effect could result from the grassland scenario providing a more novel encoding task than those used as a control (i.e., moving house or pleasantness ratings). This account would explain why other novel scenarios, such as survival in space or fending off a zombie attack, would also generate the survival processing advantage. However, the empirical evidence for this explanation is limited and further research would be required to explore whether the novel nature is partially or solely responsible for the elevated levels of recall. Interestingly, the evidence presented here suggests the survival processing advantage does not only favour scenarios that are evolutionary salient, but can also be transposed to other survival situations.

A further area of research that has challenged the effectiveness of survival processing explored the role of planning, which has been widely studied in its role of guiding human memory (e.g., Klein, 2007). Klein, Robertson and Delton (2010) have proposed that a pivotal role of human memory is to permit the maintenance of information about past events in order for this information to be used to resolve future concerns. To empirically address this question, Klein et al. (2010) conducted an experiment where they compared recall performance between participants who had either encoded items with regards to the likelihood that they had taken the item on a past camping trip (past), how likely the item would be at a campsite if they went on a trip now (atemporal), how likely they would be to take the item on a camping trip they were planning for the future (planning), or how relevant the item was for their survival if they were stranded in a forest (survival). The results of the study demonstrated that significantly more items were recalled when the planning scenario had been employed during the encoding task. However, the survival task yielded the second best performance, showing significantly higher recall than the past condition but statistically comparable levels of recall when compared to the atemporal condition. While this is clear evidence of higher recall performance when the planning scenario had been used, it is important to note that the average recall across all four conditions differed by less than two recalled items. Therefore, while performance was significantly higher, the mean difference was comparatively small (especially given that Nairne et al. (2007) reported improved recall performance of between approximately 2.4 and 6 items, depending on the experiment design and condition employed as a control). An important consideration here is that it is unlikely that processing an item for its survival properties does not actually include an element of planning. For instance, if you consider the word 'string' in a survival context, it is likely that you would rate the item's relevance for survival by considering its possible functions (e.g., building tools, trapping animals or building a shelter). Thus, it is difficult to completely separate the planning and survival processes. In an attempt to tease these processes apart, Klein, Robertson and Delton (2011) devised three encoding scenarios: these were survival with planning, survival without planning and planning without survival. The results of the study revealed no significant difference in memory performance between survival with planning and planning without survival, although both scenarios produced significantly better performance than survival without planning. Klein et al. (2011) suggest this provides evidence that planning is a pivotal component of the survival processing scenario's success. However, other evidence suggests that planning cannot explain the entirety of the survival processing effect, as survival processing has been shown to produce higher recall than hypothetical planning tasks (such as planning a bank heist or burglary) alone (Kang et al., 2008).

The evidence presented here has demonstrated that while there is a wealth of research supporting the survival processing effect, there are still considerable questions regarding the mechanism that generates the effect. What appears to be evident is that survival processing seems to be a relatively robust effect that produces a higher proportion of recall than a number of other well-established encoding tasks, and the observed benefit is also maintained across time in healthy adults. However, all the research considered thus far has explored survival processing in younger adults with intact cognition. Thus, an important question is whether survival processing is still effective in aging populations, and whether it can be used as a tool to help assist in the preservation of memory.

8.3   Survival processing and aging populations

Despite the vast amount of research exploring the parameters of the survival processing effect, there has been comparatively little research investigating whether the effect is still prevalent in older adults. The first study to probe age effects in survival processing was reported by Nouchi (2012). Nouchi (2012) aimed to explore the role of elaboration (i.e., focusing on the meaning of information to be recalled, such as relating the item to a past experience or a logical inference) in the survival processing effect. It has been suggested that older adults show reduced performance elaboration tasks (Burke & Light, 1981; Eysenck, 1974). By this token, if the survival processing effect were solely based upon effective elaboration, then the survival processing advantage would be reduced in older adults. Nouchi (2012) asked 16 younger adults (mean age = 20.19, SD = 1.06) and 16 older adults with intact cognitive function (Mini Mental State Examination score = 28.8, SD = 1.2, mean age = 70.32, SD = 3.31) to rate 18 items with regards to their relevance to their survival in a foreign grassland, and 18 items in a self-referential encoding task (rating items with regards to how easily they bring to mind an important experience from their own life). The results indicated that while the younger adults recalled significantly more items than the older adults, there was a significant survival processing advantage observed within both age groups. Nouchi (2012) concluded that elaboration was not the mechanism driving the survival processing effect. Despite some methodological limitations – for example, there was no attempt to compare performance on a memory task that is known to require elaboration to test for a baseline difference between the groups – this was the first study to demonstrate the survival processing advantage in older adults with intact cognitive function.

Not all of the evidence has supported the presence of the survival processing effect in older adults. Stillman, Coane, Profaci, Howard and Howard (2013) also explored the elaboration hypothesis in older adults. They hypothesised that if survival processing was driven by the elaboration process, it should be reduced or eliminated in older adults, as changes in cognitive ability associated with aging may limit the ability for older adults to make use of an elaborative encoding mechanism. To further test this hypothesis, they also asked one group of younger adults to complete a concurrent task (counting the frequency of high or low toned beeps) around the traditional encoding tasks. This aimed to reduce the attentional resources of the younger adults to a similar level to those of the older adults. The study subsequently had three participant conditions (younger adult full attention, younger adult with divided attention and older adults) and two encoding conditions (each participant either encoding the words using an ancestral survival task or the moving task employed by Nairne et al. (2007)). The results indicated the survival processing advantage was present in the younger adults with both full and divided attention (although overall recall was higher in the full attention condition, as would be expected). More interestingly, however, the older adults' data revealed that significantly more words had been recalled in the moving condition than the survival condition, failing to replicate the survival processing effect in older adults. Surprisingly, this effect was replicated in two further experiments using both a between and within participant design (to ensure the effect was not the result of a misbalance in performance between groups), meaning that Stillman et al. (2013) found no evidence of the survival processing advantage. Yang, Lau and Truong (2014) argued that the control condition (moving scenario) employed by Sillman et al. (2013) was not well matched to the survival processing scenario in terms of valence and arousal and may have subsequently masked potential survival processing effects in older adults. They explored the survival processing effect with conditions that had been controlled in terms of arousal, valence, novelty and familiarity. They compared survival in a foreign grassland, survival on a mountain and a cruise holiday (Experiment 1) and survival on a mountain versus winning the lottery (Experiment 2) and found evidence of the survival processing effect in both young and old adults in both experiments. Interestingly, the retrieval observed in the mountain survival scenario was moderately higher than that observed in the grassland scenario, although this difference did not prove to be statistically significant. This finding could support the hypothesis that the failure to observe the survival processing effect reported by Sillman et al. (2013) was simply the result of a poorly matched control task.

Pandeirada, Pinho and Faria (2014) also explored survival processing effects in older populations, but their study focused on the difference between a group of older adults with normal cognitive function and a group of older adults with lower cognitive function (with a mean Mini Mental State Examination score of 21.88, SD = 1.2 in the lower cognitive function group and 28.47, SD = 1.2 in the normal cognitive function group). All participants were aged between 50 and 70 years of age, with similar age ranges across the groups (M = 62.76, SD = 5.38; and M = 61.59, SD = 6.29, respectively), and were asked to rate 16 nouns with regards to their relevance to survival in the foreign grassland scenario and 16 to their relevance in the moving scenario. The results indicated a significantly lower proportion of recall in the patients with lower cognitive function than observed in the participants with normal cognitive function, which is not surprising. More interestingly, both groups displayed evidence of the survival processing advantage, with significantly more items being recalled when survival processing had been employed than when the items had been rated in the moving scenario. This finding directly conflicts with the findings of Sillman et al. (2013), who demonstrated no benefit of survival processing in older adults when compared to the moving scenario. It also suggests that the failure to demonstrate the survival processing effect in Sillman et al. (2013) was not simply the result of a poorly matched control scenario, as proposed by Yang et al. (2014), as Pandeirada et al. (2014) demonstrated the survival processing advantage when using the moving scenario as a control. As such, further research would be required to understand why the discrepancy outlined in Sillman et al. (2013) was observed.

To the author's knowledge, so far, only four studies have investigated the survival processing effect in older adults. The majority of these studies have shown the effect to be robust and is still effective in older populations and participants with lower cognitive function (Nouchi, 2012; Pandeirada et al., 2014; Yang et al., 2014). However, it is important to note that not all studies have found evidence that supports the benefit of survival processing in this age range (Sillman et al., 2013), so while the evidence in favour of survival processing being effective in older adults is compelling, it is far from conclusive, and further research would be beneficial to further explore the phenomenon.

8.4 Can survival processing be employed to aid the preservation of memory?

This chapter has briefly summarised the evidence put forward exploring the survival processing effect. Since Nairne et al. (2007), there has been an influx of research that has explored the effect and the parameters of this advantage. The majority of this research has shown the survival processing advantage to be a robust phenomenon, although it is important to note that not all of the evidence presented has supported the survival processing effect (e.g., Klein, 2012; Klein et al., 2011; Sillman et al., 2013). The central aim of this chapter was to consider the potential application of the survival processing effect, essentially addressing the question, 'can the survival processing effect be utilised to help preserve memory?' The remainder of this chapter will now consider this question.

It is clear from the research evidence that the survival processing is a particularly effective encoding task (for instance, Bröder et al., 2011; Kang et al., 2008; Nairne et al., 2007) and that the mnemonic advantage generated is maintained across time for a minimum of 48 hours after encoding (Raymaekers et al., 2014). The survival processing effect can also be transposed from lists of words to benefit other types of stimuli such as pictures (Otgaar et al., 2010), the recall of location information (Nairne et al., 2012), and other encoding environments (Kostic et al., 2012). All of this evidence provides a solid foundation that would suggest that survival processing could be used as a memory intervention in people who suffer from lower levels of memory performance. Indeed, this suggestion is further strengthened by the evidence of advantage in older adults (Nouchi, 2012; Yang et al., 2014) and, more importantly, older adults with mild cognitive impairment (Pandeirada et al., 2014).

There are also a number of questions that have been raised regarding the survival processing effect; for instance, it does not appear to function as well when people are considering survival in a modern (albeit foreign) city. This is a potential concern when considering survival processing as an intervention because a modern city is most likely to be the environment in which survival processing would be employed. While this could represent a problem, memory performance in the modern survival scenario has been shown to be more effective than pleasantness ratings (Nairne & Pandeirada, 2010), but not the moving scenario or the survival in the foreign grassland scenario. This suggests that while considering survival in a modern context may provide a boost in memory performance, it would not be to the same extent as that observed in the grassland and this in turn could reduce the effectiveness of an intervention. There have also been a number of studies that have shown the importance of planning in survival processing (Klein, 2012; Klein et al., 2011). While these studies have not always shown survival processing to produce superior recall when compared to a planning condition, they have demonstrated the importance of planning within the survival processing scenario (Klein et al., 2011). Thus, this evidence would promote the need to directly include an element of planning in any scenario used as a potential intervention.

The evidence presented here suggests the potential of survival processing for promoting memory performance. If a task could incorporate the key components of survival processing, such as an element of planning, elaboration and a novel way of processing information, it could be predicted to be a useful 'tool' in the preservation of memory. For instance, if a participant was asked to consider how relevant a group of items on a shopping list were to their survival at that point in time and to consider the implications for their future use/survival, the participant would need to consider each item on the list with regards to their immediate survival-promoting properties, their self-relevance and they would also need to engage in an element of future planning. Based on the research evidence presented here, it would be anticipated that this would be an effective encoding mechanism to allow the individual to successfully recall more items from their shopping list than other encoding paradigms. However, this is currently speculative and while it is clear that survival processing has the potential to effectively contribute to the preservation of memory, further research is required to fully ascertain the extent to which it can be employed in everyday life.

References

Abel, M., & Bäuml, K.T. (2013). Adaptive Memory: The influence of sleep and wake delay on the survival-processing effect. *Journal of Cognitive Psychology, 25,* 917–924.

Bröder, A., Krüger, N., & Schütte, S. (2011). The survival processing memory effect should generalise to source memory, but it doesn't. *Psychology, 2,* 896–901.

Burke, D.M., & Light, L.L. (1981). Memory and aging: The role of retrieval processes. *Psychological Bulletin, 90,* 513–546.

Burns, D.J., Burns, S.A., & Hwang, A.J. (2011). Adaptive memory: Determining the proximate mechanisms responsible for the memorial advantages of survival processing. *Journal of Experimental Psychology: Learning Memory and Cognition, 37,* 206–218.

Craik, F.I., & Lockhart, R.S. (1972). Levels of processing: A framework for memory research. *Journal of Verbal Learning and Verbal Behavior, 11*, 671–684.

Eysenck, M.W. (1974). Age differences in incidental learning. *Developmental Psychology, 10*, 936–941.

Godden, D.R., & Baddeley, A.D. (1975). Context-dependent memory in two natural environments: On land and underwater. *British Journal of psychology, 66*, 325–331.

Howe, M.L., & Otgaar, H. (2013). Proximate mechanisms and the development of adaptive memory. *Current Directions in Psychological Science, 22*, 16–22.

Kang, A.H.K., McDermott, K.B., & Cohen, S.M. (2008). The mnemonic advantage of processing fitness-relevant information. *Memory & Cognition, 36*, 1151–1156.

Klein, S.B. (2007). Phylogeny and evolution: Implications for understanding the nature of a memory system. In H.L. Roediger, Y. Dudai, & S.M. Fitzpatrick (Eds.), *Science of memory: Concepts* (pp. 377–381). Oxford, UK: Oxford University Press.

Klein, S.B. (2012). A role for self-reverential processing in tasks requiring participants to imagine survival on the Savannah. *Journal of Experimental Psychology: Learning, Memory, and Cognition, 38*, 1234–1242.

Klein, S.B., Robertson, T.E., & Delton, A.W. (2010). Facing the future: Memory as an evolved system for planning future acts. *Memory and Cognition, 38*, 13–22.

Klein, S.B., Robertson, T.E., & Delton, A.W. (2011). The future-orientation of memory: Planning as a key component mediating the high levels of recall found with survival processing. *Memory, 19*, 121–139.

Kostic, B., McFarlan, C.C., & Cleary, A. M. (2012). Extensions of the survival advantage in memory: Examining the role of ancestral context and implied social isolation. *Journal of Experimental Psychology: Learning, Memory, and Cognition, 38*, 1091–1098.

Nairne, J. S. (2005). The functionalist agenda in memory research. In A. F. Healy (Ed.), *Experimental psychology and its applications* (pp. 115–126). Washington, DC: American Psychological Association.

Nairne, J.S., & Pandeirada, J.N.S. (2010). Adaptive memory: Ancestral priorities and the mnemonic value of survival processing. *Cognitive Psychology, 61*, 1–22.

Nairne, J.S., Pandeirada, J.N.S., Gregory, K.J., & Van Arsdall, J.E. (2009). Adaptive memory: Fitness relevance and the hunter-gatherer mind. *Psychological Science, 20*, 740–746.

Nairne, J.S., Pandeirada, J.N.S., & Thompson, S.R. (2008). Adaptive memory: The comparative value of survival processing. *Psychological Science, 19*, 176–180.

Nairne, J.S., Thompson, S.R., & Pandeirada, J.N.S. (2007). Adaptive memory: Survival processing enhances retention. *Journal of Experimental Psychology: Learning, Memory, and Cognition, 33*, 263–273.

Nairne, J.S., VanArsdall, J.E., Pandeirada, J.N.S., & Blunt, J.R. (2012). Adaptive memory: Enhanced location memory after survival processing. *Journal of Experimental Psychology: Learning, Memory, and Cognition, 38*, 495–501.

Nouchi, R.U.I. (2012). The effect of aging on the memory enhancement of the survival judgment task. *Japanese Psychological Research, 54*, 210–217.

Nouchi, R., & Kawashima, R. (2012). Effect of the survival judgement task on memory performance in subclinically depressed people. *Frontiers in Psychology, 3*, 114.

Otgaar, H., Smeets, T., Merckelback, H., Jelicic, M., Verschuere, B., Galliot, A., & van Riel, L. (2011). Adaptive memory: Stereotype activation is not enough. *Memory & Cognition, 39*, 1033–1041.

Otgaar, H., Smeets, T., & van Bergen, S. (2010). Picturing survival memories: Enhanced memory after fitness-relevant processing occurs for verbal and visual stimuli. *Memory & Cognition, 38*, 23–28.

Packman, J.L., & Battig, W.P. (1978). Effects of different kinds of semantic processing on memory for words. *Memory & Cognition, 6,* 502–508.

Pandeirada, J.N.S., Pinho, M.S., & Faria, A.L. (2014). The mark of adaptive memory in healthy and cognitively impaired older adults and elderly. *Japanese Psychological Research, 56,* 168–179.

Raymaekers, L.H.C., Otgaar, H., & Smeets, T. (2014). The longevity of adaptive memory: Evidence for the mnemonic advantages of survival processing 24 and 48 hours later. *Memory, 22,* 19–25.

Roediger, H. L., & Karpicke, J.D. (2006). Test-enhanced learning: Taking memory tests improves long term retention. *Psychological Science, 17,* 249–255.

Seamon, J.G., Bohn, J.M., Coddington, I.E., Ebling, M.C., Grund, E.M., Haring, C.T., . . . Siddique, A.H. (2012). Can survival processing enhance story memory? Testing the generalizability of the adaptive memory framework. *Journal of Experimental Psychology: Learning, Memory, and Cognition, 38,* 1045–1056.

Sillman, C.M., Coane, J.H., Profaci, C.P., Howard Jr, J.H., & Howard, D.V. (2013). The effects of healthy aging on the mnemonic benefit of survival processing. *Memory & Cognition, 42,* 175–185.

Soderstrom, N.C., & McCabe, D.P. (2011). Are survival processing memory advantages based on ancestral priorities? *Pyschonomic Bulletin Review, 18,* 564–569.

Symons, C.S., & Johnson, B.T. (1997). The self-reference effect in memory: A meta-analysis. *Psychological Bulletin, 121,* 371–394.

Tulving, E. (2002). Episodic memory: From mind to brain. *Annual Review of Psychology, 53,* 1–25.

Weinstein, Y., Bugg, J.M., & Roediger, H.L. (2008). Can the survival recall advantage be explained by basic memory processes? *Memory & Cognition, 36,* 913–919.

Yang, L., Lau, K.P., & Truong, L. (2014). The survival effect in memory: Does it hold into old age and non-ancestral scenarios? *PloS ONE, 9,* e95792.

9

THE EFFECTS OF AGING AND EXERCISE ON RECOLLECTION AND FAMILIARITY BASED MEMORY PROCESSES

Richard J. Tunney, Harriet A. Allen, Charlotte Bonardi and Holly Blake

9.1 Introduction

In common with many other European countries, the United Kingdom has an aging population. The percentage of people aged 65 or older has increased from 15% in 1985 to 17% in 2010, but is set to increase rapidly to a projected 25% of the population in 2035 (Office for National Statistics, 2012). Over a similar period, the number of centenarians has increased from 2,500 in 1980 to 12,640 in 2010 (Office for National Statistics, 2011). Cognitive decline is a normal part of aging, but memory can be more sensitive to age than other aspects (Cullum et al., 2000). It is well established that as people age, although still able to recognize others as familiar, they are less likely to retrieve details such as their name or why they are familiar (the *butcher-on-the-bus* phenomenon). A general decline in grey matter volume, resulting from lower synaptic densities rather than cell death, is the likely cause of cognitive decline (Hedden & Gabrieli, 2004). In particular, a more rapid decline in hippocampal volume compared to associated areas is likely to result in noticeable effects on declarative or episodic memory compared to familiarity based memory. Research with both humans and animals suggests that this is due to a relative decline in functioning of the hippocampus, and that this structure is responsible for recollection, while familiarity based processes are mediated in adjacent regions such as the rhinal cortex. Selective decline in the ability to retrieve contextual information is one of the more debilitating effects of age on memory, and so it is crucial to find ways of ameliorating this process. Although many studies indicate that even brief exercise interventions can enhance performance on a number of neuro-psychological tests of cognitive function, the precise mechanisms underlying these effects are unclear. One intriguing possibility stems from evidence that physical activity produces synaptogenesis and neurogenesis in the hippocampus – which might ameliorate or reverse the age-related decline in hippocampal function thought to impair the recollection process. In this chapter, we review the evidence for this hypothesis using data from both rodent and human studies.

9.2   Effects of aging on recall, recollection and familiarity based memory

A result frequently found is that older adults have greater impairments in recall or recollection than they do in familiarity or recognition judgements (see also Chapters 3, 4 and 7). This finding has been replicated using multiple methods of measurement. For instance, using the subjective 'remember/know' method (see Chapter 7), Parkin and Walter (1992) observed that older adults made a similar number of correct recognitions of retrieved items labelled as 'know' but fewer 'remember' judgements than younger adults. This reduction of remember judgements was correlated with reduced performance on tests that are thought to measure frontal or executive function.

One issue with using the remember/know methodology in older adults, however, is that some studies have reported that older adults also present impairments in metacognition (Souchay, Isingrini, & Espagnet, 2000). Metacognition refers to the ability of one individual to monitor and control her or his own cognitive ability. If this ability is impaired, it becomes difficult to discriminate whether the overall deficit is due to loss of memory *per se*, or loss of the metacognitive ability to subjectively distinguish between remembered and known events.

Nevertheless, other methods for discriminating between recollection and recognition also show reduction in recollection and maintained familiarity in older adults. Performance in recall tasks is reduced relatively more in older adults than performance in recognition tasks (for a review, see Yonelinas, 2002). Performance also declines on associative memory and source memory tasks (e.g., Naveh-Benjamin, 2000; Yonelinas, 2002).

Deficits in recall with age are usually presumed to be at the level of encoding, rather than at retrieval, and are associated with reduced performance on tests of 'frontal' or executive function (Yonelinas, 2002). Therefore, it is expected that recall performance in older adults can be improved by changes at the encoding stage (see Chapter 8). For example, Park, Smith, Morrell, Puglisi and Dudley (1990) instructed participants to remember pairs of images; older adults were poorer (compared to younger adults) at recalling unrelated pairings, but better when the pictures showed interacting pairs or pairs with related meanings (see also Grady, 2000).

It is not clear, however, whether the loss of recall reflects an absolute impairment or a tendency to fail to engage appropriate encoding, or retrieval, strategies. It has been shown that even when an item is not recognised at test, its presence can facilitate both repetition priming and matching based on meaning; for example, identifying an item as belonging to the same category as one encountered previously (Koutstaal, 2003).

There is a close relationship between context and explicit retrieval such as recall and recollection. For example, Mandler (1980) described the *butcher-on-the-bus* phenomenon to illustrate the independence of familiarity and recollection based memory processes. In the most widely used form, the *butcher-on-the-bus* describes a scenario in which a person's face is recognized as being *familiar*, but the recognition is not accompanied by the *recollection* of contextual details such as the person's name or occupation. Although some theoretical models might discuss these differences as an environmental context effect and the presence or absence of retrieval cues (see Chapter 9), the majority of models interpret the effect in terms of the differing characteristics of recollection and familiarity based memory processes; namely, that recollection encodes context but familiarity does not, or that the difference is one of memory strength and that context information is more easily retrieved for stronger memories such as people we know well, as opposed to acquaintances (see Chapter 3).

In two experiments, Tunney, Mullett, Moross and Gardner (2012) presented participants with pictures of faces and scenes as paired associates. At test, the faces were presented with either the previously associated scene or a different scene. In Experiment 1, participants made more remember responses to old face-scene pairs than to new face-scene pairings. Process estimates revealed that context increased the sensitivity of recollection based memory and also the sensitivity of familiarity based memory (but see Gruppuso, Lindsay, & Masson, 2007, for a slightly different result). In Experiment 2, participants were first asked to make recognition judgements for the test faces and to report their subjective experience of remembering. They were then asked to identify the context that each test face was associated with from a choice of four (i.e., 4-alternative forced-choice, 4-AFC). So if the hypothesis that recollection encodes context and familiarity does not is correct, then recognition responses for items reported as 'remembered' should be followed by more accurate context decisions for items reported as 'known'. The data confirmed this prediction, although the accuracy of context judgements associated with 'knowing' was reliably above chance, albeit lower than for 'remembered' items. This pattern of results is more consistent with a single process explanation, postulating that knowing and remembering correspond to different degrees of memory strength on a single continuum, rather than a traditional dual-process account (see Chapter 3).

Yovel and Paller (2004) report event-related potential (ERP) data consistent with a single process interpretation. The magnitude and duration of ERPs attributed to recollection were greater than those attributed to familiarity, but their forms were not qualitatively distinct, suggesting that they were produced by the same neural systems. Eldridge, Engel, Zeineh, Bookheimer and Knowlton (2005) used functional magnetic resonance imaging (*f*MRI) to probe neural activation following remember and know judgements. They observed the expected behavioural patterns in which participants could recall more contextual information for items reported as remembered than known. The *f*MRI analyses revealed that remember responses were accompanied by greater activation in the right medial temporal lobe, and in particular the subiculum subregion of the hippocampus. The CA1 and CA23DG regions also showed differential activity: CA1 activity was greater for remembered items compared to forgotten items, while the Ca23DG region showed deactivation for known items. Both remember and know responses were accompanied by increased activation in the left perirhinal cortex.

Age-related changes in the subjective experience of remembering and recollection of contextual details are paralleled by age-related changes in the underlying neural circuits. The entorhinal cortex and CA1 regions show little or no age-related decrease in volume. By contrast, those areas associated with recollection by Eldridge et al. (2005), such as the subiculum and dentate gyrus, show age-related decreases in volume (see also Hedden & Gabrieli, 2004; Small, Tsai, DeLaPaz, Mayeux, & Stern, 2002).

Although the precise relationship between recollection and familiarity based memory as single or independent processes remains a matter of empirical investigation, it is clear that there are subtly different effects of aging on tests of memory. Indeed, a selective decline in the ability to retrieve contextual information is one of the more debilitating effects of age on memory, and raises the possibility that aging might also affect the sensitivity of older adults to context as a retrieval cue. Indeed, a wide range of studies have found that memory for context appears to be particularly sensitive to aging (e.g., Spencer & Raz, 1995; Zacks, Hasher, & Li, 2000). Moreover, research with both animals and humans suggests that a decline in functioning of the hippocampus might mediate this age-related memory decline.

9.3   Recollection and familiarity in humans and rodents

Although work on animals interprets the distinction between recollection and familiarity in a slightly different theoretical context (e.g., Tam, Bonardi, & Robinson, 2015), parallels with theorising on human memory still emerge. Exposure to a target item *directly* activates its memory trace, reflecting the development of *familiarity* – meeting the butcher makes him familiar. In contrast, *recollection* occurs because the target becomes associated with its contextual details, and these associations result in *associative* activation of a memory trace – seeing the butcher, the participant recalls his name via the association between them.

However, direct memory trace activation fades with time, but familiarity does not (Tunney, 2003; 2010). Thus, some argue that familiarity also results from associative activation via *permanent* associations that form among the item's *constituent elements* during exposure. Recollection, in contrast, is solely the result of associative activation of contextual information by the target item. The environment where the target is encountered also becomes associated with its contextual information, so it is easier to recall the butcher's name in his shop than on the bus[1], and will also associatively activate the target itself – another way associative activation contributes to the familiarity effect. In short, associative activation contributes to both familiarity and recollection, but the former can also benefit from direct activation of the item's memory trace. This is reminiscent of Tunney et al.'s (2012) findings that context judgements, which rely on associative memory, were related to both remembering and knowing, although more strongly with the former.

Most familiarity tests in animals employ the Spontaneous Object Recognition (SOR) task, exploiting rodents' predisposition to explore novel objects. Animals preexposed to item A will subsequently explore A less than a novel item B – and this is taken as evidence of A's familiarity. The task becomes harder as the test is delayed because direct activation of A's memory trace dissipates; at longer delays, only indirect activation of A's memory trace by the experimental environment makes A familiar.

SOR performance is typically unaffected by hippocampal damage (e.g., Barker & Warburton, 2011; Good, Barnes, Staal, McGregor, & Honey, 2007) unless the delay before test is extended (Clark, Zola, & Squire, 2000), or the lesions large (Broadbent, Squire, & Clark, 2004). Nonetheless, we have argued that familiarity relies on (a) *direct* activation of the memory trace by the target, and *associative* activation of the memory trace by (b) constituent elements of the target, and (c) the preexposure environment. Thus, variants of the SOR task have been proposed as cleaner measures of these underlying processes. For example, in a Relative Recency (RR) task, preexposure to A and *then* B results in a preference for the less recent A. As, here, processes (b) and (c) are equated, test performance must stem from differences in (a) – direct activation of the memory trace is stronger for the more recent item. Hippocampal damage impairs RR performance (e.g., Barker & Warburton, 2011; DeVito & Eichenbaum, 2010).

In contrast, in the Object-in-Context (OIC) task, animals are exposed to four items; at test, two items exchange position, and command more exploration. Here, processes (a) and (b) are equated, so performance must stem from differences in associative activation (c). If local environmental features associate with each item during exposure, memory traces of stationary items will be more effectively activated. Hippocampal damage tends not to impair OIC performance (e.g., Barker & Warburton, 2011; DeVito & Eichenbaum, 2010; Good et al., 2007).

In summary, results from animal studies do not fully support the human findings. Evidence for hippocampal involvement is strongest for RR performance, which we argue relies on direct memory trace activation, and is thus more closely allied to familiarity. In contrast, OIC performance – a purer measure of associative memory (i.e., recollection) – is less reliably affected by hippocampal damage. However, OIC tasks are not a perfect operational parallel of recollection tasks in humans, as in OIC, the environment must activate the target item, whereas in human tasks, the opposite is the case. Moreover, in the majority of these lesion studies, the entire hippocampus was damaged, so if different parts of this structure play different roles, as was suggested above, important differences might be obscured. The handful of studies that selectively lesion different subfields suggest that CA1 might be especially critical for RR performance (Hoge & Kesner, 2007; Hunsaker, Rosenberg, & Kesner, 2008). But these findings do clearly demonstrate that the hippocampus plays a key role in performance on these memory tasks.

Studies of brain activation in humans have supported the findings of the behavioural work reviewed above. Older adults typically have different patterns of brain activation to younger adults, with brain activation in older adults being more related to familiarity based memory than for younger adults. For example, in an early study on the topic, Daselaar, Fleck, Dobbins, Madden and Cabeza (2006) indexed familiarity and recollection with confidence judgements, where low confidence correct judgements were considered to be based on familiarity and high confidence correct judgements were considered to be based on recall. They found that older adults showed more familiarity based judgements in a memory test than younger adults. Older adults also showed more brain activity on retrieval in the rhinal cortex than younger adults. Older adults also showed more functional connectivity between prefrontal cortex and rhinal cortex, whereas younger adults showed connectivity between the prefrontal cortex and the hippocampus (see also Cabeza et al., 2004).

Older adults show brain activity more consistent with familiarity based recognition and memory than with recall based memory. This would suggest that older adults would be worse at memory for associations, which appears to be the case. However, when associations are made, it also appears that older adults may use the same mechanisms as younger adults, up to a point. Miller et al. (2008) asked older and younger adults to learn face-name pairs in an associative learning task. For those older adults who performed well overall, brain activation patterns in the hippocampus and associated regions were similar to those shown by younger adults. This suggests that older adults who maintain recall based memory activate similar processes to young adults. For those older adults who did not, overall, perform well, activation in successful memory trials was associated with a different network of brain activations (including additional frontal activations).

The results above are consistent with older adults using different strategies than younger adults for many memory tasks. The reasons for this shift in strategy are unclear. One cause may be deterioration in the brain areas that underlie recollection, i.e., the hippocampus. There is a growing consensus that the hippocampus suffers atrophy or deterioration even in healthy aging (Pereira et al., 2014; Raz, 2000), although this is by no means a universal finding (Sullivan, Marsh, Mathalon, Lim, & Pfefferbaum, 1995; Sullivan & Pfefferbaum, 2014). One reason for the discrepant findings could be that hippocampus volume decline is not linear. Hippocampus volume has been shown to decline non-linearly, with a sharp decline starting somewhere between 60 and 80 but with relative preservation until that point (Pfefferbaum et al., 2013). This is in contrast to a relatively steady decline of more frontal areas.

Age-related declines in memory formation have also been attributed to failures of encoding. In a classic study, Grady et al. (1995) showed that older adults, compared to younger adults, failed to activate the hippocampus at encoding, but presented greater activity in the prefrontal cortex at retrieval, thus confirming that an age-related strategic shift may have been occurring. These findings, however, do not resolve the question of whether these age-related performance changes are due to a decline in the overall recall capacity, or to a genuine strategic shift from one strategy to another. That is, although the ability to use recall effectively is maintained, since encoding is more difficult, such ability is generally not used. Similarly, the ability to use recall memory might be maintained but losses in other executive functions might mean that the necessary processes tend not to be evoked.

9.4   Exercise and cognitive function

The importance of exercise for physical and cognitive function is well-known. Promoting physical activity is important across the lifespan, but in older adults, there are significant implications for the maintenance of functional ability, independence and health-related quality of life. Physical activity is thought to be protective against cognitive decline, and can generate improvements in cognitive function. Indeed, protective effects of physical activity against cognitive impairment have been observed regardless of the way in which activity levels are measured (e.g., Acti-Graph accelerometer, self-report or doubly labelled water; Steinberg et al., 2014).

The link between exercise and cognitive function has been demonstrated in a range of populations, including healthy middle-aged adults, healthy older adults and adults with mild cognitive impairments (a risk factor for the development of Alzheimer's disease). The precise nature of this link is still under investigation, although the beneficial effects of physical exercise on memory and executive function seem to be well-established (Colcombe & Kramer, 2003), and studies have investigated domain-specific effects of physical activity on cognition, and detected improvements in a wide range of cognitive functions, including executive function, memory, processing speed, and attention (Buchman, Boyle, Leurgans, Barnes, & Bennett, 2011; Lautenschlager et al., 2008; Scarmeas et al., 2011; Wang et al., 2014; Wang, Luo, Barnes, Sano, & Yaffe, 2013).

Overall, this area of research is rapidly progressing, and exercise in older adults has been shown to improve task-related cognitive function, brain connectivity and regional brain volume (Voss, Nagamatsu, Liu-Ambrose, & Kramer, 2011). Our understanding of the biological mechanisms involved in the impact of exercise on cognitive function suggests that there are likely to be changes at the molecular, vascular, synaptic and neural levels (Lista & Sorrentino, 2010). These changes in brain health and cognitive function have been demonstrated in a wealth of human studies. For example, in middle-aged, cognitively healthy adults considered to be at risk of developing Alzheimer's disease (AD) because of the presence of bio-markers, greater cardiorespiratory fitness was associated with increased grey matter volumes in several brain regions that are implicated in AD (including the hippocampus, amygdala, precuneus, supramarginal gyrus and rostral middle frontal gyrus), and those with greater fitness had better cognitive performance on tests of verbal learning and memory, speed and flexibility, and visuo-spatial ability (Boots et al., 2014). Researchers have been adopting new techniques to investigate neural adaptability and efficiency during cognitive processing. Using multiscale entropy analysis (MSE) of electronencephalography (EEG), a recent study indicated that physically active older adults have better accuracy on both visuo-spatial attention and working memory conditions relative to their sedentary counterparts (Wang et al., 2014). Finally, current research on brain microstructural integrity has found that in old, community dwelling adults, being exercise active may help to preserve brain micro-structural integrity in memory-related networks (Tian et al., 2014).

Some light on the mechanisms that might underlie these changes comes from work on animals. Although numerous changes in brain chemistry and cellular degeneration are likely to result from advancing age, brain-derived neurotrophic factor (BDNF) is present in relatively high concentrations in the hippocampus and cortex, and shows significant age-related changes in concentration (Erickson, Miller, & Roecklein, 2012; Voss et al., 2013). Lower concentrations of serum BDNF are found in older adults and Alzheimer's patients with more severe cognitive impairment (Laske et al., 2011), and BDNF is found in reduced concentrations in the hippocampi of older animals (Silhol, Bonnichon, Rage, & Tapia-Arancibia, 2005). Lower concentrations of BDNF in cerebrospinal fluid are predictive of memory performance and hippocampal volume (Li et al., 2009). Given the key relationship between lower BDNF hippocampal volume and memory performance, it seems reasonable to assume that any intervention that increases BDNF might be beneficial, and indeed exercise (in the form of voluntary wheel-running) has consistently been shown to increase hippocampal BDNF levels in rats (e.g., Ploughman et al., 2005; Vaynman, Ying, & Gomez-Pinilla, 2004), and has also been shown to improve performance on tests of spatial learning and memory (e.g., Van Praag, Shubert, Zhao, & Gage, 2005; Vaynman et al., 2004). Likewise, regular aerobic exercise increases BDNF in humans, and can result in improved memory performance (Erickson et al., 2012). In rodents, this type of exercise has also been related to increased cell proliferation in the hippocampus, and selective increases in cerebral blood volume, which is related to reduction in age-related decline in cell proliferation, and neurogenesis in the dentate gyrus (e.g., Kronenberg et al., 2006; Pereira et al., 2014; Van Praag et al., 2005). In older humans, levels of aerobic fitness correlate with hippocampal volume (Erickson et al., 2012), and one intriguing study shows that increased levels of BDNF associated with exercise improved rodent's performance in the Morris water maze (Vaynman et al., 2004), suggesting that the effect of the exercise improved context-dependent learning.

Perhaps the most optimistic set of results are those that show that exercise has a prophylactic effect on age-related memory decline. In humans, exercise is firmly associated with a decreased risk of mild cognitive impairment (Geda et al., 2010). In rodents, increased levels of insulin-like growth factor 1 (IGF-1) that result from treadmill exercise (although not voluntary wheel-running)[2] reduce the effects of neurotoxins on the hippocampus (Ploughman et al., 2005).

Despite rapid advances in knowledge, at present, the precise causal mechanisms for each of the neurocognitive changes that follow exercise have not yet been fully determined. Furthermore, the best form of physical exercise to generate improvement remains unclear. Previous research has strongly advocated a link between aerobic fitness and cognitive function; one possible mechanism for this might be the increased energy expenditure resulting from moderately vigorous physical activity, since community based research with cognitive intact elderly women has shown that those with the highest exercise frequency and who expended the most kilocalories were least likely to experience cognitive decline (Yaffe, Barnes, Nevitt, Lui, & Covinsky, 2001). Randomised trials have also shown that high-intensity, progressive resistance training can improve global cognitive function, and executive functioning over 18 months (Singh et al., 2014). Benefits of combination training (e.g., combining aerobic and resistance exercise) have also been shown (Snowden et al., 2011).

Nevertheless, it is still unclear which approaches to exercise are most important for targeting particular cognitive functions. Research studies often include interventions that are based on aerobic exercise and/or resistance training at various intensities. Exercise in older age is a complex issue, since poor physical function and chronic disease can preclude the participation of many older adults in structured or higher-intensity exercise training programmes. While increased aerobic fitness and resistance training have been associated with the prevention or delay of cognitive decline, this is not always feasible in some settings since the majority of older adults are sedentary and many have difficulty with engagement in, and maintenance of, exercise programmes. For healthcare practitioners, promotion of age-appropriate, easily accessible and socially engaging physical activities is therefore paramount.

As such, there is an emerging body of research that focuses on the relationship between non-exercise, lifestyle physical activities (e.g., 'mind-body' approaches; or encouraging active lifestyles) and whether they have similarly beneficial effects on neurocognitive outcomes. For example, moderate-intensity low-impact forms of physical activity that are based on cognitive enrichment 'mind-body' strategies (such as Tai Chi) have shown potential for improvement in measures of executive function, language, learning and/or memory (Blake & Hawley, 2012; Miller & Taylor-Piliae, 2014). Studies of objectively measured habitual physical activity behaviour have shown that a greater amount, duration and frequency of daily walking activity may be associated with larger hippocampal volume in older women (Varma, Chuang, Harris, Tan, & Carlson, 2014).

While it is generally agreed that physical exercise maintains or improves cognitive function, further work is required to fully understand both the causal mechanisms for observed cognitive changes and the type, dose and intensity of exercise that is required to generate clinically significant changes in cognition. Although further research will reveal the underlying mechanisms by which exercise can ameliorate cognitive decline in the elderly, the research is sufficiently clear to convey the message that exercise can have significant benefits on the mental life of the elderly.

Notes

1 Context may also allow selective retrieval of associative information that was acquired in its presence. Thus, the association between the butcher's appearance and his name may be more readily retrieved in the context in which it was acquired (in the butcher's shop) than in others (such as on the bus).

2 The effects of voluntary and forced wheel running on these measures often differs, and this may in part be attributed to the added stress associated with the latter procedure (Carruthers, Zampieri, & Damiano, 2014).

References

Barker, G. R. I., & Warburton, E. C. (2011). When is the hippocampus involved in recognition memory? *The Journal of Neuroscience, 31*(29), 10721–10731.

Blake, H., & Hawley, H. (2012). The effects of Tai Chi exercise on physical and psychological health of older people. *Current Aging Science: Special Issue: Physical Activity, Exercise and Ageing, 5*, 19–27.

Boots, E. A., Schultz, S. A., Oh, J. M., Larson, J., Edwards, D., Cook, D., . . . Carlsson, C. M. (2014). Cardiorespiratory fitness is associated with brain structure, cognition, and mood in a middle-aged cohort at risk for Alzheimer's disease. *Brain Imaging and Behavior, 10*(4), 1–11.

Broadbent, N. J., Squire, L. R., & Clark, R. E. (2004). Spatial memory, recognition memory, and the hippocampus. *Proceedings of the National Academy of Sciences of the United States of America, 101*(40), 14515–14520.

Buchman, A. S., Boyle, P. A., Leurgans, S. E., Barnes, L. L., & Bennett, D. A. (2011). Cognitive function is associated with the development of mobility impairments in community-dwelling elders. *The American Journal of Geriatric Psychiatry, 19*(6), 571–580.

Cabeza, R., Daselaar, S. M., Dolcos, F., Prince, S. E., Budde, M., & Nyberg, L. (2004). Task-independent and task-specific age effects on brain activity during working memory, visual attention and episodic retrieval. *Cerebral Cortex, 14*(4), 364–375.

Carruthers, K., Zampieri, C., & Damiano, D. (2014). Relating motor and cognitive interventions in animals and humans. *Translational Neuroscience, 5*(4), 227–238.

Clark, R. E., Zola, S. M., & Squire, L. R. (2000). Impaired recognition memory in rats after damage to the hippocampus. *The Journal of Neuroscience, 20*(23), 8853–8860.

Colcombe, S., & Kramer, A. F. (2003). Fitness effects on the cognitive function of older adults a meta-analytic study. *Psychological Science, 14*(2), 125–130.

Cullum, S., Huppert, F. A., McGee, M., Dening, T., Ahmed, A., Paykel, E. S., & Brayne, C. (2000). Decline across different domains of cognitive function in normal ageing: Results of a longitudinal population-based study using CAMCOG. *International Journal of Geriatric Psychiatry, 15*(9), 853–862.

Daselaar, S. M., Fleck, M. S., Dobbins, I. G., Madden, D. J., & Cabeza, R. (2006). Effects of healthy aging on hippocampal and rhinal memory functions: An event-related fMRI study. *Cerebral Cortex, 16*(12), 1771–1782.

DeVito, L. M., & Eichenbaum, H. (2010). Distinct contributions of the hippocampus and medial prefrontal cortex to the "what–where–when" components of episodic-like memory in mice. *Behavioural Brain Research, 215*(2), 318–325.

Eldridge, L.L., Engel, S. A., Zeineh, M. M., Bookheimer, S.Y., & Knowlton, B. J. (2005). A dissociation of encoding and retreival processes in the human hippocampus. *Journal of Neuroscience, 25*, 3280–3286.

Erickson, K. I., Miller, D. L., & Roecklein, K. A. (2012). The Aging Hippocampus Interactions between Exercise, Depression, and BDNF. *The Neuroscientist, 18*(1), 82–97.

Geda, Y. E., Roberts, R. O., Knopman, D. S., Christianson, T. J. H., Pankratz, S. V., Ivnik, R. J., . . . Rocca, W. A. (2010). Physical exercise, aging, and mild cognitive impairment: A population-based study. *Archives of Neurology, 67*(1), 80–86.

Good, M. A., Barnes, P., Staal, V., McGregor, A., & Honey, R. C. (2007). Context—but not familiarity—dependent forms of object recognition are impaired following excitotoxic hippocampal lesions in rats. *Behavioral Neuroscience, 121*(1), 218.

Grady, C. L. (2000). Functional brain imaging and age-related changes in cognition. *Biological Psychology, 54*(1), 259–281.

Grady, C. L., McIntosh, A. R., Horwitz, B., Maisog, J. M., Ungerleider, L. G., Mentis, M. J., ... Haxby, J.V. (1995). Age-related reductions in human recognition memory due to impaired encoding. *Science, 269*(5221), 218–221.

Gruppuso, V., Lindsay, D. S., & Masson, M.E.J. (2007). I'd know that face anywhere. *Psychonomic Bulletin & Review, 14*, 1085–1089.

Hedden, T., & Gabrieli, J. D. E. (2004). Insights into the ageing mind: A view from cognitive neuroscience. *Nature Reviews Neuroscience, 5*(2), 87–96.

Hoge, J., & Kesner, R. P. (2007). Role of CA3 and CA1 subregions of the dorsal hippocampus on temporal processing of objects. *Neurobiology of Learning and Memory, 88*(2), 225–231.

Hunsaker, M. R., Rosenberg, J. S., & Kesner, R. P. (2008). The role of the dentate gyrus, CA3a, b, and CA3c for detecting spatial and environmental novelty. *Hippocampus, 18*(10), 1064–1073.

Koutstaal, W. (2003). Older adults encode – but do not always use – Perceptual details intentional versus unintentional effects of detail on memory judgments. *Psychological Science, 14*(2), 189–193.

Kronenberg, G., Bick-Sander, A., Bunk, E., Wolf, C., Ehninger, D., & Kempermann, G. (2006). Physical exercise prevents age-related decline in precursor cell activity in the mouse dentate gyrus. *Neurobiology of Aging, 27*(10), 1505–1513.

Laske, C., Stellos, K., Hoffmann, N., Stransky, E., Straten, G., Eschweiler, G. W., & Leyhe, T. (2011). Higher BDNF serum levels predict slower cognitive decline in Alzheimer's disease patients. *The International Journal of Neuropsychopharmacology, 14*(03), 399–404.

Lautenschlager, N. T., Cox, K. L., Flicker, L., Foster, J. K., van Bockxmeer, F. M., Xiao, J., ... Almeida, O. P. (2008). Effect of physical activity on cognitive function in older adults at risk for Alzheimer disease: A randomized trial. *JAMA, 300*(9), 1027–1037.

Li, G., Peskind, E. R., Millard, S. P., Chi, P., Sokal, I., Yu, C-E., ... Montine, T. J. (2009). Cerebrospinal fluid concentration of brain-derived neurotrophic factor and cognitive function in non-demented subjects. *PLoS ONE, 4*(5), e5424.

Lista, I., & Sorrentino, G. (2010). Biological mechanisms of physical activity in preventing cognitive decline. *Cellular and Molecular Neurobiology, 30*(4), 493–503.

Mandler, G. (1980). Recognizing: The judgement of previous occurrence. *Psychological Review, 87*, 252–271.

Miller, S. L., Celone, K., DePeau, K., Diamond, E., Dickerson, B. C., Rentz, D., ... Sperling, R. A. (2008). Age-related memory impairment associated with loss of parietal deactivation but preserved hippocampal activation. *Proceedings of the National Academy of Sciences, 105*(6), 2181–2186.

Miller, S. M., & Taylor-Piliae, R. E. (2014). Effects of Tai Chi on cognitive function in community-dwelling older adults: A review. *Geriatric Nursing, 35*(1), 9–19.

Naveh-Benjamin, M. (2000). Adult age differences in memory performance: Tests of an associative deficit hypothesis. *Journal of Experimental Psychology: Learning, Memory, and Cognition, 26*(5), 1170.

Office for National Statistics. (2011). *Estimates of centenarians in the UK, 2010.* HMSO.

Office for National Statistics. (2012). *Population ageing in the United Kingdom, its constituent countries and the European Union.* HMSO.

Park, D. C., Smith, A. D., Morrell, R. W., Puglisi, J. T., & Dudley, W. N. (1990). Effects of contextual integration on recall of pictures by older adults. *Journal of Gerontology, 45*(2), P52-P57.

Parkin, A. J., & Walter, B. M. (1992). Recollective experience, normal aging, and frontal dysfunction. *Psychology and Aging, 7*, 270–298.

Pereira, J. B., Valls-Pedret, C., Ros, E., Palacios, E., Falcon, C., Bargalo, N., . . . Junque, C. (2014). Regional vulnerability of hippocampal subfields to aging measured by structural and functional diffusion MRI. *Hippocampus, 24*, 403–414.

Pfefferbaum, A., Rohlfing, T., Rosenbloom, M. J., Chu, W., Colrain, I. M., & Sullivan, E. V. (2013). Variation in longitudinal trajectories of regional brain volumes of healthy men and women (ages 10 to 85 years) measured with atlas-based parcellation of MRI. *Neuroimage, 65*, 176–193.

Ploughman, M., Granter-Button, S., Chernenko, G., Tucker, B. A., Mearow, K. M., & Corbett, D. (2005). Endurance exercise regimens induce differential effects on brain-derived neurotrophic factor, synapsin-I and insulin-like growth factor I after focal ischemia. *Neuroscience, 136*(4), 991–1001.

Raz, N. (2000). Aging of the brain and its impact on cognitive performance: Integration of structural and functional findings. In F. I. M. Craik & T.A. Salthouse (Eds.), *The handbook of aging and cognition – II* (pp. 1–90). Mahwah, NJ: LEA.

Scarmeas, N., Luchsinger, J. A., Brickman, A. M., Cosentino, S., Schupf, N., Xin-Tang, M., . . . Stern, Y. (2011). Physical activity and Alzheimer disease course. *The American Journal of Geriatric Psychiatry, 19*(5), 471–481.

Silhol, M., Bonnichon, V., Rage, F., & Tapia-Arancibia, L. (2005). Age-related changes in brain-derived neurotrophic factor and tyrosine kinase receptor isoforms in the hippocampus and hypothalamus in male rats. *Neuroscience, 132*(3), 613–624.

Singh, M. A. F., Gates, N., Saigal, N., Wilson, G. C., Meiklejohn, J., Brodaty, H., . . . Suo, C. (2014). The Study of Mental and Resistance Training (SMART) Study – resistance training and/or cognitive training in mild cognitive impairment: A randomized, double-blind, double-sham controlled trial. *Journal of the American Medical Directors Association, 15*(12), 873–880.

Small, S. A., Tsai, W. Y., DeLaPaz, R., Mayeux, R., & Stern, Y. (2002). Imaging hippocampal function across the human life span: Is memory decline normal or not? *Annals of Neurology, 51*(3), 290–295.

Snowden, M., Steinman, L., Mochan, K., Grodstein, F., Prohaska, T. R., Thurman, D. J., . . . Zweiback, D. J. (2011). Effect of exercise on cognitive performance in community-dwelling older adults: Review of intervention trials and recommendations for public health practice and research. *Journal of the American Geriatrics Society, 59*(4), 704–716.

Souchay, C., Isingrini, M., & Espagnet, L. (2000). Aging, episodic memory feeling-of-knowing, and frontal functioning. *Neuropsychology, 14*(2), 299.

Spencer, W. D., & Raz, N. (1995). Differential effects of aging on memory for content and context: A meta analysis. *Psychology & Aging, 10*, 527–539.

Steinberg, S. I., Sammel, M. D., Harel, B. T., Schembri, A., Policastro, C., Bogner, H. R., . . . Arnold, S. (2014). Exercise, sedentary pastimes, and cognitive performance in healthy older adults. *American journal of Alzheimer's disease and other dementias, 30*(3), 290–298. doi:10.1177/1533317514545615

Sullivan, E. V., Marsh, L., Mathalon, D. H., Lim, K. O., & Pfefferbaum, A. (1995). Age-related decline in MRI volumes of temporal lobe gray matter but not hippocampus. *Neurobiology of Aging, 16*(4), 591–606.

Sullivan, E. V., & Pfefferbaum, A. (2014). Neuroradiological characterization of normal adult ageing. *British Journal of Radiology, 80*, S99–S114.

Tam, S. K. E., Bonardi, C., & Robinson, J. (2015). Relative recency influences object-in-context memory. *Behavioural Brain Research, 281*, 250–257.

Tian, Q., Erickson, K. I., Simonsick, E. M., Aizenstein, H. J., Glynn, N. W., Boudreau, R. M., . . . Harris, T. B. (2014). Physical activity predicts microstructural integrity in memory-related networks in very old adults. *The Journals of Gerontology Series A: Biological Sciences and Medical Sciences, 69*(10), 1284–1290.

Tunney, R. J. (2003). Implicit and explicit knowledge decay at different rates: A dissociation between priming and recogntion in artificial grammar learning. *Experimental Psychology, 50,* 124–130.

Tunney, R. J. (2010). Do changes in the subjective experience of recognition over time suggest independent processes? *British Journal of Mathematical and Statistical Psychology, 63,* 43–62.

Tunney, R. J., Mullett, T. L., Moross, C. J., & Gardner, A. (2012). Does the butcher-on-the-bus phenomenon require a dual-process explanation? A signal detection analysis. *Frontiers in Cognitive Science, 3,* 1–11.

Van Praag, H., Shubert, T., Zhao, C., & Gage, F. H. (2005). Exercise enhances learning and hippocampal neurogenesis in aged mice. *The Journal of Neuroscience, 25*(38), 8680–8685.

Varma, V. R., Chuang, Y. F., Harris, G. C., Tan, E. J., & Carlson, M. C. (2014). Low-intensity daily walking activity is associated with greater hippocampal volume in older adults. *Hippocampus, 25*(5), 605–615. doi:10.1002/hipo.22397

Vaynman, S., Ying, Z., & Gomez-Pinilla, F. (2004). Hippocampal BDNF mediates the efficacy of exercise on synaptic plasticity and cognition. *European Journal of Neuroscience, 20*(10), 2580–2590.

Voss, M. W., Erickson, K. I., Prakash, R. S., Chaddock, L., Kim, J. S., Alves, H., . . . Mailey, E. L. (2013). Neurobiological markers of exercise-related brain plasticity in older adults. *Brain, Behavior, and Immunity, 28,* 90–99.

Voss, M. W., Nagamatsu, L. S., Liu-Ambrose, T., & Kramer, A. F. (2011). Exercise, brain, and cognition across the life span. *Journal of Applied Physiology, 111*(5), 1505–1513.

Wang, C-H., Tsai, C-L., Tseng, P., Yang, A. C., Lo, M-T., Peng, C-K., . . . Liang, W-K. (2014). The association of physical activity to neural adaptability during visuo-spatial processing in healthy elderly adults: A multiscale entropy analysis. *Brain and Cognition, 92,* 73–83.

Wang, S., Luo, X., Barnes, D., Sano, M., & Yaffe, K. (2013). Physical activity and risk of cognitive impairment among oldest-old women. *The American Journal of Geriatric Psychiatry, 22*(11), 1149–1157.

Yaffe, K., Barnes, D., Nevitt, M., Lui, L-Y., & Covinsky, K. (2001). A prospective study of physical activity and cognitive decline in elderly women: Women who walk. *Archives of Internal Medicine, 161*(14), 1703–1708.

Yonelinas, A. P. (2002). The nature of recollection and familiarity: A review of 30 years of research. *Journal of Memory and Language, 46,* 441–517.

Yovel, G., & Paller, K. A. (2004). The neural basis of the butcher-on-the-bus phenomenon: When a face seems familiar but is not remembered. *Neuroimage, 21,* 789–800.

Zacks, R. T., Hasher, L., & Li, K. Z. (2000). Human memory. In F. I. M. Craik & T. A. Salthouse (Eds.), *The Handbook of Aging and Cognition* (pp. 293–358). Mahwah, NJ: Erlbaum Associates.

10

MEMORY TRAINING FOR OLDER ADULTS

A review with recommendations for clinicians

Robin L. West and Carla M. Strickland-Hughes

10.1 Introduction

Cognitive training programs for older adults span a very wide range of research, from case studies with people with dementia to extensive individual practice of specific information processing skills, and from comprehensive group training programs for healthy seniors to broad approaches that increase cognitive engagement. A primary target of these cognitive interventions is memory improvement. Improved memory is a key aim for several reasons. Foremost, as an integral process involved in everyday experience, memory capacity may affect older individuals' ability to live independently (Fisher, 2012; Montegjo, Montenegro, Fernández, & Maestú, 2012; Stine-Morrow & Basak, 2011). Older adults themselves recognize the importance of memory, and have fears concerning memory loss (Dark-Freudeman, West, & Viverito, 2006). In part, these fears are realistic because cross-sectional and longitudinal studies report age-related declines in working memory, learning of new associations (see Chapter 3), and encoding of new long-term memories (Mather, 2010; McDaniel, Einstein, & Jacoby, 2008). Thus, memory is emphasized in training because it is essential, valued, and at risk for decline.

Our purpose in this chapter is to first review the literature on memory training, focusing on healthy seniors with no significant memory impairment. We consider memory training outcomes as well as maintenance of training gains over time. Although it is very clear that physical activity has cognitive benefits, Chapter 9 in this volume provides an overview of that work. Here we focus on mental activities and behavioral programs that foster memory success. Following the literature overview, we make practical, research-based recommendations for scholars and clinicians with respect to those methods and approaches to training that are most likely to yield success.

10.2   Memory training outcomes

10.2.1   *Improved memory performance*

A long-accepted body of work establishes that older adults benefit from memory training when comparing memory performance following an intervention to performance on a pretest (Berry, Hastings, West, Lee, & Cavanaugh, 2010; Gross et al., 2012). At the same time, well-documented practice effects suggest that memory improvement will occur simply from retaking memory assessments (Ball et al., 2002; Hertzog, Kramer, Wilson, & Lindenberger, 2009). Therefore, this review focuses only on those intervention studies that compare pretest to posttest gains of trainees to control groups, who do not participate in the memory training. Control groups may be inactive/wait-list participants (completing assessments and nothing else) or active groups (participating in different activities, matched to the intervention by frequency, duration, social engagement, etc.) designed to act as placebo controls (Boot, Simons, Stothart, & Stutts, 2013; Zehnder, Martin, Altgassen, & Clare, 2009).

Meta-analyses have confirmed greater pretest to posttest gains for older memory trainees compared to active and inactive control groups. Training gains are greater for interventions that incorporate pretraining, such as relaxation or attention exercises, and gains are greater for group training compared to programs training adults individually (Verhaeghen, Marcoen, & Goossens, 1992). These earlier findings were replicated more recently, showing significant differences in pretest to posttest memory gains for trainees versus controls (estimated effect size was 0.31 standard deviations). Training gains were not affected by age of participant or specific trained strategy, although programs employing multiple strategies were more effective than those focused on training a single strategy (Gross et al., 2012).

Three experimental studies will be highlighted here as examples of memory intervention: the Advanced Cognitive Training for Independent and Vital Elderly (ACTIVE) trial, the Everyday Memory Clinic (EMC), and a theater arts program. The first study, ACTIVE, represents a randomized clinical trial conducted with older adults ($N = 2,832$) in six different U.S. cities. Posttest outcomes were assessed immediately as well as repeatedly over time. Participants were assigned to training in memory, reasoning, or speed of processing, with each training program serving as an active control for the other types of training. The focus of the memory training was verbal episodic memory (e.g., list or story recall); trainees completed 10 weekly sessions of 60–75 minutes of learning (first five sessions) and then practicing (last five sessions) strategies, such as association and imagery. More than a quarter of memory trainees demonstrated reliable improvement in verbal episodic memory immediately following the intervention, and memory trainees outperformed the other groups on the verbal memory tasks one and two years later (Ball et al., 2002). Plus, verbatim recall of stories was higher for memory versus non-memory trainees immediately following training (Sisco, Marsiske, Gross, & Rebok, 2013).

The second study of note is EMC, a five-week multifactorial intervention emphasizing self-regulatory beliefs. Adults over 50 learned and practiced five strategies in weekly group meetings with extensive homework (West, Bagwell, & Dark-Freudeman, 2008) or learned the same strategies in a self-help format (Hastings & West, 2009). EMC was designed to enhance memory self-efficacy (confidence in one's memory ability) through enactive mastery (e.g., trainees focused on easier strategies and tasks first), vicarious experience (e.g., strategy modeling), verbal persuasion (e.g., positively framed feedback), and anxiety reduction (e.g., emphasis on self-set goals rather than high memory scores). Compared to controls, EMC trainees demonstrated improved name and story recall, and more effective strategy usage after training and at follow-up testing (West et al., 2008). Active trainees, classified by attendance, homework completion, and in-class participation, demonstrated greater training gains than both inactive trainees and the control group (Bagwell & West, 2008).

Several innovative approaches have evaluated the potential memory benefits of cognitive activity from programs emphasizing naturalistic, community-based engagement (Carlson et al., 2008; 2009; Stine-Morrow et al., 2014; see also Chapter 11). For example, Noice and colleagues designed a program to improve memory in the context of a four-week theater arts program. Episodic memory gains for older adult trainees exceeded that of inactive control groups and groups trained in other arts programs (i.e., visual arts or singing; Noice & Noice, 2006; 2009; 2013; Noice, Noice, & Staines, 2004). The program demonstrated gains in samples of independently living older adults (Noice et al., 2004), residents of long-term care facilities (Noice & Noice, 2006), and less affluent adults residing in subsidized, low-income, retirement homes (Noice & Noice, 2009). Importantly, Noice and Noice (2013) replicated memory gains even when training was administered by others (a retirement home activity director and a professional acting teacher), demonstrating widespread feasibility of this particular approach to intervention.

10.2.2 Transfer and practical impact

10.2.2.1 Broader gains from training

Researchers agree that intervention programs lead to memory gains on the trained tasks. But training can be far more beneficial if it also leads to broader cognitive change, active lifestyles, and improved well-being (Hertzog et al., 2009; Stine-Morrow & Basak, 2011). One criticism of cognitive interventions for older adults is the "generalist assumption" that researchers may assume far-reaching benefits from specific training, when the observed benefits are actually rather narrow (McDaniel & Bugg, 2012; Salthouse, 2006). It is true that there is little evidence that memory training on one set of tasks generalizes to other kinds of memory or to real-world memory gains, but there is some evidence of transfer across fairly similar memory tasks (Berry et al., 2010). Further, there are indications that training does transfer to other important outcomes.

For example, older adults, compared to younger adults, are less likely to spontaneously or successfully employ mnemonics (McDaniel & Bugg, 2012). Yet,

ACTIVE study trainees improved in their use of memory strategies immediately following training, and these gains were maintained over five years and were closely related to memory ability (Gross & Rebok, 2011). Additionally, participation in the ACTIVE trial predicted improved activities of daily living after five years, although these effects were not evident immediately following training (Rebok et al., 2014; Willis et al., 2006). With increased evidence of plasticity, even in late life, engaged lifestyles and participation in cognitive interventions may promote neurogenesis (Park & Bischof, 2013). Indeed, increased neural activation during cognitive tasks was found in a subsample of participants from the Experience Corps study, a community-based program in which older adults volunteered in literacy projects in elementary schools (Carlson et al., 2009). Other memory training programs have demonstrated reductions in depression and loneliness (Cohen-Mansfield et al., 2014), and depression is a known risk-factor for dementia (Ownby, Crocco, Acevedo, Vineeth, & Loewenstein, 2006; Pomara et al., 2012). In addition, self-evaluative change is an important non-trained outcome for cognitive interventions.

10.2.2.2   Change in self-evaluative beliefs

In the broad sense, self-evaluative beliefs relate positively to quality of life (Montegjo et al., 2012), relate negatively to depression (Floyd & Scogin, 1997), and predict mortality in late life (Wiest, Schüz, & Wurm, 2013). More specifically, memory beliefs correlate positively with memory performance (Beaudoin & Desrichard, 2011; Crumley, Stetler, & Horhota, 2014; Valentijn et al., 2006). Theoretically, positive self-evaluative beliefs should foster greater engagement in cognitively stimulating activities (Bandura, 1997), which would certainly have important practical consequences, given the association between cognitive activity and performance (Hertzog et al., 2009).

Some time ago, a meta-analysis by Floyd and Scogin (1997) revealed a small but significant effect ($d = .19$) of memory training on subjective memory; that is, assessments of own memory functioning. Further, gains in subjective memory seemed to be enhanced by pretraining and interventions focused on changing attitudes. Across subsequent literature, training sometimes led to improved memory self-ratings without changing performance on most trained tasks, or evidence showed improved performance without change in beliefs (cf. Rapp, Brenes, & Marsh, 2002; Valentijn et al., 2005; Woolverton, Scogin, Shackelford, Black, & Duke, 2001). Three recent studies illustrate a strong relationship between self-evaluation and training.

The EMC intervention yielded significant changes in memory self-efficacy (MSE) and control beliefs for memory (believing that improvement can derive from one's own efforts). In contrast, the wait-list control group demonstrated modest *declines* in beliefs (West et al., 2008). MSE was a significant predictor of episodic memory performance at follow-up, and change in MSE was a direct predictor of training gains (West & Hastings, 2011). The ACTIVE study also assessed beliefs. Five years following the ACTIVE intervention, the memory trainees were less likely than other groups to report significant declines in the *chance* control scale (i.e., believing that your performance outcomes are driven by chance; Wolinsky et al., 2009). Finally, Cohen-Mansfield and colleagues (2014) compared three different interventions offered to older adults with subjective memory complaints: health promotion classes, ACTIVE memory training, and a participation/book club on strategies. All groups showed improved performance, but only the memory group improved in reported memory complaints.

10.2.2.3   Transfer to cognitive outcomes

Results from cognitive training via computer or video games show promise for cognitive transfer (Kueider, Parisi, Gross, & Rebok, 2012). Video games elicit extended practice of core processes such as working memory, visual attention, and speed of processing (Hertzog et al., 2009). In a meta-analysis comparing pretest to posttest gains for older adults trained with video games to performance of control groups, video-game training enhanced memory, reaction time, attention, and general cognition (Toril, Reales, & Ballesteros, 2014). Core skill training (e.g., working memory practice) has led to transfer to other types of cognition, but rarely to other types of memory (Morrison & Chein, 2011).

Transfer or generalization of training has been explored for decades, with limited transfer shown to occur between different types of memory tasks. However, it is likely that more positive evidence for transfer would be observed if interventions were designed with conceptual models for transfer in mind (Barnett & Ceci, 2002; Hering, Rendell, Rose, Schnitzspahn, & Kliegel, 2014; Zelinski, 2009). Clearly, when looking at transfer of training, it is valuable to consider benefits that extend beyond memory per se to broader abilities, beliefs, and neurological and mental health outcomes. In turn, these outcomes may promote a positively engaged, healthy cognitive lifestyle and potential maintenance of gains.

10.2.3   Long-term maintenance

Memory interventions with older people demonstrate promise for maximizing memory and promoting positive self-evaluative beliefs. Although evidence on long-term maintenance is lacking, follow-ups have been conducted at one month (West et al., 2008), one year (Ball et al., 2002), two years (Bottiroli, Cavallini, & Vecchi, 2008), and three years (Scogin & Bienas, 1988; Stigsdotter-Neely & Bäckman, 1993) after initial training, with mixed results. The majority of intervention studies examine gains cross-sectionally and do not offer extensive evaluation of outcomes over time, particularly more than one year later (Gross et al., 2012). Consequently, little is known about long-term maintenance of benefits from memory training.

The ACTIVE trial was the first memory program to assess long-term outcomes, up to 10 years after training (Rebok et al., 2014). A subset of memory trainees completed four booster sessions (follow-up training intended to promote maintenance of gains) about one year after initial training. Analyses of these long-term data showed that memory trainees demonstrated improved memory, relative to active controls, up to five years following the study (Willis et al., 2006). Interestingly, this gain was unaffected by participation in booster sessions (Rebok et al., 2013), and no memory training or booster effects were significant 10 years following the program (Rebok et al., 2014).

Hertzog and colleagues (2009) have proposed that cognitive interventions are unlikely to function like vaccines, protecting against decline and potentially requiring periodic boosters, but rather like a physical activity intervention, wherein continuing exercise is necessary for maintenance of performance gains. While the data on ACTIVE maintenance is hopeful, that evidence cannot confirm Hertzog's proposition regarding the benefits of training. Cognitive interventions may indeed yield meaningful long-term benefits to the extent they improve related outcomes, such as enhanced self-evaluative beliefs, neurogenesis, or elevated cognitive engagement in everyday life, but this awaits further longitudinal research.

10.3   Recommended approaches to training

As a practical matter, there are countless ways that memory training can be done. Six decades of research on training for older adults, however, indicates that particular approaches are likely to be most effective. The two most important questions are *what* and *how* to train. The following recommendations derive from a "best practices" review of training (West, 2010), as well as discussions at a recent cognitive training workshop (American Institute for Research, 2014).

10.3.1   Metamemory

Metamemory represents a person's knowledge about memory, including knowledge about how memory works and knowledge about one's own memory skill (Hertzog & Hultsch, 2000). In working with older adults, it is extremely useful to present knowledge about how memory works, and, in particular, explanations about the aging process and memory (Troyer, 2001). Older adults have many memory fears (Dark-Freudeman et al., 2006; Hertzog et al., 2009), and just providing information about normal age-related declines may relieve stress in older adults who may worry excessively about dementia, or ruminate over each memory failure (Hess, Auman, Colcombe, & Rahhal, 2003; Valentijn et al., 2005; Welch & West, 1995).

Research has also suggested that training in monitoring skills can be beneficial (Dunlosky, Kubat-Silman, & Hertzog, 2003). For example, if a person knows that a name or a password has been sufficiently studied, then he/she can cease strategic encoding effort without problematic consequences. Dunlosky and Hertzog have developed a paradigm for training of monitoring skills (Hertzog & Dunlosky, 2012) and demonstrated its effectiveness in at-home as well as in-laboratory settings (Bailey, Dunlosky, & Hertzog, 2010). Their research suggests that, once trained for a particular memory task, self-monitoring can sometimes be transferred to other memory tasks (Cavallini, Dunlosky, Bottiroli, Hertzog, & Vecchi, 2010). If true, this will be an important approach to use in future training studies.

10.3.2 Self-evaluative beliefs

It is not surprising that there has been considerable interest in self-evaluation in the training literature (West, Welch, & Yassuda, 2000), as age differences in beliefs about one's own memory are a prevalent finding in aging research (Berry et al., 2010), and the relationship between beliefs and performance increases with age (Blanchard-Fields, Horhota, & Mienaltowski, 2008). Attempts to alter memory self-evaluation have been part of memory training research for decades, but, until recently, the research showed modest success, as noted above. Recent evidence from experimental studies demonstrates that self-evaluative beliefs might not only be changed by memory training, but may actually regulate performance benefits from training, through moderation and mediational processes (Miller & Lachman, 1999; Payne et al., 2012; West & Hastings, 2011).

Methodological factors may explain variations across studies. Some researchers have assessed individuals' confidence in their current capacity ("I can recall names"), using measures such as the Metamemory in Adulthood (MIA) capacity subscale (Dixon, Hultsch, & Hertzog, 1988) or the Memory Self-Efficacy Questionnaire-4 (West, Thorn, & Bagwell, 2003). Others have emphasized more general assessments of beliefs ("My memory is not very good"; "My memory is worse than it used to be"). While training gains may encourage people to feel more confident about improvement on specific tasks, training may not change older adults' opinions that their memory has declined from youth or that their memory could still benefit from more training. Thus, questionnaires that tap into more specific capacity or ability ratings are more likely to show change as a function of training than general memory ratings.

Looking only at more specific capacity measures, past research shows that MSE predicts current (Stine-Morrow, Shake, Miles, & Noh, 2006) as well as future performance (Valentijn et al., 2006), and is related to the motivational gains observed when participants are given memory goals or feedback (Strickland-Hughes, West, Smith, & Ebner, under review; West, Ebner, & Hastings, 2013). As noted earlier, MSE predicted memory gains in the EMC study (West & Hastings, 2011). Additionally, trainees with higher initial levels of MSE allocated more time to training and benefited more from an inductive reasoning intervention (Payne et al., 2012).

Considering the collective evidence, self-evaluative beliefs can be viewed as important antecedents and consequences of cognitive intervention. Thus, measures of MSE or current capacity (using the MIA) are recommended for investigators interested in assessing memory self-ratings. Assessments of self-reported memory are also useful for clinicians looking at the impact of clinical programs. In the absence of change in self-rated performance following training, it is likely that trainees will not be sufficiently motivated to continue the considerable effort that maintenance of training gains may require.

10.3.3 Strategies and practice

Most training programs for older adults do not focus on self-monitoring or self-evaluative beliefs. They focus on strategy training, and the strategies that are most often taught are encoding techniques, specifically association, categorical organization, imagery, and methods specific to text or number recall (see Derwinger, Stigsdotter, MacDonald, & Bäckman, 2005; Gross et al., 2012; Meyer & Poon, 2004; West, 1995; West et al., 2008).

One issue often debated is whether training should focus on unfamiliar or familiar strategies. For example, organization is a strategy that older adults generally know (e.g., how to organize a shopping list into meats, beverages, dairy products, etc.). Working on this familiar strategy then focuses trainees on extensive practice, so that they can organize items quickly and effectively. An alternative methodology is to enhance the ability of older adults to use techniques that they rarely use in everyday life. Mental imagery would be an example of that kind of strategy (Verhaeghen & Marcoen, 1996; West, 1995; West et al., 2008). Interestingly, there is some suggestion that the benefits may be similar for learning new strategies and practicing known techniques (Bailey et al., 2010). In a more extensive training program, instructors might want to first emphasize well-known strategies to promote positive motivation in trainees and later move on to less familiar, more complex strategies (West et al., 2008).

It is often assumed that training-related gains occur because trainees are using the newly learned strategies, but this assumption is rarely tested due to the difficulty in implementing think-aloud procedures and in assessing internal cognitive processes directly (West et al., 2000). Most of the data we have on strategy use comes either from objective assessments of clustering or subjective self-reports of strategy use. For example, strategy use in the EMC was assessed using detailed checklists. Although trainees employed more strategies than controls at posttest, detailed analyses revealed that they used the simpler techniques or focused only on the easier components of the more complex methods practiced in training (West et al., 2008). Thus, trainees likely use only some of what they have been taught. However, they probably also benefit from general changes in information processing, such as paying greater attention, and being more motivated to concentrate on to-be-remembered items after training.

Many laboratories are now focused on training specific subcomponents of memory through repeated practice (Borella, Carretti, Riboldi, & de Beni, 2010; Jaeggi, Buschkuehl, Shah, & Jonides, 2014; Karbach & Verhaeghen, 2014; Morrison & Chein, 2011; see also Chapter 4), in tasks such as visual attention or working memory. This is also the approach commonly used in commercial software (see Shipstead, Redick, & Engle, 2012; Zelinksi et al., 2011). It has been clear for decades that older adults show plasticity and perform better on those skills that are explicitly trained (Cohen-Mansfield et al., 2014; Verhaeghen, 2000; West, 1995), and we can confidently say that untrained control groups show significant improvements from repeated practice with memory assessments (Ball et al., 2002; Gross et al., 2012; Hertzog et al., 2009). At the same time, it is not clear that repeated practice of component subskills can provide significant general benefits for memory in the laboratory or in daily life (Buschkuehl et al., 2008; Dahlin, Stigsdotter-Neely, Larsson, Bäckman, & Nyberg, 2008; Harrison et al., 2013). Nevertheless, these programs have built-in motivational mechanisms that are valuable (e.g., providing positively framed feedback, showing that the person's "memory age" is getting younger as they improve, or raising the difficulty level gradually to ensure that the tasks remain challenging over time) because they encourage trainees to continue to engage in effortful cognitive activity (Hertzog et al., 2009). However, the benefits of core skill practice for improving episodic memory remain unclear.

Overall, then, training of strategies (one or many; familiar or novel) and extended practice may be beneficial. Training multiple, rather than single, strategies may be more effective in improving memory performance, but no single strategy seems more effective than others (Gross et al., 2012). Therefore, to increase training impact, we recommend selecting strategies most relevant to the desired outcome and offering instructions in more than one technique. To understand and maximize practical impact, scholars should continue to evaluate how strategies are actually being utilized in everyday life.

10.3.4   Social effects in training

Should training programs for seniors be designed for individuals or for groups? We strongly recommend the group approach. An early meta-analysis of training outcomes (Verhaeghen et al., 1992) demonstrated that group training has a larger effect size than individual training. There are several reasons to encourage a group approach. First, training for individuals tends to focus on single strategies or single core skills. In contrast, group training programs tend to be more comprehensive, offering not only strategy training, but also a focus on attention, beliefs about memory, and/or factual education about the aging process. These additional components, present in a multifactorial training program, seem to represent value-added (Gross et al., 2012).

A second reason that group programs may be more beneficial has to do with their potential social effects (Stine-Morrow, Parisi, Morrow, Greene, & Park, 2007; Stine-Morrow et al., 2014). In groups of seniors, it is likely that trainees will discover that their limitations are not as severe as those of other trainees, and that they are not alone in struggling in particular memory situations. This has the side benefit of making individuals much less anxious, and anything that helps older individuals to be less stressed about memory is beneficial (Hess et al., 2003; Welch & West, 1995). Interestingly, the social factors in training are considered so valuable that many researchers design studies with a social control group (Charness, 2007; Noice, Noice, & Kramer, 2014; Park et al., 2014) or compare groups that receive different forms of training, in order to control for the social elements of training (Ball et al., 2002; Cohen-Mansfield et al., 2014; Stine-Morrow et al., 2014).

Another important point to note is that many older adults are unwilling or uninterested in training as a solo learning exercise. Research shows, for example, that the greatest hindrance for older adult participation in lifelong learning programs is the lack of a "partner" in the class (Ostiguy, Hopp, & MacNeil, 1998). More specifically, drop-out rates are larger for older adults when they are randomly assigned to a self-taught program rather than to group training (Hastings & West,

2009). This preference exists even though self-taught programs often result in substantial benefit to trainees (Andrewes, Kinsella, & Murphy, 1996; Hastings & West, 2009; Stine-Morrow et al., 2014).

Several researchers are using group engagement paradigms for enhanced cognition; that is, offering broad social-cognitive engagement through senior volunteering in schools or school-like cognitive team activities (Hertzog et al., 2009; Park et al., 2014; Rebok, Carlson, & Langbaum, 2007; Stine-Morrow et al., 2007; Stine-Morrow et al., 2014). It is often assumed that the social elements of such activities contribute to the motivation to maintain participation over extended periods of time. It is too early to tell if these engagement-style programs will yield long-term memory benefits for participants, but preliminary reports are promising (cf. Carlson et al., 2008; 2009; Park et al., 2014; Stine-Morrow et al., 2014).

10.3.5   Real-world skills

The majority of training programs to date have focused on laboratory test performance. More recent paradigms using repeated practice have an even narrower focus, working to improve a specific sub-skill (Hertzog et al., 2009; Karbach & Verhaeghen, 2014; Morrison & Chein, 2011). As noted above, attempts to show that these two methodologies provide broad everyday memory benefits have typically failed, although there is evidence that practice in core skills may generalize to reasoning or executive functioning (Borella et al., 2010; Karbach & Verhaeghen, 2014; Morrison & Chein, 2011). Given that transfer of training from one memory task to another is seen only rarely (West & Crook, 1992; Willis et al., 2006), and that the observed transfer is typically what would be characterized as near transfer (to a task similar to the one trained), it would be logical for scientists to focus their training efforts directly on those real-world skills that older adults seek to improve (Stigsdotter-Neely, 2000). For example, teach older adults to remember names, to retain passwords, or to recall procedural knowledge needed for smart phones or computers. In other words, if transfer is not likely to occur, training should focus on the common memory concerns of older adults (American Institute for Research, 2014; Fisher, 2012). In fact, in the absence of a comprehensive training program to offer to clients, clinicians could just recommend that older adults practice repeatedly on those memory skills that they wish to improve. More research-based recommendations about specific ways to maximize the benefits of such practice would be helpful. Along those lines, there has been some interest in developing strategies to aid in prospective memory (Hering et al., 2014; Kliegel, Altgassen, Hering, & Rose, 2011), an important everyday skill (McDaniel & Bugg, 2012). A number of investigators have also suggested that it would be helpful to teach older adults how to make effective use of external aids in their everyday life (Craik et al., 2007; Hering et al., 2014; Kliegel, Martin, McDaniel, Einstein, & Moor, 2007; Shum, Fleming, Gill, Gullo, & Strong, 2011), which would expand training beyond the existing emphasis on promotion of internal memory processing.

10.4   Conclusions

Memory is a valued skill, important for older individuals' quality of life and ability to live independently. Yet, some memory processes are known to decline as a part of normal aging. Therefore, cognitive interventions, and specifically memory training, have been of interest to experimenters and clinicians for over six decades. When evaluating training programs that include control groups while examining pretest to posttest change in memory, several key points emerge.

First, training can effectively enhance episodic memory performance for healthy, older adults. Gains are greater when participants train in groups, and when multiple, rather than single, strategies are trained. Interventions currently focus on determining how to promote the practical impact of training, either through extension of training benefits to non-trained tasks, focusing on component sub-skills of memory processing, or by encouraging real-world engagement in cognition. While interventions typically do not succeed in enhancing non-trained memory tasks, modest research evidence suggests that the benefits of training may transfer to non-cognitive, real-world benefits and may have lasting impact.

Based on the reviewed research, we made several recommendations. One successful approach is a multifactorial group training program that includes multiple strategies and added information on topics such as normal aging, attention, metacognition, relaxation or self-evaluative memory beliefs. However, as practice and testing effects are well-documented, encouraging older adults to intensively practice the skills most important to them may be an effective alternative to elaborate training. Recent research focusing on self-monitoring, self-efficacy, and community-based engagement suggests that these approaches also have great potential. In short, there is compelling evidence that memory training will improve memory performance, at least in the short run, and growing evidence that its impact may be considerably broader.

References

American Institute for Research. (2014, November). *Cognitive Training Workshop.* Washington, DC.

Andrewes, D.G., Kinsella, G., & Murphy, M. (1996). Using a memory handbook to improve everyday memory in community-dwelling older adults with memory complaints. *Experimental Aging Research, 22*(3), 305–322. doi:10.1080/03610739608254013

Bagwell, D.K., & West, R.L. (2008). Assessing compliance: Active versus inactive trainees in a memory intervention. *Clinical Interventions in Aging, 3*(2), 371–382. doi:10.2147/CIA.S1413

Bailey, H., Dunlosky, J., & Hertzog, C. (2010). Metacognitive training at home: Does it improve older adults' learning? *Gerontology, 56*(4), 414–420. doi:10.1159/000266030

Ball, K., Berch, D.B., Helmers, K.F., Jobe, J.B., Leveck, M.D., Marsiske, M., . . . Willis, S.L. (2002). Effects of cognitive training interventions with older adults: A randomized controlled trial. *Journal of the American Medical Association, 288*(18), 2271–2281. doi:10.1001/jama.288.18.2271

Ball, K., Edwards, J.D., & Ross, L.A. (2007). The impact of speed of processing training on cognitive and everyday functions. *The Journals of Gerontology, Series B: Psychological Sciences and Social Sciences, 62*(Special Issue 1), 19–31. doi:10.1093/geronb/62.special_issue_1.19

Bandura, A. (1997). *Self-efficacy: The exercise of control.* New York: W.H. Freeman.

Barnett, S.M., & Ceci, S.J. (2002). When and where do we apply what we learn? A taxonomy for far transfer. *Psychological Bulletin, 128*(4), 612–637. doi:10.1037/0033-2909.128.4.612

Beaudoin, M., & Desrichard, O. (2011). Are memory self-efficacy and memory performance related? A meta-analysis. *Psychological Bulletin, 137*(2), 211–241. doi:10.1037/a0022106

Berry, J., Hastings, E., West, R., Lee, C., & Cavanaugh, J.C. (2010). Memory aging: Deficits, beliefs, and interventions. In J.C. Cavanaugh, C.K. Cavanaugh, J. Berry, & R. West (Eds.), *Aging in America, vol. 1. Psychological aspects of aging* (pp. 255–299). Santa Barbara, CA: Praeger Press.

Blanchard-Fields, F., Horhota, M., & Mienaltowski, A. (2008). Social context and cognition. In S. Hofer & D. Alwin (Eds.), *Handbook on cognitive aging: Interdisciplinary perspectives* (pp. 614–628). Thousand Oaks, CA: Sage Publications. doi:10.4135/9781412976589

Boot, W.R., Simons, D.J., Stothart, C., & Stutts, C. (2013). The pervasive problem with placebos in psychology: Why active control groups are not sufficient to rule out placebo effects. *Perspectives on Psychological Science, 8*(4), 445–454. doi:10.1177/1745691613491271

Borella, E., Carretti, B., Riboldi, F., & de Beni, R. (2010). Working memory training in older adults: Evidence of transfer and maintenance effects. *Psychology and Aging, 25*(4), 767–778. doi:10.1037/a0020683

Bottiroli, S., Cavallini, E., & Vecchi, T. (2008). Long-term effects of memory training in the elderly: A longitudinal study. *Archives of Gerontology and Geriatrics, 47*(2), 277–289. doi:10.1016/j.archger.2007/08.101

Buschkuehl, M., Jaeggi, S.M., Hutchison, S., Perrig-Chiello, P., Däpp, C., Müller, M., . . . Perrig, W.J. (2008). Impact of working memory training on memory performance in old-old adults. *Psychology and Aging, 23*(4), 743–753. doi:10.1037/a0014342

Carlson, M.C., Erickson, K.I., Kramer, A.F., Voss, M.W., Bolea, N., Mielke, M., . . . Fried, L.P. (2009). Evidence for neurocognitive plasticity in at-risk older adults: The Experience Corps program. *The Journals of Gerontology, Series A: Biological Sciences and Medical Sciences, 64*(12), 1275–1282. doi:10.1093/Gerona/glp117

Carlson, M.C., Saczynski, J.S., Rebok, G.W., Seeman, T., Glass, T.A., McGill, S., . . . Fried, L.P. (2008). Exploring the effects of an "everyday" activity program on executive function and memory in older adults: Experience Corps. *The Gerontologist, 48*(6), 793–801. doi:10.1093/geront/48.6.793

Cavallini, E., Dunlosky, J., Bottiroli, S., Hertzog, C., & Vecchi, T. (2010). Promoting transfer in memory training for older adults. *Aging, Clinical, and Experimental Research, 22*(4), 314–323. doi:10.3275/6704

Charness, N. (Ed.). (2007). Cognitive interventions and aging [Special issue]. *The Journals of Gerontology, Series B: Psychological Sciences and Social Sciences, 62*(Special Issue 1).

Cohen-Mansfield, J., Cohen, R., Buettner, L., Eyal, N., Jakobovits, H., Rebok, G., . . . Sternberg, S. (2014). Interventions for older persons reporting memory difficulties: A randomized controlled pilot study. *International Journal of Geriatric Psychiatry, 30*(5), 478–486. doi:10.1002/gps.4164

Craik, F.I.M., Winocur, G., Palmer, H., Binns, M.A., Edwards, M., Bridges, K., . . . Stuss, D.T. (2007). Cognitive rehabilitation in the elderly: Effects on memory. *Journal of the International Neuropsychological Society, 13*(1), 132–142. doi:10.1017/S1355617707070166

Crumley, J.J., Stetler, C.A., & Horhota, M. (2014). Examining the relationship between subjective and objective memory performance in older adults: A meta-analysis. *Psychology and Aging, 29*(2), 250–263. doi:10.1037/a0035908

Dahlin, E., Stigsdotter-Neely, A., Larsson, A., Bäckman, L., & Nyberg, L. (2008). Transfer of learning after updating training mediated by the striatum. *Science, 320*(5882), 1510–1512. doi:10.1126/science.1155466

Dark-Freudeman, A., West, R.L., & Viverito, K. (2006). Future selves and aging: Older adults' fears about memory. *Educational Gerontology, 32*(2), 85–109. doi:10.1080/03601270500388125

Derwinger, A., Stigsdotter-Neely, A., MacDonald, S., & Bäckman, L. (2005). Forgetting numbers in old age: Strategy and learning speed matter. *Gerontology, 51*(4), 277–284. doi:10.1159/000085124

Dixon, R.A., Hultsch, D.F., & Hertzog, C. (1988). The Metamemory in Adulthood (MIA) questionnaire. *Psychopharmacology Bulletin, 24*(4), 671–688.

Dunlosky, J., Kubat-Silman, A., & Hertzog, C. (2003). Training metacognitive skills improves older adults' self-paced associative learning. *Psychology and Aging, 18*(4), 340–345. doi:10.1037/0882-7974.18.2.340

Fisher, R. (Ed.). (2012). Target article and commentaries. *Journal of Applied Research in Memory and Cognition, 1*(1). doi:10.1016/j.jarmac.2012.01.001

Floyd, M., & Scogin, F. (1997). Effects of memory training on the subjective memory functioning and mental health of older adults: A meta-analysis. *Psychology and Aging, 12*(1), 150–161. doi:10.1037/0882-7974.12.1.150

Gross, A.L., Parisi, J.M., Spira, A.P., Kueider, A. M., Ko, J.Y., Saczynski, J.S., . . . Rebok, G.W. (2012). Memory training interventions for older adults: A meta-analysis. *Aging and Mental Health, 16*(6), 722–734. doi:10.1080/13607863.2012.667783

Gross, A.L., & Rebok, G.W. (2011). Memory training and strategy use in older adults: Results from the ACTIVE study. *Psychology and Aging, 26*(3), 503–517. doi:10.1037/a0022687

Harrison, T.L., Shipstead, Z., Hicks, K.L., Hambrick, D.Z., Redick, T. S., & Engle, R.W. (2013). Working memory training may increase working memory capacity but not fluid intelligence. *Psychological Science, 24*(12), 2409–2419. doi:10.1177/0956797613492984

Hastings, E.C., & West, R.L. (2009). The relative success of a self-help and a group-based memory training program for older adults. *Psychology and Aging, 24*(3), 586–594. doi:10.1037/a0016951

Hering, A., Rendell, P.G., Rose, N.S., Schnitzspahn, K.M., & Kliegel, M. (2014). Prospective memory training in older adults and its relevance for successful aging. *Psychological Research, 78*(6), 892–904.

Hertzog, C., & Dunlosky, J. (2012). Metacognitive approaches can promote transfer of training: Comment on McDaniel and Bugg. *Journal of Applied Research in Memory and Cognition, 1*(1). doi:10.1016/j.jarmac.2012.01.003

Hertzog, C., & Hultsch, D.F. (2000). Metacognition in adulthood and old age. In F.I.M. Craik & T.A. Salthouse (Eds.), *The handbook of aging and cognition* (2nd edition, pp. 417–466). Mahwah, NJ: Erlbaum.

Hertzog, C., Kramer, A.F., Wilson, R.S., & Lindenberger, U. (2009). Enrichment effects on adult cognitive development: Can the functional capacity of older adults be preserved and enhanced? *Psychological Science in the Public Interest, 9*(1), 1–65. doi:10.1111/j.1539-6053.2009.01034.x

Hess, T.M., Auman, C., Colcombe, S.J., & Rahhal, T.A. (2003). The impact of stereotype threat on age differences in memory performance. *Journal of Gerontology: Psychological Sciences, 58B*(1), 3–11. doi:10.1093/geronb/58.1.P3

Hill, R.D., Campbell, B.W., Foxley, D., & Lindsay, S. (1997). Effectiveness of the number-consonant mnemonic for retention of numeric material in community-dwelling older adults. *Experimental Aging Research, 23*(3). 275–286. doi:10.1080/03610739708254284

Jaeggi, S.M., Buschkuehl, M., Shah, P., & Jonides, J. (2014). The role of individual differences in cognition training and transfer. *Memory and Cognition, 42*(3), 464–480. doi:10.3758/s13421-013-0364-z

Karbach, J., & Verhaeghen, P. (2014). Making working memory work: A meta-analysis of executive-control and working memory training in older adults. *Psychological Science, 25*(11), 2027–2037. doi:10.1177/0956797614548725

Kliegel, M., Altgassen, M., Hering, A., & Rose, N. (2011). A process-model based approach to prospective memory impairment in Parkinson's disease. *Neuropsychologia, 49*, 2166–2177. doi:10.1016/j.neuropsychologia.2011.01.024

Kliegel, M., Martin, M., McDaniel, M.A., Einstein, G.L., & Moor, C. (2007). Realizing complex delayed intentions in young and old adults: The role of planning aids. *Memory and Cognition, 35*(7), 1735–1746. doi:10.3758/bf03193506

Kueider, A. M., Parisi, J.M., Gross, A.L., & Rebok, G.W. (2012). Computerized cognitive training with older adults: A systematic review. *PLoS ONE, 7*(7), e40588. doi:10.1371/journal.pone.0040588

Mather, M. (2010). Aging and cognition. *Wiley Interdisciplinary Reviews: Cognitive Science, 1*(3), 346–362.

McDaniel, M.A., & Bugg, J. (2012). Memory training interventions: What has been forgotten? *Journal of Applied Research in Memory and Cognition, 1*(1). doi:10.1016/j.jarmac.2012.11.002

McDaniel, M.A., Einstein, G.O., & Jacoby, L.L. (2008). New considerations in aging and memory: The glass may be half full. In F.I.M Craik & T. Salthouse (Eds.), *The handbook of aging and cognition* (3rd edition, pp. 251–301). New York, NY: Psychology Press.

Meyer, B.J.F., & Poon, L.W. (2004). Effects of structure strategy training and signaling on recall of text. In R.B. Ruddell & N.J. Unrau (Eds.), *Theoretical models and processes of reading* (5th edition, pp. 810–851). Neward, DE: International Reading Association.

Miller, L.M.S., & Lachman, M.E. (1999). The sense of control and cognitive aging: Toward a model of mediational processes. In T.M. Hess & F. Blanchard-Fields (Eds.), *Social cognition and aging* (pp. 17–41). San Diego: Academic Press.

Montegjo, P., Montenegro, M., Fernández, M.A., & Maestú, F. (2012). Memory complaints in the elderly: Quality of life and daily living activities. A population based study. *Archives of Gerontology and Geriatrics, 54*, 298–304. doi:10.1016/j.archger.2011.05.021

Morrison, A., & Chein, J.M. (2011). Does working memory training work? The promise and challenges of enhancing cognition by training working memory. *Psychonomic Bulletin and Review, 18*(1), 46–60. doi:10.3758/s13423-010-0034-0

Noice, H., & Noice, T. (2006). A theatrical intervention to improve cognition in intact residents of long term care facilities. *Clinical Gerontologist, 29*(3), 59–76. doi:10.1300/J018v29n03_05

Noice, H., & Noice, T. (2009). An arts intervention for older adults living in subsidized retirement homes. *Aging, Neuropsychology, and Cognition: A Journal on Normal and Dysfunctional Development, 16*(1), 56–79. doi:10.1080/13825580802233400

Noice, H., & Noice, T. (2013). Extending the reach of an evidence-based theatrical intervention. *Experimental Aging Research, 39*(4), 398–418. doi:10.1080/0361073X.2013.808116

Noice, T., Noice, H., & Kramer, A. (2014). Participatory arts for older adults: A review of benefits and challenges. *The Gerontologist, 54*(5), 741–753. doi:10.1093/geront/gnt138

Noice, H., Noice, T., & Staines, G. (2004). A short-term intervention to enhance cognitive and affective functioning in older adults. *Journal of Aging and Health, 16*(4), 562–585. doi:10.1177/0898264304265819

Ostiguy, L., Hopp, R., & MacNeil, R. (1998). Participation in lifelong learning programs by older adults. *Ageing International, 24*(2–3), 10–32. doi:10.1007/s12126-998-1002-0

Ownby, R.L., Crocco, E., Acevedo, A., Vineeth, J., & Loewenstein, D. (2006). Depression and risk for Alzheimer disease: Systematic review, meta-analysis, and metaregression analysis. *Archives of General Psychiatry, 63*(5), 530–538. doi:10.1001/archpsyc.63.5.530

Park, D. C., & Bischof, G.N. (2013). The aging mind: Neuroplasticity in response to cognitive training. *Dialogues in Clinical Neuroscience, 15*(1), 109–119.

Park, D. C., Lodi-Smith, J., Drew, L., Haber, S., Hebrank, A., Bischof, G.N., & Aamodt, W. (2014). The impact of sustained engagement on cognitive function in older adults: The Synapse Project. *Psychological Science, 25*(1), 103–112. doi:10.1177/0956797613499592

Payne, B.R., Jackson, J.J., Hill, P.L., Gao, X., Roberts, B.W., & Stine-Morrow, E.A.L. (2012). Memory self-efficacy predicts responsiveness to inductive reasoning training in older adults. *The Journals of Gerontology, Series B: Psychological Sciences and Social Sciences, 67*(1), 27–35. doi:10.1093/geronb/gbr073

Pomara, N., Bruno, D., Sarreal, A.S., Hernando, R.T., Nierenberg, J., Petkova, E., . . . Blennow, K. (2012). Lower CSF amyloid beta peptides and higher F2-isoprostanes in cognitively intact elderly individuals with major depressive disorder. *American Journal of Psychiatry, 169*(5), 523–530.

Rapp, S., Brenes, G., & Marsh, A.P. (2002). Memory enhancement training for older adults with mild cognitive impairment: A preliminary study. *Aging and Mental Health, 6*(1), 5–11. doi:10.1080/13607860120101077

Rebok, G.W., Ball, K., Guey, L.T., Jones, R.N., Kim, H-Y., King, J.W., . . . Willis, S.L. (2014). Ten-year effects of the Advanced Cognitive Training for Independent and Vital Elderly cognitive training trail on cognition and everyday functioning in older adults. *Journal of the American Geriatrics Society, 62*(1), 16–24. doi:10.1111/jgs.12607

Rebok, G.W., Carlson, M.C., & Langbaum, J.B.S. (2007). Training and maintaining memory abilities in healthy older adults: Traditional and novel approaches. *The Journals of Gerontology, Series B: Psychological and Social Sciences, 62* (Special Issue), 53–61. doi:10.1093/geronb/62.special_issue_1.53

Rebok, G.W., Langbaum, J.B.S., Jones, R.N., Gross, A.L., Parisi, J.M., Spira, A.P., . . . Brandt, J. (2013). Memory training in the ACTIVE study: How much is needed and who benefits? *Journal of Aging and Health, 25*(8 Suppl), 21S–42S. doi:10.1177/0898264312461937

Salthouse, T.A. (2006). Mental exercise and mental aging: Evaluating the validity of the "use it or lose it" hypothesis. *Perspectives on Psychological Science, 1*(1), 68–87. doi:10.1111/j.1745-6916.2006.00005.x

Scogin, F., & Bienias, J.L. (1988). A three-year follow-up of older adult participants in a memory-skills training program. *Psychology and Aging, 3*(4), 334–337. doi:10.1037/0882-7974.3.4.334

Shipstead, Z., Redick, T.S., & Engle, R.W. (2012). Is working memory training effective? *Psychological Bulletin, 138*(4), 628–654. doi:10.1037/a0027473

Shum, D., Fleming, J., Gill, H., Gullo, M., & Strong, J. (2011). A randomized controlled trial of prospective memory rehabilitation in adults with traumatic brain injury. *Journal of Rehabilitation Medicine, 43*, 216–233. doi:10.2340/16501977-0647

Sisco, S., Marsiske, M., Gross, A.L., & Rebok, G.W. (2013). The influence of cognitive training on older adults' recall for short stories. *Journal of Aging and Health, 25*(8S), 230S–248S. doi:10.1177/0898264313501386

Stigsdotter-Neely, A. (2000). Multifactorial memory training in normal aging: In search of memory improvement beyond the ordinary. In R.D. Hill, L. Bäckman, & A. Stigsdotter-Neely (Eds). *Cognitive rehabilitation in old age* (pp. 63–80). New York: Oxford University Press.

Stigsdotter-Neely, A., & Bäckman, L. (1993). Long-term maintenance of gains from memory training in older adults: Two 3-year follow-up studies. *Journal of Gerontology: Psychological Sciences, 48*(5), 232–237. doi:10.1093/geronj/45.8.P233

Stine-Morrow, E.A.L., & Basak, C. (2011). Cognitive interventions. In K.W. Schaie & S.L. Willis (Eds.), *Handbook of the psychology of aging* (7th edition, pp. 153–170). New York: Elsevier.

Stine-Morrow, E.A.L., Parisi, J.M., Morrow, D.G., Greene, J., & Park, D. C. (2007). An engagement model of cognitive optimization through adulthood. *The Journals of Gerontology, Series B: Psychological and Social Sciences, 62* (Special Issue), 62–69. doi:10.1093/geronb/62.special_issue_1.62

Stine-Morrow, E.A.L., Payne, B.R., Hill, P., Jackson, J., Roberts, B., Kramer, A., . . . Parisi, J.M. (2014). Training versus engagement as paths to cognitive optimization with aging. *Psychology and Aging, 29*(4), 891–906.

Stine-Morrow, E.A.L., Shake, M.C., Miles, J.R., & Noh, S.R. (2006). Adult age differences in the effects of goals on self-regulated sentence processing. *Psychology and Aging, 21*(4), 790–803. doi:10.1037/0882-7974.21.4.790

Strickland-Hughes, C.M., West, R.L., Smith, K.A., & Ebner, N.C. (under review). False feedback and beliefs influence name recall in younger and older adults. *Cognition.*

Toril, P., Reales, J.M., & Ballesteros, S. (2014). Video game training enhances cognition of older adults: A meta-analytic study. *Psychology and Aging, 29*(3), 706–716. doi:10.1037/a0037507

Troyer, A.K. (2001). Improving memory knowledge, satisfaction, and functioning via an education and intervention program for older adults. *Aging, Neuropsychology, and Cognition: A Journal on Normal and Dysfunctional Development, 8*(4), 256–268. doi:10.1076/anec.8.4.256.5642

Valentijn, S.A.M., Hill, R.D., Van Hooren, S.A.H., Bosma, H., Van Boxtel, M.P.J., Jolles, J., & Ponds, R.W.H.M. (2006). Memory self-efficacy predicts memory performance: Results from a 6-year follow-up study. *Psychology and Aging, 21*, 165–172. doi:10.1037/0882-7974.21.2.165

Valentijn, S.A.M., van Hooren, S.A.H., Bosma, H., Touw, D.M., Jolles, J., van Boxtel, M.P.J., & Ponds, R.W.H.M. (2005). The effect of two types of memory training on subjective and objective memory performance in healthy individuals aged 55 years and older: A randomized controlled trial. *Patient Education and Counseling, 57*(1), 106–114. doi:10.1016/j.pec.2005.05.002

Verhaeghen, P. (2000). The interplay of growth and decline: Theoretical and empirical aspects of plasticity of intellectual and memory performance in normal old age. In R.D. Hill, L. Bäckman, & A. Stigsdotter-Neely (Eds.), *Cognitive rehabilitation in old age* (pp. 3–22). New York: Oxford University Press.

Verhaeghen, P., & Marcoen, A. (1996). On the mechanisms of plasticity in young and older adults after instruction in the method of loci: Evidence for an amplification model. *Psychology and Aging, 11*(1), 164–178. doi:10.1037/0882-7974.11.1.164

Verhaeghen, P., Marcoen, A., & Goossens, L. (1992). Improving memory performance in the aged through mnemonic training: A meta-analytic study. *Psychology and Aging, 7*(2), 242–251. doi:10.1037/0882-7974.7.2.242

Welch, D. C., & West, R. L. (1995). Self-efficacy and mastery: Its application to issues of environmental control, cognition, and aging. *Developmental Review, 15*(2), 150–171.

West, R.L. (1995). Compensatory strategies for age-associated memory impairment (AAMI). In A. D. Baddeley, B.A. Wilson, & F.N. Watts (Eds.), *Handbook of memory disorders* (pp. 481–500). London: John Wiley.

West, R.L. (2010, June 10). Memory training for healthy seniors. [Webinar for MindAlert Series]. *American Society on Aging.* Retrieved from http://www.screencast.com/users/Am_Soc_on_Aging/folders/MindAlert/media/7502324a-4736-4f7b-87b5-07f3a356f3f4

West, R.L., Bagwell, D.K., & Dark-Freudeman, A. (2008). Self-efficacy and memory aging: The impact of a memory intervention based on self-efficacy. *Aging, Neuropsychology, and Cognition, 15*(3), 302–329. doi:10.1080/13825580701440510

West, R.L., & Crook, T.H. (1992). Video training of imagery for mature adults. *Applied Cognitive Psychology, 6*(4), 307–320. doi:10.1002/acp.2350060404

West, R.L., Ebner, N.C., & Hastings, E.C. (2013). Linking goals and aging: Experimental and life-span approaches. In E. Locke & G. Latham (Eds.), *New developments in goal setting and task performance* (pp. 439–459). New York: Psychology Press.

West, R.L., & Hastings, E.C. (2011). Self-regulation and recall: Growth curve modeling of intervention outcomes for older adults. *Psychology and Aging, 26*(4). 803–812. doi:10.1037/a0023784

West, R.L., Thorn, R.M., & Bagwell, D.K. (2003). Memory performance and beliefs as a function of goal setting and aging. *Psychology and Aging, 18*(1), 111–125. doi:10.1037/0882-7874.18.1.111

West, R.L., Welch, D. C., & Yassuda, M.S. (2000). Innovative approaches to memory training for older adults. In R.D. Hill, L. Bäckman, & A.S. Neely (Eds.), *Cognitive rehabilitation in old age* (pp. 81–105). Oxford, UK: Oxford University Press.

Wiest, M., Schüz, B., & Wurm, S. (2013). Life satisfaction and feeling in control: Indicators of successful aging predict mortality in old age. *Journal of Health Psychology 18*(9), 1199–1208. doi:10.1177/1359105312459099

Willis, S.L., Tennstedt, S.L., Marsiske, M., Ball, K., Elias, J., Koepke, K.M., . . . Wright, E. (2006). Long-term effects of cognitive training on everyday functional outcomes in older adults. *Journal of the American Medical Association, 296*(23), 2805–2814. doi:10.1001/jama.296.23.2805

Wolinsky, F.D., Vander Weg, M.W., Martin, R., Unverzagt, F.W., Willis, S.L., Marsiske, M., . . . Tennstedt, S.L. (2009). Does cognitive training improve internal locus of control among older adults? *The Journals of Gerontology, Series B: Psychological Sciences and Social Sciences, 65*(5), 597–598. doi:10.1093/geronb/gbp117

Woolverton, M., Scogin, F., Shackelford, J., Black, S., & Duke, L. (2001). Problem-targeted memory training for older adults. *Aging, Neuropsychology, and Cognition, 8*(4), 241–255. doi:10.1076/anec.8.4.241.5637

Zehnder, F., Martin, M., Altgassen, M., & Clare, L. (2009). Memory training effects in old age as markers of plasticity: A meta-analysis. *Restorative Neurology and Neuroscience, 27*(5), 507–520. doi:10.3233/RNN-2009-0491

Zelinski, E.M. (2009). Far transfer in cognitive training of older adults. *Restorative Neurology and Neuroscience, 27*(5), 455–471. doi:10.3233/RNN-2009-0495

Zelinski, E.M., Spina, L.A., Yaffe, K., Ruff, R., Kennison, R.F., Mahncke, H.W., & Smith, G.E. (2011). Improvement in memory with plasticity-based adaptive cognitive training: Results of the 3-month follow-up. *Journal of the American Geriatrics Society, 59*(2), 258–265. doi:10.1111/j.1532-5415.2010.03277.x

PART IV

Facing the memory challenge in dementia

11

KEEPING MEMORIES ALIVE

Creativity in dementia care, alternatives to pharmacotherapy

Niamh Malone and Donna Redgrave

In Locke's (1689) thesis 'the person is not constituted by a biography but by a remembered biography'.

(qtd. in Hacking, 1996, p. 81)

11.1   Introduction

The human need, both to acknowledge life in the process of being lived and to remember, was a central preoccupation of the philosophical writings of the 17th century English scholar John Locke. This preoccupation has re-emerged in the form of questions around available procedures and methods to enhance memory preservation in contemporary society and, in the specific context addressed here, for people living with dementia. This chapter explores the efficacy of arts interventions in dementia care, with particular consideration given to how the employment of the arts in health supports person-centred care (Kitwood, 1997) and facilitates methods to enhance memory preservation.

While there is a considerable body of medical research on dementia (First & Tasman, 2010), this chapter takes a social perspective, considering how arts interventions may enhance the communicative capacities of persons living with dementia, strengthening selfhood and identity and ultimately enhancing well-being. The pioneering work of the late Tom Kitwood (1997), articulated in theories of person-centred care and personhood, offers an analytical framework that will be applied to the case study considered below. The chapter begins with a brief acknowledgement of the key features of dementia, understood as a medical condition, and the practical consequences of this approach, with an eye specifically to the British context. Following an overview of the development and role of the creative arts in health care, and notes on person-centred care, identity and memory, two forms of artistic practice – Reminiscence Theatre and Imaginary Theatre – come into focus. A case study tracking the emergence of Imaginary Theatre as a development of Reminiscence Theatre is selected from a portfolio of work by *RMD Memory Matters Theatre Company*, evidencing some benefits of arts interventions in care plans for people living with dementia.

11.2   Dementia in context

Dementia is an umbrella term for a cluster of more than 200 diseases associated with the human brain. It is progressive, has no known cure, is the fifth leading cause of death and the most feared disease among people over 65, one in three of whom will develop dementia (Elliott et al., 2014). The most commonly diagnosed form of dementia is Alzheimer's disease, followed by vascular dementia. In 2014, dementia was a global epidemic affecting 44.4 million people, a figure set to triple by 2050, at a cost to the global economy of £350 billion. The World Health Organization (WHO) Report *Dementia: A Public Health Priority* (2012) stated that "The total number of new cases of dementia each year worldwide is nearly 7.7 million, implying one new case every four seconds" (p. 11). While dementia most commonly affects older people, people as young as 27 have been diagnosed.

In the United Kingdom alone, dementia currently affects 800,000 people, rising to one million by 2050. With current costs estimated at £23 billion, Prime Minister David Cameron pledged a "drive by the UK to discover new drugs and treatment that could slow down the onset of dementia or even deliver a cure by 2025" (Department of Health and Prime Minister's Office, 2014). His undertaking responds to the recommendations of the 2013 G8 Dementia Summit.

11.3   The development and implementation of the creative arts in health care settings

The historical evolution of medical practice in Western society proceeds in close parallel with scientific developments both in medical procedures and advances in technological support. Brodzinski (2010) charts the development of a biomedical model of practice, driven by research in the natural sciences, emerging as early as the European Renaissance. She describes Harvey's theory of the biomedical model (1628), based on the fundamental assumption that the human form was ultimately a machine, as a "dualistic, mechanistic, reductionist, empirical, interventionist" (Brodzinski, 2010, p. 4) approach. From that time, through the Enlightenment, and up until the mid to late 20th century, health was seen ultimately as an absence of disease, assessed using evaluative measures based primarily on empirical, scientific markers.

During the late 1960s and early 70s, coinciding with what Kershaw (1991) refers to as a 'counter-cultural revolution' in Western society, there was a considerable shift in people's attitudes towards health, and the 'illness' perspective was challenged by a 'health' perspective. According to Brodzinski (2010, p. 4), an exploration took place of how the physical body was attuned to social, emotional and spiritual factors, which ultimately became recognised as 'the social model' of health. While presence of a disease or condition continues to be recognised and treated, this model places a significant emphasis on the cumulative impact on individual health factors such as income level, housing quality, educational opportunities and access to social networks.

This shift in perspective from medical to social conceptions of health had a parallel in arts practice, where Kershaw's (1991) counter-cultural revolution saw the implementation of arts projects specifically tailored to address social issues. Prentki and Preston (2009) suggest that applied theatre practices, which emerged during this era, were implemented for clear sociological reasons, beyond perceived benefits of exposure to an art form per se: "for both practitioners and participants there may often be an overt, political desire to use the process of theatre in the service of social and community change" (p. 9).

As the social model of health emphasised psychological aspects alongside external, environmental factors in contributing holistically to a person's state of well-being, claims made for therapeutic outcomes of arts practices, in the form of social interventions, achieved credibility. From the late 20th century, a wide range of health care provisions actively incorporated 'arts in health' programmes. Senior (cited in Brodzinski, 2010) notes that "by 1983, 65 British hospitals were funding some sort of arts provision and by 1992, there were at least 300 projects around the country" (p. 8). As artistic intervention programmes began to mushroom throughout the country, by the turn of the 21st century, the beneficial relationship between arts and health care was recognised in government policy, and 2004 became a watershed year, during which a *Public Health White Paper* was published, the Department of Health produced *Arts in Health* – a review of existing projects – and Arts Council England announced a National Arts in Health Strategy.

A decade later, 'Arts in Health' is recognised as a significant field of practice within the applied arts spectrum. Arts interventionist companies have become commonplace throughout Western society, and many are interdisciplinary in focus, with drama, music, visual art and dance/movement among the most popular art forms employed in the service of health care. This chapter now considers a UK case study, the work of *RMD Memory Matters,* a theatre company situated in the northwest of England and Wales, which employs the arts in the service of health.

11.4   Person-centred care, identity and memory

RMD Memory Matters practices person-centred care founded on the concept of personhood (Kitwood, 1997). Personhood is defined as "a standing or status that is bestowed upon one human being, by others, in the context of relationship and social being. It implies recognition, respect and trust" (Kitwood, 1997, p. 8). These principles are extended to persons living with dementia through considerate care structures with the ultimate goal to enhance well-being. Kitwood's ethical stance and holistic practice sets out to counter what he calls "the malignant social psychology" (1997, p. 4) model of care, which focuses on the medical condition and the cognitive decline of the individual, rather than acknowledging the 'unique subjectivity' of the person. Kitwood's model of practice begins by asking how persons living with dementia experience life and relationships. This approach seeks to validate the behaviours and feelings of the person as they are presented, and strives to understand any behavioural incidents that may be deemed irrational or problematic. Kitwood (1997) argues that such a positive approach enables "a dialectical interplay in which the social psychology works to offset the process of neurological decline" (p. 5). Kitwood's overarching practice is referred to as Dementia Care Mapping, which is "a serious attempt to take the standpoint of the person with dementia, using a combination of empathy and observation skills" (1997, p. 4). Kitwood's care mapping is part of a multi-disciplinary approach to dementia care, which seeks to lower dependency on pharmacotherapy interventions, the preferred weapon of what he refers to as the 'chemical cosh' industry. Arts intervention, as the selected case study will show, can play a significant role in the implementation of a 'Dementia Care Map' for individuals living with dementia. Kitwood (1997, p. 82) lists six requirements for person-centred care to be implemented successfully, which include love, comfort, attachment, inclusion, occupation and identity. While each of these requirements inform the approach adopted by *RMD Memory Matters* when designing and implementing art intervention programmes for people living with dementia, understanding how dementia impacts a person's identity is of particular concern.

From a medical perspective, dementia is commonly associated with loss of a sense of individual autonomy, causing a considerable weakening of a personal sense of identity and purpose. According to Backhaus (2011, p. 194), focusing on the bio-medical paradigm of dementia, which emphasises a decline in cognitive abilities, contributes to a state of 'de-selfing' for the person living with dementia. Preserving a sense of identity as the condition progresses can be particularly challenging for persons living with dementia, as the task is greatly compromised by progressive memory loss, and growing difficulties in communicating effectively with family members, peers and carers. Bevins (2008, p. 8) suggests that memory is "an essential prerequisite for identity" and understandings of self are partly dependent on an ability to locate oneself in one's past experiences. He draws on Atchley's (1989; as cited in Bevin, 2008, p. 8) *continuity theory*, which proposes that, in times of transition, ageing adults are motivated towards "both inner psychological continuity and the maintenance of existing external structures (e.g., group memberships)". As the severity of the disease increases, many people are moved into residential care, dislocated from family, friends and established social encounters, and thus psychological and social continuity are disrupted. Continuity theory foregrounds the importance of 'autobiographical memory' in enabling individuals to construct consistent life stories "to perceive ourselves as the same person in the present as in the past" (Bevins, 2008, p. 8). This approach complements the principles of person-centred care, where care procedures are grounded in respect for the integrity of individuals, and their sense of identity. Continuity theory is central to the development of Reminiscence Theatre as a form of arts intervention, which we will argue in this chapter is a powerful tool in the struggle to strengthen social identities among persons living with dementia.

11.5   Arts practices in dementia care

> One of the ironies of our times is that our society removes people [living with dementia] from everything that nourishes them – their homes, neighbourhoods, and roles in the family, confines them to institutions, then has to contrive 'activities' to fill up all that emptiness.
>
> (Zoutewelle-Morris, 2011, p. 40)

While care homes typically arrange an array of activities for their residents, ranging from flower arranging to yoga, this section considers the role of arts interventions in the service of dementia care. *RMD Memory Matters Theatre Company* responds to Zoutewelle-Morris's implied demand for the provision of high quality person-centred activities in residential care facilities, specifically, by designing and delivering customized interactive and stimulating arts activities.

Kasayka and Hill (2001) suggest that "the core functions of healing arts therapies in the care of persons with dementia are the reclamation, the regeneration and the celebration of the human spirit" (p. 9), all of which complement Kitwood's person-centred care. They emphasise the strength of arts experiences in aiding communication, creating joyous and playful environments while extending a sense of accomplishment to people. It is important to note that while 'arts in community', 'arts therapies' and 'arts activities' are all strongly connected and work towards similar objectives, they also differ in specific ways from what is considered here. According to White (2009, p. 3), arts in community health operates outside of acute health care settings and is identifiable by its use of participatory arts to promote health. Zoutewelle-Morris (2011) summarises arts therapy as using "diagnosis and planned intervention to cure or lighten symptoms. Art activity uses creative skills to generate a sense of enjoyment, satisfaction and companionship through a moment of engagement without trying to change the person or condition" (p. 173). What connects all of these approaches is the desire to enhance the well-being of people living with dementia, providing emotional relief and opportunities for personal expression. Kasayka and Hill (2001, p. 10) refer to Sandel's (1992) summary of key outcomes of arts therapies when employed, which are applicable to most arts interventions:

1   increasing orientation and activation
2   facilitating reminiscence and remembering
3   increasing self-understanding and acceptance
4   developing meaningful interpersonal relationships
5   building communal spirit

Sandel's findings support Zoutewelle-Morris's (2011) insistence that arts interventions are most effective when they are used to "communicate, validate and support that person where she is, as she is" (p. 13). She emphasises the need for art facilitators to enter the world inhabited by a person with dementia, whether fictitious or real in that moment. At the core of all arts intervention is social interaction, and Putman (summarised in White, 2009) argues that the actual "*positive* contributions to health made by social integration and social support rival in strength the detrimental contributions of well-established biomedical risk factors" (p. 3).

While arts intervention is an umbrella term, encompassing a wide range of diverse practices, Reminiscence Theatre and Imaginary Theatre provide examples of how the creative interventions support progressive sociological developments in dementia care.

11.5.1   Arts practices in dementia care

> The sharing of stories is a medium through which people who are ill can transcend their experience of illness so that their humanness is affirmed.
>
> (Ryan & Schindel-Martin, 2011, p. 3)

Reminiscence Theatre is a recognised practice in the field of Applied Theatre, and, since the turn of the century, has a significant presence in 'arts in health'. Pam Schweitzer (2007, p. 11) states that in Reminiscence Theatre,

> [t]he exercise of memory, accessed by reminiscence and recall and the interplay of imagination provides the basis for creating theatrical and musical representations as well as exhibitions of individuals' and groups' lived experiences.

The process of reminiscing and encouraging care home residents with dementia to recall personal stories in a supportive environment, very often sharing them with peers, contributes towards reinforcing and strengthening identities and affirming their positions within former and current locations (Ryan & Schindel-Martin, 2011). The process of publicly voicing and sharing stories also promotes and strengthens communication and relations between residents. Continuity Theory affirms that the stimulation of 'autobiographical memory' by this form of arts intervention enhances person's sense of self. *RMD Memory Matters'* Reminiscence Theatre processes are designed to achieve all five outcomes of Sandel's summary as referred to earlier, thereby fostering personhood as recognised by Kitwood (1997).

'Imaginary Theatre' is an emerging, original form of structured storytelling practice that was facilitated by *RMD Memory Matters Theatre Company (RMD MMTC)* in the context of the *Never Ending Story* project. While it could be argued that imagination is central to any kind of arts activity, 'Imaginary Theatre' as a practice developed by *RMD MMTC* places particular emphasis on the necessity to enter into the lived world of the resident(s), whether fictitious or real, to encourage them to communicate, verbally or non-verbally, so as to articulate the story of the world as they experience it in their minds. This approach extends Reminiscence Theatre strategies to encourage both memory recall/preservation and general cognition. Imaginary Theatre champions the *process* of the artistic intervention as opposed to the end *product*, emphasising the present. Episodes of Imaginary Theatre involve residents in peer interaction, imaginative stimulation, listening and a selection of communication avenues (verbal, somatic, aural and visual). The creative events that make up Imaginary Theatre are initiated by a participant facilitator, who takes responsibility for including and involving all present as co-creators of fictions offered by individual group members. Specifically, as in the case study that follows, a facilitator may introduce a 'pre-text' – an object, image or topic – designed to excite the interest of group members, whose responses he/she then structures towards creative exploration of the social worlds they recall. Imaginary Theatre may be considered a form of Applied Theatre practice that invites residents to escape the institutional confines of the nursing home, and move deliberately into different times and places. This approach introduces and fosters what Killick (2013) refers to as 'playfulness' in dementia care, where play is understood as "the unfettering of the mind and body; it is without purposefulness; it welcomes the unexpected" (p. 12). It is when a carer/arts facilitator purposefully enters into the 'world' of the person living with dementia that the 'unexpected' is enabled.

Imaginary Theatre complements established arts intervention practices such as *narrative thematic conversation* (Ryan & Schindel-Martin, 2011, p. 11), which encourages narrative construction through the creation of poetry, storytelling or visual art, and is closely related to Silverstone's *guided fantasies*, which encourages the resident "to follow a fantasy in his or her imagination and then talk about it" (2009, p. 23). People living with dementia have varying capabilities for maintaining narrative coherence, and the fact that in Imaginary Theatre, formal coherence is not completely necessary opens up possibilities for anyone to enter the process. This form of practice gives "a fullness of living where imagination, intuition and the creative impulse share parity of esteem with cognitive ability and analytical thought" (Thorne, cited in Silverstone, 2009, p. 12). The creative environment needed to facilitate Imaginary Theatre practice conforms to Harnett's (2014) 'respite spaces', as, while workshops are conducted within care home settings, spaces are 'playfully framed' and the connotations of usual institutional functions are temporarily removed. Harnett raises the possibility of residents themselves gaining confidence and capacity to initiate 'respite spaces' where imaginative and reminiscence-based dialogue can be deliberated upon, without interventions from carers and/or arts facilitators.

11.5.2   Case study

RMD Memory Matters Theatre Company (est. 2010) piloted a project called *Never Ending Story* in dementia care settings across North Wales in 2014. *Never Ending*

Story was a creative storytelling project using elements of drama, reminiscence, music, movement, visual arts and craft in a multi-disciplinary context for people with dementia and their care workers in residential settings. The project aimed to engage, communicate and create a sense of identity in an imaginative and socially inclusive environment. By autumn 2014, 40 people with dementia and 20 care staff participated, and the final project placement involved 50 people with dementia and 26 care staff. On completion (January 2015), 136 participants had been involved. The project was designed to run for 10 weeks, with each session being two hours in duration, and the following case study arose from this work.

Never Ending Story used a multi-disciplinary approach to connect creatively with each person in their world, seeking to transform the lived and immediate experience for people living with dementia. In parallel with creative interaction with residents, *Never Ending Story* provided an inclusive training platform for care workers, focused on altering the dementia care environment into a conducive, productive and playful space.

The project worked on stimulating the imagination of each resident, in keeping with Kitwood's (1997, p. 83/84) philosophy that:

> To have an *identity* is to know who one is, in cognition and in feeling. It means having a sense of continuity with the past; and hence a "narrative", a story to present to others. It also involves creating some kind of consistency across the different roles and contexts of a person's life.

Through the presentation of a selection of stimuli, cues were given to the residents to promote imaginative cognitive action, where past events or imaginary narratives were communicated and further explored. Stimuli included visual (images), aural (music, spoken word) and tactile (objects/props/costumes), all of which were connected through a theme chosen weekly, such as Seaside, Travel, Olympics, Love and Marriage, Going Out, Funfair and Music Hall. Each session was recorded, and stories generated by residents were included in a booklet presented to the residents at the end of the project.

Typically, Imaginary Theatre invites group members to work collectively towards creating a story. In the *Never Ending Story* project, the *Travel* theme resulted in one of the residents, Matilda (name changed for reasons of confidentiality), responding directly to stimuli presented in the session (flags, hats, maps, music, etc.), asking the group: "Has anybody here seen Kelly? Kelly from the Isle of Man?" Matilda's imaginative impulse inspired the whole group to enter an imaginary world to find Kelly, in an example of what Silverstone (2009) refers to as 'guided fantasies'. As the workshop progressed and the narrative developed, Matilda, who initiated the episode, ended up finding and marrying Kelly, commenting: "Gosh! I didn't think I'd be doing that today!" Matilda was presumably moved by a specific item within the range of stimuli and the creative space that prompted her to ask about Kelly. The question (has anybody seen. . .) is actually a phrase out of a song by Florrie Ford, which Matilda appeared to have recalled in the moment created by the collection of objects presented.

In this example, the imaginative framework created by the workshop content and structure affirms Killick's (2013) insistence on the power of 'playfulness' in dementia care, while also supporting Harnett's (2014) concept of 'playful framing', where a facilitator enters another's imaginative world, neutralising institutionalised norms, which otherwise dominate the setting, and creating a 'respite space', in which residents initiate purposeful imaginative episodes. In anonymised evaluations, care workers commented on how, in contrast to an 'often frustrated situation'

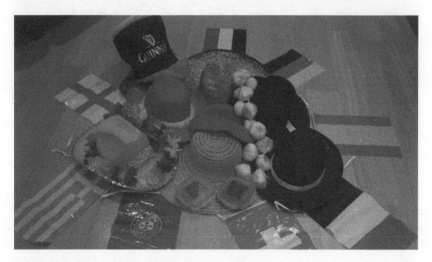

FIGURE 11.1 Props used for week themed 'Travel'.

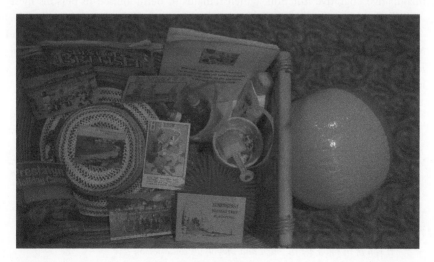

FIGURE 11.2 Props used for week themed 'Seaside'.

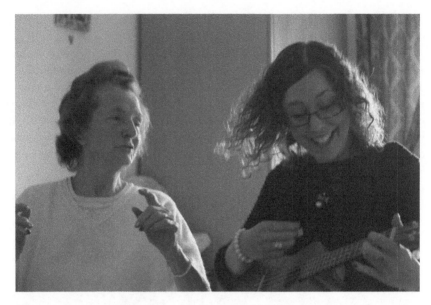

FIGURE 11.3 Donna Redgrave in participant facilitator role.

observed when residents were kept in the space without arts intervention, they could now see the real benefits of employing Imaginary Theatre strategies to create an inclusive space, alive with social meaning. The Kelly episode was directed from within by the residents themselves, temporarily transforming an institutional care environment into a creative hub of imaginative activity, fostering personal senses of self, encouraging social interactions and demonstrating the capacity for imaginative cognitive function, which remains to be mobilised in persons living with dementia.

Another workshop within the *Never Ending Story* programme, titled 'Love and Marriage', drew on what Ryan and Schindel-Martin (2011, p. 11) refer to as *narrative thematic conversation*. As a collaborative exercise, the group decided to write a love letter from 'Lovers' Lane', which read:

> *My dearest Charlie,*
> *I really enjoyed that dance*
> *and I wouldn't mind if you would take me for afternoon tea at the Ritz.*
> *I have fallen head over heels for you!*
> *We'll meet again,*
> *Don't know where,*
> *Don't know when,*
> *But I know we'll meet again some sunny day!*
> *If you're in town get in touch and maybe we could fall in love*
> *All my love*

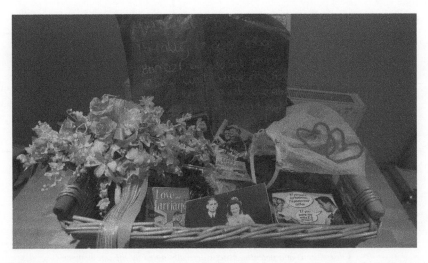

FIGURE 11.4   Props, including the group-composed poem, for the week themed 'Love and Marriage'.

Collaborating to compose this letter was an important step towards a collective sense of well-being among the residents involved, and nurtured a celebratory environment in which work produced by participants is welcomed, shared, discussed and valued from a positive and caring perspective.

These two short examples of particular workshops from within the *Never Ending Story* project demonstrate how Imaginary Theatre, an interactive arts intervention, applies the insights and principles of Kitwood's (1997) person-centred care practice. Imaginary Theatre strategies, developed and delivered by the arts facilitator, Ms Donna Redgrave, were designed to be re-employed by the carers once the project reached its completion. Through active observation and participation over the duration of the project, carers were supported to acquire confidence and 'creative framing skills' to continue to deliver Imaginary Theatre in group and individual sessions. This staff development dimension was a crucial part of the work, enabling carers to keep imaginary scenarios 'in play' within a resident community, which can contribute to reducing agitation, confusion and anxiety among participants. By opting for a creative framework of person-centred care, *RMD MMTC* seeks to mitigate, or avoid altogether, such damaging and stressful scenarios. The following responses, recorded during the evaluation process for the *Never Ending Story* project, give a clear sense of how these effects appear in practice.

While the full, formal evaluation of the *Never Ending Story* project is pending at the time of writing, responses documented so far, from residents, care workers and managements of care homes involved, testify to the potential benefits of structured arts interventions in conjunction with person-centred care.

TABLE 11.1 Evaluation feedback notes, *Never Ending Story* project, 2014

Feedback from residents (people living with dementia):

'I can't thank you enough for bringing us friends all together here, I can tell you I will never ever forget this day'

'Thank you, you have really taken me away from this place, I have enjoyed some time away, I'll never forget you'

'Everybody being together, being part of something'

'My gosh that brought it all back!'

'I have truly enjoyed myself, I mean that from the heart'

Feedback from carers:

'NES has made such a difference to the home'

'What a wealth of ideas to be going on with'

'Simple but effective'

'Residents have a lot of history and stories to tell, and now time to tell their story'

'You don't need a lot of expensive props but a lot of enthusiasm'

Observations and potential benefits formally noted by the care home:
- People are eating better
- Residents' moods are more positive on days that *RMD MMTC* visits
- Residents are sleeping better
- A significant decrease in agitation in residents and reduction in pharmacological interventions, particularly on the days that *RMD MMTC* visits

---

11.6 Conclusion

> Empowering someone is different from helping them because it approaches them from their strengths and not their limitations.
>
> (Zoutewelle-Morris, 2011, p. 24)

Arts intervention programmes have evolved over recent decades as a direct challenge to reductionist tendencies apparent in the bio-medical model of treatment, which, more often than not, fails to acknowledge the psychosocial make-up of persons living with dementia. The employment of arts interventions in the care of people living with dementia contributes significantly to the growth in a humanistic approach to care, which focuses on the individual living with dementia as opposed to the disease, enabling them to maintain a dignified and valued social status (George, Stuckey, & Whitehead, 2013, p. 837).

The authors of this chapter argue on the basis of the case study considered here that the emergent, original form of Imaginary Theatre has clear potential to play a very useful role in enabling and supporting person-centred care and progressive sociological care strategies.

References

Atchley, R. C. (1989). A continuity theory of normal aging. *The Gerontological Society of America, 26*(2), 183–190.

Backhaus, P. (2011). *Communication in elderly care: Cross-cultural perspectives,* London: Continuum.

Bevins, A. (2008). *Memory, identity and well-being: Preserving selfhood in dementia.* Doctoral Thesis, University of Exeter, UK.

Brodzinski, E. (2010). *Theatre in health and care.* Basingstoke: Palgrave Macmillan.

Department of Health and Prime Minister's Office. (2014). UK commits to new action to find breakthrough on dementia. Retrieved from https://www.gov.uk/government/news/uk-commits-to-new-action-to-find-breakthrough-on-dementia

Elliott, M., Harrington, J., Moore, K., Davis, S., Kupeli, N., Vickerstaff, V., . . . Jones, L. (2014). A protocol for an exploratory phase I mixed-methods study of enhanced integrated care for care home residents with advanced dementia: The compassion intervention. *BMJ Open, 4*(6), e005661.

First, M. B., & Tasman, A. (2010). *Clinical guide to the diagnosis and treatment of mental disorders* (2nd edition). Oxford: Wiley-Blackwell.

George, D. R., Stuckey, H. L., & Whitehead, M. M. (2013). An arts-based intervention at a nursing home to improve medical students' attitudes toward persons with dementia. *Academic Medicine, 88*(6).

Hacking, I. (1996). Memory sciences, memory politics. In P. Antze & M. Lambek (Eds.), *Tense past: Cultural essays in trauma and memory* (pp. 67–88). London: Routledge.

Harnett, T. (2014). Framing spaces in places: Creating "respite space" in dementia care settings. *Dementia, 13*(3), 396–411.

Innes, A., & Hatfield, K. (2001). *Healing arts therapies and person-centered dementia care.* London: Jessica Kingsley Publishers.

Kasayka, R. E., & Hill, H. (2001). Introduction. In A. Innes & K. Hatfield (Eds.), *Healing arts therapies and person-centered dementia care.* London: Jessica Kingsley Publishers.

Kershaw, B. (1991). *The politics of performance: Radical theatre as cultural intervention.* London: Routledge.

Killick, J. (2013). *Playfulness and dementia: A practical guide.* London: Jessica Kingsley Publishers.

Kitwood, T. (1997). *Dementia reconsidered: The person comes first.* Buckingham: Open University Press.

Prentki, T., & Preston, S. (2009). *The applied theatre reader.* London: Routledge.

Ryan, E. B, & Schindel-Martin, L. (2011). Using narrative arts to foster personhood in dementia. In P. Backhaus (Ed.), *Communication in elderly care.* London: Continuum Press.

Sandel, S. L. (1992). *Dance movement therapy and the elderly.* Hearing Testimony to the US Special Committee on Aging, 18 June.

Schweitzer, P. (2007). *Reminiscence theatre: Making theatre from memories.* London: Jessica Kingsley Publishers.

Silverstone, L. (2009). *Art therapy exercises.* London: Jessica Kingsley Publishers.

White, M. (2009). *Arts development in community health.* Oxon: Radcliffe Publishing Ltd.

World Health Organization. (2012). *Dementia: A public health priority.* Geneva, Switzerland: WHO.

Zoutewelle-Morris, S. (2011). *Chocolate rain, 100 ideas for a creative approach to activities in dementia care.* London: Hawkers Publications Ltd.

12

REMEMBERING TO REMEMBER

The living lab approach to meeting the everyday challenges of people living with dementia

Grahame Smith

12.1   Introduction

The everyday challenges of living with dementia can adversely impact an individual's ability to be independent. By supporting the individual to co-create solutions to these everyday challenges, it is possible to develop solutions to these challenges that are sustainable (Woods, Smith, Pendleton, & Parker, 2013). An example of this cooperative approach is the *living lab*, part of the Innovate Dementia project at Liverpool John Moores University, which is working in partnership with a local mental health NHS Trust. The living lab provides a pragmatic research environment where people living with dementia co-design, co-create, co-produce, and customise real life solutions to their everyday challenges (Woods et al., 2013). As a specific work stream, this approach has started to explore how the development of an 'external technological scaffold' can significantly assist an individual in the early stages of dementia to 'remember to remember' – in turn, this could promote independence and reduce social isolation (Dobbins, Merabti, Fergus, & Llewellyn-Jones, 2014; Pea, 2004). This chapter will explore how this specific work was undertaken and also highlight ongoing work within this area.

12.2   Listening to people living with dementia

Living with dementia can be challenging and at times overwhelming for both the person with dementia and their caregiver, but with the right support, living well with dementia can become a reality rather than just an aspiration. It is estimated that there are over 800,000 people with dementia in the UK. Of this number, 17,000 are estimated to be under the age of 65 (Alzheimer's Society, 2014). Some studies argue that these figures are an underestimation due to the difficulties people experience in receiving a diagnosis (Alzheimer's Society, 2014;

Woods et al., 2013). As people are living longer, it is predicted also that the incidence of dementia will double by 2030, and more than triple by 2050 (Woods et al., 2013; WHO & ADI, 2012). On this basis, the challenge for society is to ensure that current and future dementia care delivery is fit for purpose, and have a greater emphasis on improving the quality of life and wellbeing of those living with dementia (Department of Health, 2009). The Innovate Dementia project has established transnational living labs "in order to test and evaluate innovative dementia care models, focusing specifically on key elements of integrated care; intelligent lightning, nutrition and exercise, living environment with social and aesthetic conditions, and models of assistance for persons with dementia and their carers" (Woods et al., 2013, p. 6).

To develop these models, we have to understand that dementia is a syndrome that is progressive in nature, and that it has an adverse impact upon multiple higher cortical functions, including memory (Budson, 2014; Woods et al., 2013). Enabling people with dementia to remember through the use of technology is on the increase (see also Chapter 15) – this type of technology can externally aid a person's memory and enhance emotional wellbeing through promoting a person's independence (Dobbins et al., 2014; Lauriks et al., 2007). Taking this into account, our team has been developing a memory enabling technology that was co-designed and co-created by people living with dementia with the aim of assisting an individual to live well with dementia (Dobbins et al., 2014; Woods et al., 2013). The use of assistive technologies within the dementia field has been criticised for not meeting the real needs of the user, something the project team wanted to address (Lauriks et al., 2007; Pedell, Beh, Mozuna, & Duong, 2013). For this technology to be readily adopted by the people with dementia, it needs to be 'easy to use and useful', and, in addition, the users, people living with dementia, need to be centrally involved in the design process (Pedell et al., 2013).

A way of doing this, especially when designing something new or innovative, is to create a working environment that engenders a real life understanding of the users' needs (Ståhlbröst & Bergvall-Kåreborn, 2011). To engender this understanding, the project team first listened to people living with dementia as they talked about their everyday challenges (Bracken & Thomas, 2005; Estey-Burtt & Baldwin, 2014). This phase of the project allowed the project team to begin co-designing a specific solution to the challenges of people living with dementia (Bergvall-Kåreborn & Ståhlbröst, 2010).

12.3   Pragmatic approach

The Innovate Dementia project is a European (Interreg IVB) funded project, which started in April 2012, and is aiming to:

•   Evaluate how innovative approaches in dementia care are utilised across north-west Europe, highlighting best practice and future areas of research and development

- Create collaborations that bring people living with dementia together with health and social care, academia, and business; this is called a 'triple helix' approach, in which to share and enhance each other's knowledge, expertise, and performance
- Influence the development of health innovation, new technologies, and lifestyles to prevent the development of dementia and enable people to live well with dementia
- Establish 'living labs' in order to test and evaluate innovative dementia care models

(Woods et al., 2013, p. 6)

Health and social care practitioners, on a daily basis, have to innovate, especially in the case of resources becoming scarce and care becoming more complex, while at the same time, they are expected to continue to deliver high quality care (Wilson, Whitaker, & Whitford, 2012). All members of the project team have a health or social care practitioner background. However, in order for the innovation within the project to be sustainable, there has to be a robust structure that places the involvement of people living with dementia at the centre of the process (Woods et al., 2013). On this basis, the project framed the innovation process within a notional structure called a living lab:

> A Living Lab is a user-centric innovation milieu built on every-day practice and research, with an approach that facilitates user influence in open and distributed innovation processes engaging all relevant partners in real-life contexts, aiming to create sustainable values.
>
> *(Bergvall-Kåreborn & Ståhlbröst, 2010, p. 191)*

The project's living lab collaboratively utilises the knowledge and expertise of all partners, including people living with dementia, in a way that shared learning takes place (Bergvall-Kåreborn, Ihlström Eriksson, Ståhlbröst, & Svensson, 2009). The living lab approach first emerged from an information communication technology background but is now used more widely, including within a health and social care context, though this is the first time it has been specifically utilised within the field of dementia (Bergvall-Kåreborn, Ihlström Eriksson et al., 2009). Philosophically, a living lab is pragmatic in its approach, which is akin to the philosophical pragmatism of Richard Rorty. Within the project, the ideas and practices that arise from the collaborative process are valued in terms of their 'usefulness, workability, and practicality' (Reason, 2003; Reason & Bradbury, 2001). The mediating factor is how these ideas and practices or solutions address the everyday challenges of people living with dementia (Woods et al., 2013). A solution may be a service delivery change or a technological innovation (e.g., a mobile app); this solution, unlike traditional design processes, is then co-created by people living with dementia to determine whether it really does meet the target users' needs. At an application level, the living lab approach has the characteristics of action research, emphasising 'practical knowing through a participatory process', or, as in the living lab's case, a collaborative process that is user-centric (Reason, 2003; Reason & Bradbury, 2001). This collaborative process is, in effect, a large open innovation group that coordinates the work of smaller groups, the progress of which is regularly monitored.

The open innovation group creates a space in which to innovate, explore, and validate potential solutions to the challenge of living everyday with dementia; it also brings interested parties together in a triple helix arrangement: academia, business, and the health and social care sector (Etzkowitz & Leydesdorff, 1997). The limitation of the triple helix approach is that it does not refer directly to the user. On this basis, the Innovate Dementia project should be referred to as a quadruple helix, which has all of the properties of a triple helix and is enhanced by being driven by the real needs of people living with dementia (Dewsbury & Linskell, 2011; Woods et al., 2013). It was agreed that before the project work began in earnest, the 'generic' definition for a living lab needed to be fit for the project's purpose; the following working definition was agreed upon:

> [A] pragmatic research environment which openly engages all relevant partners with an emphasis on improving the real-life care of people living with dementia through the use of economically viable and sustainable innovations.
> *(Woods et al., 2013, pp. 13–14)*

Further, it was recognised that to utilise a living lab approach within the dementia field gives this living lab a unique status, but more importantly, a unique responsibility especially in the case of working with a group of individuals who can be vulnerable (Estey-Burtt & Baldwin, 2014; Smith, 2012b). Taking this into consideration, the work of the project and the governance of its work not only interface explicitly with the relevant ethical frameworks, but it is also underpinned by an agreed principled approach as follows (Bergvall-Kåreborn, Holst, & Ståhlbröst, 2009):

- Continuity
- Openness
- Realism
- Empowerment of users
- Spontaneity

12.4 The challenges of living with dementia

Dementia is described as a long-term and progressive condition that impacts adversely upon a person's cognitive functioning, their emotional control, mood, social behaviour, and their social functioning (Woods et al., 2013; WHO, 1993). Dementia is a general classifying term that is sub-divided into different types, the most common being Alzheimer's disease dementia (Commission of the European

Communities, 2009; NCCMH, 2007; NICE & SCIE, 2006; WHO, 1993; Woods et al., 2013). It is important to recognise that dementia, whatever the type, will affect people in different and very personal ways and that the development of any type of assistive technology in the dementia field needs to take this into account (Woods et al., 2013). In addition to this, a technological solution also needs to take into account that the effective management of dementia is no longer based on symptom control alone, but it also need focus on improving the quality of life of the person with dementia (Woods et al., 2013). The challenge for the project was therefore to co-design a solution that was not only memory enabling but also person-centred with a focus on supporting people with dementia to func-tion as independently as possible (Kitwood, 1997; Woods, 2004; Woods et al., 2013).

To address this challenge, the project team in the early stages of the project arranged an open innovation group that in essence was a listening exercise with a focus on both clearly identifying the everyday challenges of living with dementia and also identifying needs that were not being fully met (Lauriks et al., 2007). Another goal was to ensure that the unique voice of people living with dementia was captured in a way that was relevant and also grounded within reality (Bracken & Thomas, 2005; Estey-Burtt & Baldwin, 2014; McLaughlin, 2006). This process gen-erated a list of themes; Table 12.1 is a summary of these themes – the everyday challenges of people in the early stages of dementia.

TABLE 12.1 Everyday challenges of people in the early stages of dementia

• Not being orientated to time and day	• May lose a word or be unable to name an object
• Difficulty in using household appliances, including phones and remote controls	• Problems remembering to carry out daily tasks
• Feeling unsafe when going for a walk or going to the shops	• Problems remembering to eat and drink, or remembering that you have already done that
• Being distressed by 'cold calling'	• Difficulty when using public transport
• Not knowing how to keep in contact	• Not always feeling independent
• Struggles to interact	• Feeling frustrated when events are unplanned
• Shopping can be difficult due to the regular re-arranging of aisles	• Signage can be confusing
• Not always remembering to look at memory prompts, such as sticky notes	• Medications keep changing and it can be difficult to remember which ones need to be taken
• It can be difficult to remember to take medication	• Being dependent on carers to remember to take medication and/or eat
• Feeling that technology can be scary	• Problems remembering where things should go or where they are; worries about losing stuff

12.5   User-led solutions

Historically, research funding in the dementia field has been significantly lower than in other long-term conditions. This is now changing and there is an increasing focus on promoting dementia research within the UK (Woods et al., 2013) and worldwide. Initiatives such as the UK Prime Minister's dementia challenge, which has a focus on delivering major improvements in dementia care and research, have started to drive this change (Woods et al., 2013). Building on these initiatives, the project team was keen to ensure that a proposed memory enabling solution was grounded in reality in ways that the solution could be used to improve the quality of life of people living with dementia (Lauriks et al., 2007; McLaughlin, 2006).

A limitation of formal care delivery is that it can lack flexibility; this in part is maybe why people living with dementia report that needs are not fully met, and assistive technology that is co-designed and co-created by people living with dementia is one way of addressing this concern (Lauriks et al., 2007). When looking for solutions, it is important to recognise that people living with dementia may not know what solutions already exist, and if they are technological solutions, they may not know the potential benefits of using such technology (Pedell et al., 2013).

Introducing technology to the care delivery process is a challenge, as even the use of technological approaches needs to be evidence-based. Moreover, evidence-based practice may be a dominant approach, but it only provides one narrow perspective, which can be a limited way of understanding the challenges of living with dementia (Bracken & Thomas, 2005; Estey-Burtt & Baldwin, 2014; Smith, 2012a). This is why the project team utilised a multiple meaning approach, working with both the evidence and also the narrative of the person living with dementia (Estey-Burtt & Baldwin, 2014; Johnson, Onwuegbuzie, & Turner, 2007; Smith, 2012a). Care solutions, even if they are technological, should be clinically effective and, where possible, evidenced-based, but they should also consider any inherent user's values and meanings (Bracken & Thomas, 2005; Smith, 2012a). Capturing the voice of people living with dementia was the first stage of the co-design process. Before moving onto the second stage, a cross-checking process took place to ensure that the team's understanding of a shared experience was the same as the person who shared the experience, so that the true meaning of the experience of the person with dementia was preserved (Johnson et al., 2007; Smith 2012a). This cross-checking process meant that the whole of the person was valued irrespective of their age or condition, thus ensuring a person-centred approach (Parker, 2012).

After the checking process was complete, the second stage was to consider potential solutions. Once again, this process required that people living with dementia were actively engaged as equal partners (Weber, 2011). The living lab structure ensures that there is a concerted effort throughout to explore and value the experiences of people with dementia in a way that is both collaborative and person-centred (McKeown, Clarke, & Repper, 2006). The strength of people living with dementia being centrally involved in co-creating solutions is that through

TABLE 12.2 Potential solutions

• Remote control that is voiced controlled	• Proximity sensors
• An alarm pendant that feels non-stigmatising by being covert rather than overt	• Reminders of how to use domestic devices
• Coordinating care website for informal carer	• Sensory technology (e.g., to detect things like hydration)
• Retro-fitted domestic appliances that are smart but easy to use	• Immersive spaces to trigger memories and engagement
• Technology to remind who you have already phoned	• Quick dial phone with 'pictorial' representation
• Reminder that a device needs charging	• Automatic messages to carers that a task has been completed
• Wearable GPS – supports going out and finding your way home	• Technology that can be integrated into own things; tracking devices
• Alert on a gate	• Simplified version of Google Maps
• Wall mounted reminders device	• Personalised design of technology
• Simplify technology – having help to operate and set up	• Easy to use Skype
• Monitor blood pressure and temperature remotely	• Smart doors with cues
• Smart tags for keys – tell you where they are	• Smart alarm clocks that switch themselves off
• Smart TV reminders – 'ticket taping' with important messages	• In case of emergency – information on phone
• Speaking clock that uses a familiar voice	• Devices that flash or have an alarm to catch your attention
• Messages on a smart device that remind you to complete daily tasks	• Smart medication box with automatic dispenser
• All reminding technologies are integrated throughout the home	• Smart devices such as a kettle with instructions 'how to make tea'

this process, the eventual solution is more likely to be useful, useable, and compatible with real needs (McKeown et al., 2006; Woods et al., 2013). From a research perspective, the living lab approach meets a simple measure of good involvement in that people with dementia are consulted, collaborated with, and feel in control (Evans & Jones, 2004; Hanley et al., 2004). Table 12.2 is a summarised list of potential solutions that were identified.

12.6   Memory enabling

After the solution stage was complete, the information was checked through the open innovation group process. The next stage was for the open innovation group to decide on the type of technology they wanted to co-design and co-create. To assist the decision-making process, the group was given the opportunity to explore different types of existing technology. What was interesting at this stage was how surprised people with dementia were that assistive technology was easier to use than first thought, and using this approach broke down a number of barriers related to the use of technology (Lauriks et al., 2007). The project also made clear that, currently, assistive technologies are carer-centric and this was an opportunity to focus on technology that has been developed specifically for people with dementia to be supported by their informal carers (Olsson, Engstrom, Skovdahl, & Lampic, 2012).

The group wanted to co-create a memory enabling technology; this was not surprising, as memory difficulties are a common feature of dementia (Budson, 2014; Dobbins et al., 2014; Parker, 2012). Members of the group who were diagnosed with dementia were already engaging with their local dementia care pathway, including using psychological-based memory enabling approaches with a focus on facilitated reflection on cognitive functions through an organised programme (Parker, 2012). The emphasis of this work, which is group-based, is to assist the person to be as independent as possible (Kitwood, 1997; Parker, 2012). Taking this into consideration, it was recognised that co-creating a memory enabling technology was not a replacement for this type of activity, but would instead complement it in an integrated way, thus possibly becoming a part of the person's care pathway (Dobbins et al., 2014; Lauriks et al., 2007; Pea, 2004). There are a number of devices available that prompt memory, but most have not been co-designed and co-created by people with dementia, and are 'owned' by the carer (Lauriks et al., 2007; Nugent, 2007).

Any assistive technology has its limitations where a person with dementia is capable of using a device, and the device can only compensate for some impairments, so it cannot be a standalone device (Lauriks et al., 2007). Devices are more useful or have a more positive impact when the user has specific training – by co-creating the device, the person with dementia would be very familiar with how it worked (Mate-Kole et al., 2007). The informal care-giver also needed to be involved, not as the owner of the technology, but as the partner in its use (Olsson et al., 2012). Generally, where assistive technology can be seen to be useful in the day-to-day care delivery process, the response from people living with dementia is positive (Landau et al., 2009). The next stage was to create a co-designed brief using the information accrued so far. The group agreed that the technology should have the following qualities:

- Has both visual and audio prompts and cues
- Needs to be an everyday object – e.g., phone, TV
- It has to be habit forming: used on an everyday basis and becomes part of the person's daily life
- Needs to be recognisable as an object but also, if using audio, needs to have a familiar voice
- Cost of adapting existing technology needs to be considered
- Needs to be adaptive to the person's lifestyle and in relation to changes in their condition
- Needs to be adaptive to a person's tastes

- It has to be easy to use – intuitive and accessible
- The prompt has to be congruent to time and the person's actions – remembering to remember
- More than one person may be involved in the remembering process
- Has to be interactive and part of an integrative solution – carer network
- Reminder should not be static – needs to catch the attention

The group also decided that the technology should be used for the following three priorities:

1   Medication reminders
2   Remembering to eat – the right diet
3   Remembering to be active, daily tasks and routine, being safe, preventing social isolation, promote independence

We now had a co-designed brief, but to co-create this technology, we needed to engage with a business. We asked people living with dementia how the right business should be selected. Taking the group's views into consideration, it was decided, through a tendering process, that each interested business would be interviewed through a 'pitching process' (Clark, 2008). The challenge set out in the brief was to develop a memory enabling technology that positively manages risk, is empowering, and is specifically designed for a person with dementia (Pea, 2004; Woods et al., 2013). Further, it was agreed that the solution should be a software solution with most of the qualities set out in the 'qualities list'. It should also, where possible, meet the three priorities.

Each tendering business was interviewed by a panel comprising of members of the project team, including people living with dementia (Clark, 2008). The final say on which proposal was successful resided with the people with dementia sitting on the panel (Bracken & Thomas, 2005; Clark, 2008).

12.7   Conclusion

Since the tendering process, the successful business has worked with a group of 20 participants who are living with dementia in its early stages. Framed by the strong collaborative process of the living lab, the group have met for a minimum of six fortnightly co-creation sessions, and their progress has been monitored and supported by the large open innovation group (Woods et al., 2013). The memory enabling technology, which will be a smart device app, is ready to be launched in 2015, followed by a period of evaluation. Overall, the process of co-design through to co-creation (see Figure 12.1) has engendered a sense of shared ownership, increasing the chances of the innovation, and truly meeting the real needs of people living with dementia (Woods et al., 2013).

Championing the real needs of people living with dementia through this pragmatic research approach – a living lab – not only increases the project's chances of

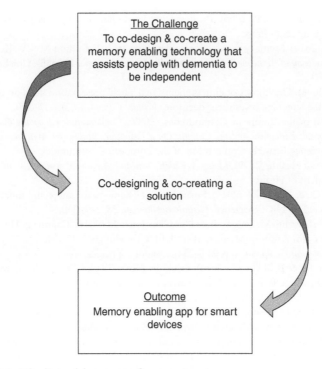

FIGURE 12.1 The living lab process of co-creation.

success, it also benefits people living with dementia by (Bracken & Thomas, 2005; Estey-Burtt & Baldwin, 2014; McLaughlin, 2006):

- Having a research process that is relevant to the needs of people living with dementia and is grounded in their reality
- Strengthening the voice of people living with dementia and capturing their unique perspective

References

Alzheimer's Society. (2014). *Dementia UK* (2nd edition). London: Alzheimer's Society.

Bergvall-Kåreborn, B., Holst, M., & Ståhlbröst, A. (2009). Concept Design with a Living Lab Approach. *42nd Hawaii International Conference on System Sciences*. Retrieved from https://pure.ltu.se/portal/files/2637469/Article.pdf

Bergvall-Kåreborn, B., Ihlström Eriksson, C., Ståhlbröst, A., & Svensson, J. (2009). A Milieu for Innovation: Defining Living Labs. *2nd ISPIM Innovation Symposium, New York, NY*. Retrieved from http://pure.ltu.se/portal/en/persons/anna-staahlbroest(b08416df-93dc-46c1-bd12–8f96767e1b4d)/publications.html?page=2

Bergvall-Kåreborn, B., & Ståhlbröst, A. (2010). Living Lab: An Open and User-Centric Design Approach. In D. Haftor & A. Mirijamdotter (Eds.), *Information and Communication Technologies, Society and Human Beings: Theory and framework* (pp. 190–207). London: IGI Global.

Bracken, P., & Thomas, P. (2005). *Postpsychiatry: Mental health in a postmodern world*. Oxford: Oxford University Press.

Budson, A. (2014). Memory dysfunction in dementia. In A. E. Budson & N. W. Kowall (Eds.), *The Handbook of Alzheimer's Disease and other Dementias* (pp. 315–335). Chichester: Wiley Blackwell.

Clark, C. (2008). The impact of entrepreneurs' oral 'pitch' presentation skills on business angels' initial screening investment decisions. *Venture Capital, 10*(3), 257–279.

Commission of the European Communities. (2009). *Communication from the Commission to the European Parliament and the Council: On a European initiative on Alzheimer's disease and other dementias*. Brussels: Commission of the European Communities.

Department of Health. (2009). *Living Well with Dementia: A national dementia strategy*. London: Department of Health.

Dewsbury, G., & Linskell, J. (2011). Smart home technology for safety and functional independence: The UK experience. *NeuroRehabilitation, 28,* 249–260.

Dobbins, C., Merabti, M., Fergus, P., & Llewellyn-Jones, D. (2014). Capturing Human Digital Memories for Assisting Memory Recall. In S. Fairclough & K. Gilleade (Eds.), *Advances in Physiological Computing* (pp. 211–234). London: Springer.

Estey-Burtt, B., & Baldwin, C. (2014). Ethics in dementia care: Storied lives, storied ethics. In M. Downs & B. Bowers (Eds.), *Excellence in Dementia Care* (2nd edition, pp. 53–65). Maidenhead: Open University Press.

Etzkowitz, H., & Leydesdorff, L. (Eds.). (1997). *Universities in the Global Knowledge Economy: A triple helix of university-industry-government relations*. London: Cassell.

Evans, C., & Jones, R. (2004). Engagement and empowerment, research and relevance: Comments on user-controlled research. *Research, Policy and Planning, 22*(2), 5–13.

Hanley, B., Bradburn, J., Barnes, M., Evans, C., Goodare, H., Kelson, M., . . . Wallcraft, J. (2004). *Involving the Public in NHS, Public Health and Social Care Research: Briefing notes for researchers*. Eastleigh: Involve.

Johnson, R. B., Onwuegbuzie, A. J., & Turner, L. A. (2007). Toward a definition of mixed methods research. *Journal of Mixed Methods Research, 1*(2), 112–133.

Kitwood, T. (1997). *Dementia Reconsidered*. London: Open University Press.

Landau, R., Werner, S., Auslander, G. K., Shoval, N., & Heinik, J. (2009). Attitudes of family and professional care-givers towards the use of GPS for tracking patients with dementia: An exploratory study. *British Journal of Social Work, 39*(4), 670–692.

Lauriks, S., Reinersmann, A., Van der Roest, H. G., Meiland, F. J., Davies, R. J., Moelaert, F., . . . Droes, R. M. (2007). Review of ICT-based services for identified unmet needs in people with dementia. *Ageing Research Reviews, 6*(3), 223–246.

Mate-Kole, C.C., Fellows, R.P., Said, P.C., McDougal, J., Catayong, K., & Dang, V. (2007). Use of computer assisted and interactive cognitive training programs with moderate to severely demented individuals: A preliminary study. *Ageing & Mental Health, 11*(5), 483–493.

McKeown, J., Clarke, A., & Repper, J. (2006). Life story work in health and social care: Systematic literature review. *Journal of Advanced Nursing, 55*(2), 237–247.

McLaughlin, H. (2006). Involving young service users as co-researchers: Possibilities, benefits and costs. *British Journal of Social Work, 36*(8), 1395–1410.

National Collaborating Centre for Mental Health (NCCMH). (2007/2011). *Dementia: A NICESCIE Guideline on supporting people with dementia and their carers in health and social care*. National Clinical Practice Guideline Number 42: The British Psychological Society and Gaskell.

National Institute for Health and Clinical Excellence (NICE), & Social Care Institute for Excellence (SCIE). (2006). *Dementia: Supporting people with dementia and their carers in health and social care – NICE clinical guideline 42*. London: NICE & SCIE.

Nugent, C. D. (2007). Editorial: ICT in the elderly and dementia. *Aging & Mental Health*, *11*(5), 473–476.

Olsson, A., Engstrom, M., Skovdahl, K., & Lampic, C. (2012). My, your and our needs for safety and security: Relatives' reflections on using information and communication technology in dementia care. *Scandinavian Journal of Caring Sciences*, *26*, 104–112.

Parker, D. (2012). Psychological interventions and working with the older adult. In G. Smith (Ed.), *Psychological Interventions in Mental Health Nursing* (pp. 120–131). Maidenhead: Open University Press.

Pea, R. D. (2004). The social and technological dimensions of scaffolding and related theoretical concepts for learning, education, and human activity. *The Journal of the Learning Sciences*, *13*(3), 423–451.

Pedell, S., Beh, J., Mozuna, K., & Duong, S. (2013). Engaging Older Adults in Activity Group Settings: Playing Games on Touch Tablets. *OzCHI '13 Proceedings of the 25th Australian Computer-Human Interaction Conference: Augmentation, Application, Innovation, Collaboration, Adelaide*. Retrieved from http://dl.acm.org/citation.cfm?id=2541090

Reason, P. (2003). Pragmatist philosophy and action research: Readings and conversation with Richard Rorty. *Action Research*, *1*(1), 103–123.

Reason, P., & Bradbury, H. (Eds.). (2001). *Handbook of Action Research: Participative inquiry and practice*. London: Sage Publications.

Smith, G. (2012a). An introduction to psychological interventions. In G. Smith (Ed.), *Psychological Interventions in Mental Health Nursing* (pp. 1–10). Maidenhead: Open University Press.

Smith, G. (2012b). Psychological interventions within an ethical context. In G. Smith (Ed.), *Psychological Interventions in Mental Health Nursing* (pp. 143–154). Maidenhead: Open University Press.

Ståhlbröst, A., & Bergvall-Kåreborn, B. (2011). Living Labs – Real-World Experiments to Support Open Service Innovation. *eChallenges e-2011 Conference Proceedings, Florence, Italy*. Retrieved from http://pure.ltu.se/portal/en/publications/living-labs—realworld-experiments-to-support-open-service-innovation(b98e1a89-3c38-4e11-9325-3a946c845641).html

Weber, M. E. A. (2011). *Customer Co-creation in Innovations: A protocol for innovating with end users*. Eindhoven: Technische Universiteit Eindhoven.

Wilson, A., Whitaker, N., & Whitford, D. (2012). Rising to the challenge of health care reform with entrepreneurial and intrapreneurial nursing initiatives. *OJIN: The Online Journal of Issues in Nursing*, *17*(2). doi:10.3912/OJIN.Vol17No02Man05

Woods, B. (2004). Invited commentary: Nonpharmacological interventions in dementia. *Advances in Psychiatric Treatments*, *10*, 178–179.

Woods, L., Smith, G., Pendleton, J., & Parker, D. (2013). *Innovate Dementia Baseline Report: Shaping the future for people living with dementia*. Liverpool: Liverpool John Moores University.

World Health Organization (WHO). (1993). *The ICD-10 Classification of Mental and Behavioural Disorders*. Geneva: World Health Organization.

World Health Organization (WHO), & Alzheimer's Disease International (ADI). (2012). *Dementia: A public health priority*. Geneva: World Health Organization.

13

COGNITIVE APPROACHES TO ENABLING PEOPLE TO LIVE WELL WITH DEMENTIA

Sarah Jane Smith and Jan R. Oyebode

13.1   Introduction

Cognitive deficits are a hallmark feature of dementia, and have a significant impact on the quality of life for people living with dementia and their families. The notion of helping people to live well with dementia is increasingly featured on national and international public health agendas. Historically, the treatment of people with dementia was embedded in a medicalised approach, in as much as the focus was on treating what were considered to be the symptoms of dementia. These types of views have perhaps also been echoed in the media with representations of dementia focusing on deficits and on people who have been living with dementia for many years, rather than the many people who are striving to find ways to live well with early dementia. There are, of course, medical treatments that are aimed at slowing the decline; however, medications, such as actycholinesterease inhibitors, have had modest effects in clinical trials (Birks & Harvey, 2006).

Recent national and international government and policy initiatives emphasise the importance of psychosocial interventions to improve the lives of people with dementia, partly due to the modest effects of pharmacological interventions on cognition. These interventions can be broadly classified as socially orientated or cognitively orientated. This chapter will explore cognitively based interventions (cognitive stimulation, cognitive training and cognitive rehabilitation) that might be useful for supporting the well-being of people with dementia and their families, and familiarise the reader with the steps involved in developing interventions (see Chapter 10 for memory training for cognitively intact elderly populations).

The interventions we explore will be focused on enhancing the well-being of people in accordance with a person-centred approach (see also Chapters 11 and 12). Person-centred models of dementia care are aligned to a biopsycho-social approach that considers the psychosocial context of the person alongside the neuropsychological changes in understanding the lived experience of the person. Person-centred approaches necessitate individualised support that takes into account the social and psychological needs of the person in the context of the intervention. To this end, we will explore how interventions take account of the individual's needs as part of the process, how they can target the specific nature of the person's deficits and how they take account of the individual's personality and social context.

13.2   How cognitive changes impact on everyday functioning in dementia

Cognitive abilities are important for all aspects of our everyday functioning. Everyday memory refers to the types of memory that are important for the activities that we complete on a day-to-day basis, such as navigating our way to work, doing the shopping, or remembering where you parked the car. Investigations about how everyday memory works have primarily been concerned with the functional aspect of memory, i.e., what memory is for. One of the challenges for investigating how everyday memory works (and thus what happens when it stops working) is ensuring that the research is ecologically valid, i.e., the methods, materials and setting of the research approximate the real world that is being examined. Bruce (1985) stated that ecological memory research must consider how memory operates by identifying the underlying cognitive processes involved, what function it serves, and why it has evolved in this way.

There is a historical debate as to how best to investigate everyday memory function; whether to investigate everyday memory problems by conducting experiments in naturalistic settings, claimed to be more ecologically valid, or in traditional laboratory settings. Conventionally, the main difference between these approaches is methodological: traditional laboratory approaches are conducted in clinical laboratory settings using controlled methods, whereas naturalistic approaches are more ecologically representative but less scientifically controllable (Banaji & Crowder, 1989). The problem of studying everyday memory in laboratory settings is known as the real-world laboratory dilemma, the objective of everyday memory research being to maintain a balance between scientific validity and ecological validity.

Contemporary research makes less of a distinction between these approaches, with scientific investigations frequently incorporating ecological aspects in laboratory settings. Broadly, two approaches to studying everyday memory arose in response to the real-world laboratory dilemma. The first was to generalise laboratory findings to everyday settings, and the second was to identify everyday memory problems that are not currently accounted for by memory models (Baddeley, 2004). Taking the first approach, the idea was to swap stimuli that are not ecologically valid (i.e., unrelated word lists) for ecologically valid stimuli such as songs or rhymes. An example of the second approach is studying memory difficulties, such as prospective memory, i.e., our capacity to perform an action at a specified point in the future.

This is pertinent to the development of cognitive interventions since it is recommended that the combination of real-world and laboratory approaches works well in understanding of everyday memory problems in clinical populations (Baddeley, 2004).

13.2.1   Types of everyday memory

There are different types of everyday memory that are important for everyday functioning and can be affected by the clinical changes of dementia. As an introduction, here we consider autobiographical memory, prospective memory and meta-memory. It is important to understand the impact of dementia on these cognitive functions, so that interventions can be targeted to compensate.

Autobiographical memory (AM) has been defined as the ability to remember past events from one's own life (Kopelman, Wilson, & Baddeley, 1989). Williams, Conway and Cohen (2008) assert that AM has several functions: a directive function (using memories of past events to guide and direct our future behaviour), a social function (to build and maintain friendships by sharing personal narratives) and a self function (to build and maintain personal identity). As such, AM is of fundamental significance for the self, emotions and the experience of personhood (i.e., enduring as an individual over time; Conway & Pleydell-Pearce, 2000). Research has shown that degradation of AM can lead to an impaired sense of personal identity, in addition to being associated with depression (Williams et al., 2008). Investigation of AM in Alzheimer's disease (AD) has indicated that degradation of AM is related to changes in self-concept and personality (Addis & Tippet, 2004).

There is general agreement that AM consists of personal facts and personal events or incidents (Kopelman et al., 1989). Personal incident memory refers to the episodic component of autobiographical memory and includes memory for specific events located in time and space, while personal factual memory is associated with personal information that is not event-based (Conway & Pleydell-Pearce, 2000). AM is usually investigated by assessing individuals' representations of their past experiences, including the content of the experiences and their spatial-temporal context. Tulving (1985) proposed that the ability to recall past events depends on autonoetic consciousness (conscious experience accompanied by a sense of the self in the past). The factual information associated with AM (e.g., place of birth, where we live, names of friends, schools attended) is one facet of semantic memory, and has been described as personal semantics (Cermak & O'Connor, 1983; Kopelman et al., 1989) or personal autobiographical facts (Conway & Pleydell-Pearce, 2000). Unlike episodic AM (for personal events), semantic memory (for personal facts) is associated with noetic consciousness (knowledge without a sense of self in the past).

AM is affected in different ways for people with different profiles of impairments. For example, people with Alzheimer's disease (AD) typically have difficulties with recalling the episodic components of AM, particularly for recent events. AM is affected to the extent that people with AD cannot relive the experiences of their personal history, i.e., recollect past personal events in detail (Piolino et al., 2003).

TABLE 13.1 Everyday memory functions and related processes

Type of Everyday Memory	Processes Implicated
Autobiographical memory	Episodic memory (autonoetic consciousness), Semantic memory, Executive function
Prospective memory	Retrospective/Episodic memory, Executive function (e.g., inhibition, self-initiation)
Metamemory	Episodic memory, Executive function (e.g., set-shifting, updating, inhibition)

People with semantic dementia also have problems with retrieving episodic details to some extent (Piolino et al., 2003), but recent memories are better remembered than remote memories (Graham & Hodges, 1997; Hodges & Graham, 2001; Piolino et al., 2003; Snowden, Griffiths, & Neary, 1996), which may have become semanticised (consolidated) over time. People with Parkinson's disease have a slightly different profile of problems: they have difficulty accessing recent episodic memories, but this may be related to problems accessing the details rather than the integrity of episodic memory itself (Smith, Souchay, & Conway, 2010). We have presented an overview of the different cognitive processes implicated in AM in Table 13.1.

Prospective memory (PM) refers to remembering to carry out plans and intentions: this is crucial for tasks such as remembering to buy milk, keep a doctor's appointment or take medication. Estimates indicate that up to 80% of everyday memory difficulties involve PM failures (Crovitz & Daniel, 1984). Additionally, people with diminished PM function may encounter difficulties carrying out activities of daily living, which may influence quality of life (McDaniel & Einstein, 2007). In characterising PM, Einstein and McDaniel (1990) proposed that it is comprised of two components. First, a retrospective component, which refers to the ability to recall what it is you have to do and when you have to do it. Consequently, completing PM tasks relies on the retrieval of the specific actions to be performed, implicating the declarative memory system responsible for retrieving previously learned facts. However, recalling instructions is not sufficient to perform a PM task. It also necessitates interpretation of an external event as a cue to action, and/or an internal impetus to act (i.e., buying milk when you see a shop); accordingly, PM also includes a prospective component. The prospective component of PM requires self-initiation, as it necessitates that a person remembers to remember (Craik, 1986).

Einstein and McDaniel (1990) proposed an important distinction between event-based and time-based PM. Time-based PM refers to the initiation of an activity at a given time, i.e., "At 2 pm, I must take my medication", whereas event-based PM involves initiating an action in response to an external cue, i.e., "I must get a repeat prescription the next time I visit the GP". As such, PM tasks can be classified in different ways, dependent upon the PM cue that is presented (Kvavilashvili & Ellis, 1996). This diversity in the contextual demands of different PM tasks means that some are more attentionally demanding than others. The accepted view is that time-based PM tasks require more cognitive effort than event-based PM tasks (Craik, 1986; Einstein & McDaniel, 1990). In event-based tasks, the required behaviour is prompted by an external cue, e.g., responding to a given word in the context of an ongoing task (Einstein & McDaniel, 1990), whereas time-based tasks rely more on self-initiated mental processes, such as checking the time, rather than on contextual cues for the restoration of the remembering state.

Age-related differences have been observed on both event-based and time-based tasks, although the impairments are more evident in time-based than event-based tasks (D'Ydewalle, Bouckaert, & Brunfaut, 2001; Einstein, Richardson, Guynn, Cunfer, & McDaniel, 1995; Henry, MacLeod, Phillips, & Crawford, 2004). It is hypothesised that the impairments observed are due to the relation of PM tasks to resource demanding self-initiated processes, which are implicated more in time-based tasks (Prull, Gabrieli, & Bunge, 2000) and are thought to depend upon executive functioning, a cognitive ability that is affected by ageing (Bunce, 2003). Clinically, people with AD can perform poorly in PM tasks due to impairments related to the retrospective component, i.e., recalling what it is they have to do (Jones, Livner, & Backman, 2006), whereas people with more frontal-like impairments, such as Parkinson's disease, have problems with tasks requiring self initiation, i.e., time-based tasks, but can still retrieve the details of the instructions (Smith, Souchay, & Moulin, 2012).

Everyday memory also pertains to the use of memory strategies and awareness of memory (meta-memory). When planning to complete a list of chores, for example, people often start with the chore that they believe they are most likely to forget. While doing the chores, they may also have to add or cross off chores from the list as they go along. This means they must monitor their progress; deficient monitoring might lead to missing a chore or appointment, or to repetition or over-checking (Koriat, Ben-Zur, & Sheffer, 1988). Thus, effective self-management of everyday memory relies on accurate knowledge of our abilities and effective online monitoring during everyday activities so we can update our knowledge about our memory function to suit our needs.

The metamemory framework provides a conceptual model of these issues (Nelson & Narens, 1990). It suggests that memory operates on two interrelated levels: the object level (where our memory processes operate) and the meta-level (which contains our knowledge and beliefs regarding our memory function). Information is exchanged between these levels via two processes: monitoring and control. Monitoring refers to the collation of information regarding memory performance. Monitoring may be considered analogous to 'listening' through a telephone handset. Control refers to the process by which we use this information to self-regulate our performance. If an individual frequently forgets items when they are shopping, for example, they will monitor this forgetting behaviour. They can regulate their memory performance by providing themselves with cues, like a shopping list (i.e., control), which should improve their performance. This reciprocal relationship suggests that proficient memory function relies on effective metamemory function (Dunlosky & Connor, 1997; Nelson & Narens, 1990).

One way of understanding the relationship between monitoring and control processes is by using recall-readiness tasks. This procedure involves offering a list of items to learn, indicating that participants can spend as much or as little time learning the items as required. One would expect individuals to adjust their study time with regards to the ease of the items to recall; for example, the word 'dog' is an easier word to learn than 'cataclysmic', thus one would spend longer learning the word cataclysmic than dog. Using this paradigm, it has been shown that older adults have difficulty allocating extra study time to difficult tasks (Souchay & Isingrini, 2004). However, when older adults are trained to monitor their study through self-testing, they are able regulate their study time more effectively (Robinson, Hertzog, & Dunlosky, 2006).

In summary, it is useful to know more about the nature of people's everyday memory problems so that we can offer targeted support to compensate for the specific types of problems people are having. For example, if someone is frequently missing appointments, is it a) because they forget the details of the appointment or making the appointment (episodic memory), b) a problem with initiating their response to appointment time (prospective memory), or c) they have forgotten that they have difficulties remembering appointments and failed to compensate for this deficit (metamemory)? The different underlying cognitive problems may have different implications for the approaches and support that we offer.

13.3 The major types of cognitive intervention for dementia

The main approaches to improving everyday memory functioning of people with dementia are cognitive training, cognitive stimulation and cognitive rehabilitation. These are all based, at least to some extent, on the application of cognitive science. They share two underlying premises: first, that it is possible for people with dementia to improve their ability to carry out day-to-day activities and tasks through strengthening extant brain function, which may be under par due to a lack of opportunity or a lack of confidence; and second, that it is possible to achieve some new learning or re-learn formerly known information and skills despite the presence of dementia (Fernández-Ballesteros, Zamarron, Tarraga, Moya, & Iniguez, 2003). In addition, cognitive rehabilitation follows the premise that, by informed use of compensatory strategies, we can enable people to get around many problems in everyday functioning that are caused by memory or other cognitive difficulties. In this section, we describe cognitive stimulation, cognitive training and cognitive rehabilitation in a little more detail, citing the guiding principles, the application and mode of delivery and the evidence base.

13.3.1 Cognitive stimulation

Aims and principles

Cognitive stimulation aims to reduce excess disability, rebuild confidence and self-esteem, and enhance general social and cognitive functioning. It is an approach that includes elements of reality orientation (Holden & Woods, 1995), reminiscence (Woods, Spector, Jones, Orrell, & Davies, 2005) and engagement in activity. It is delivered in a social context, following person-centred values (see below). The approach did not arise from cognitive theories, but its core focus is on cognition, and several aspects of delivery are based on broad-base cognitive theory, including that cognitive activity needs to be sustained to avoid decline through disuse (for review, see Salthouse, 2006); that orientation for time, person and place provide us with necessary reference points for keeping track of our lives; that prompts to reminisce can enable people with dementia to better access long-term memories (autobiographical memory; Woods et al., 2005); and that encoding experiences through a range of modalities and senses leads to stronger memory traces (Haxby et al., 2001).

Implementation

Cognitive stimulation can be successfully facilitated by any of a range of health and social care professionals who have interpersonal skills, understanding of the approach and a fundamental appreciation of person-centred care. It is most commonly delivered in a group format with people with mild to moderate dementia on a once or twice weekly basis for 14 or more sessions of 45–75 minutes each. Each session has a characteristic format that includes an initial section, during which participants share introductions and orientate themselves to the context in terms of time, place and current affairs, followed by a longer section focused on a topic of interest that varies from week to week. This topic can be anything that connects with the lives, past and present, of the attenders: for example, fashion, food, working life or birthdays. The facilitators come prepared with materials that may trigger memories of past experiences relevant to the theme, as well as current issues concerning the theme. All attenders are invited to join in, with as much sensory and multi-modality experience as possible. If discussing fruit, for example, the facilitator might bring an orange and a lemon to the meeting so that those taking part can feel, smell and taste the items, as well as talk about them. The meetings are intended to have a social, rather than a classroom, atmosphere, which boosts confidence.

Evidence

A Cochrane review of 15 randomised controlled trials (RCTs) of cognitive stimulation therapy, and meta-analysis of results for 718 participants, confirms the benefits of this approach for cognition and quality of life in people living with dementia (Woods, Aguirre, Spector, & Orrell, 2012). Much of the UK work in the field has been conducted by a group of researchers, including Bob Woods, Aimee Spector and Martin Orrell. They have carried out a series of studies to refine, manualise and gather evidence of the impact of cognitive stimulation. Specifically, an RCT demonstrated short-term improvements on brief cognitive tests for severity of dementia (Spector et al., 2003) with later studies demonstrating benefits not only for memory, but also for naming, word-finding and comprehension, as well as quality of life (Spector, Orrell, & Woods, 2010). A recent study (Orrell et al., 2014) showed that improvements in self-rated quality of life were maintained over six months in people with dementia who had the benefit of maintenance cognitive stimulation therapy (CST) sessions on a weekly basis following an initial more intensive programme. Continuing cognitive benefits were shown on a general screening test of cognition, the Mini-Mental State Examination (Folstein, Folstein, & McHugh, 1975), in those who received CST as well as anti-dementia medication, in comparison to those who received anti-dementia drugs alone. Most recently, a study has been conducted to assess the benefits of carrying out CST with people with dementia in the home setting on a 1:1 basis led by a relative or carer (Orrell et al., 2012); however, the results of this study have not yet been published. The overall positive findings of application of CST in groups settings have led to the UK National Institute for Clinical Excellence including cognitive stimulation in its guidelines for dementia interventions (NICE, 2006).

13.3.2   Cognitive training

Aims and principles

Cognitive training consists of guided practice on a set of standard tasks designed to target and 'exercise' particular cognitive functions (such as planning, attention or memory). The principle of cognitive training is that the training should improve performance (or at least maintain function) in the targeted domain and should generalise beyond the context of the training task. The tasks are pitched at different levels of difficulty to optimise improvements in performance in line with individuals' ability; levels of difficulty can also be adjusted within the same task to reflect improvements within the task. In addition to personalisation on a difficulty level, there is also scope to personalise the cognitive training tasks themselves: for example, by practicing recalling items that have some personal relevance (Davis, Massman, & Doody, 2001).

Implementation

Cognitive training can be offered on an individual basis (e.g., Davis et al., 2001; Loewenstein, Acevedo, Czaja, & Duara, 2004) or in group sessions (Bernhardt, Maurer, & Froelich, 2002). Typically, sessions are facilitated by practitioners, but the training can also be completed individually or with support from family members (Quayhagen et al., 2000). The approaches to training are diverse, and it can be offered in a variety of formats with some tasks emulating everyday activities, some being cognitive-based paper and pencil tasks, and some being computerised or based on virtual reality (Clare, 2003).

The concept of cognitive training has been popularised in recent years with the advent of Dr Kawashima's brain training programmes, which are available on personalised and hand held computers. The objective is to improve performance on a set of tasks that reflect different cognitive skills to reduce your 'brain age'. Computerised cognitive training packages are increasingly being developed for clinical applications, and the improvements that these types of tasks elicit are also being assessed.

Evidence

The evidence for the efficacy of cognitive training is still mixed. An early review indicated that cognitive training may be useful for slowing decline in dementia (Gatz et al., 1998). A more recent review found no significant benefits of cognitive training in people with or without dementia (Bahar-Fuchs, Clare, & Woods, 2013). There were methodological limitations within the studies identified in the review, one being that the target outcome measures may not have been sensitive enough to measure the effects of the training. Indeed, there is evidence that performance can be improved on specific training tasks. Questions remain as to whether these tasks in turn offer improvements to the real-life difficulties people may be having.

Other investigations relate to the format of interventions: Lorant-Royer, Munch, Mescle and Lieury (2010) tested the benefits of a computerised brain training programme and found it did not demonstrate benefits over and above paper-based cognitive training tasks, a no training group. Other studies have shown that video-based games can develop specific cognitive capacities. Owen et al. (2010) tested 11,430 participants without dementia on online cognitive training tasks over a period of six weeks, finding that, while improvements were observed on all of the tasks that people were trained on, no evidence was found of transfer effects to other tasks.

13.3.3   Cognitive rehabilitation

Aims and principles

The aim of using cognitive rehabilitation is to improve a person's ability to successfully manage those aspects of day-to-day life that have a cognitive component and that have become impaired or abandoned by the impact of dementia on cognitive processes, thereby improving the person's quality of life and well-being. Cognitive rehabilitation includes "any intervention strategy or technique which intends to enable clients or patients, and their families, to live with, manage, by-pass, reduce or come to terms with deficits precipitated by injury to the brain" (Wilson, 1997, p. 488). The approach is applied through individually tailored interventions that employ the principles of effective learning and information processing to address specific goals in real-life settings. It involves the sophisticated application of cognitive theory and research findings to find ways of benefitting individuals with acquired brain problems, in this case dementia.

Implementation

The starting point for cognitive rehabilitation is a discussion with the person with dementia and close others involved in their care to identify whether there are specific tasks that might be addressed using the approach. Personally relevant goals can include things such as (re-)learning to use equipment (e.g., a mobile phone or microwave oven), re-learning everyday tasks (e.g., doing the shopping, baking) and (re-)learning names (e.g., grandchildren or club members). Development of the tailored intervention requires a full analysis of the difficulties a person with dementia is having with a task, as well as understanding of their cognitive strengths and weaknesses, awareness, and the environmental context and resources. This rounded understanding leads to a formulation that informs the intervention.

While many interventions are focused on memory problems, a number of other cognitive processes may also be involved and, where this is the case, need to be addressed, including attention, planning, sequencing, keeping track, object recognition, searching and spatial aspects of behaviour. The tailored intervention then draws on the latest knowledge of effective strategies for promoting whichever aspects of cognitive processing are impaired, including encoding, storage and retrieval of information. Strategies may be compensatory or restorative in nature. Those that aim to restore function or promote new learning include errorless learning, in-depth processing, spaced retrieval, active rehearsal, modelling and use of fading cues. Compensatory strategies include the use of external aids such as alarms, labels and white boards; diaries and memory wallets, instructions and checklists; and environmental adaptations. The intervention usually takes place in the environment in which the activity will be performed (for example, the person's own home) and involves about six to twelve 45–60 minute sessions depending on the complexity of the intervention and the progress of the individual. Due to its specialist nature, cognitive rehabilitation is generally undertaken by a clinical psychologist or an occupational therapist.

Evidence

Although the cognitive rehabilitation approach has been quite widely applied in clinical work with people with dementia, published research evidence is scant and often related to single case designs or small studies; therefore, more rigorous and large-scale studies are needed (Bahar-Fuchs et al., 2013; Hopper et al., 2013). In the UK, a series of studies has been conducted and published by Linda Clare (see Clare, 2008, for a summary). These have shown, for example, that for one person, being supported to learn the names of fellow attenders at a social club had the benefit of giving him continued confidence to attend, so reducing risk of social isolation (Clare, Wilson, Breen, & Hodges, 1999). In contrast to this study with a person with early dementia, cognitive rehabilitation approaches have also been successfully used to address specific issues for people with more advanced dementia living in care home settings. Bird (2001), for example, describes the combined use of external memory aids, cued recall and learning-by-doing to assist a woman with dementia to remember what she had done with her belongings.

In addition to these small-scale studies, there is also evidence of effectiveness from an RCT that a protocol-driven approach that allows individual goals to be addressed can produce benefits (Clare et al., 2010). This study compared a group of people with mild dementia who received eight sessions of goal-oriented cognitive rehabilitation, with an 'attention' control group who received relaxation therapy and a treatment as usual group. Self-rated goal performance and satisfaction were significantly improved in the cognitive rehabilitation group following intervention compared with the other two groups, and attention, memory, quality of life and mood were also better in the cognitive rehabilitation group. Following this, a larger scale study is being conducted (Clare et al., 2013).

13.4 A person-centred approach to cognitive interventions

This section will introduce some of the different dialogues that have dominated dementia care, and informed today's conceptualisation of a *person-centred* approach. It is now accepted that it is important to take a person-centred approach to the care and support provided to people with dementia (Department of Health, 2009). Therefore, cognitive interventions should strive to be person-centred in nature, and not focus on neurological impairments in isolation from other factors that influence the lived experience of the person.

The biopsychosocial approach to healthcare is the precursor to the development of person-centred care. A seminal paper by Engel (1977) made a clear and convincing case for treating an individual with any health condition within the full biological, psychological and social context of their life. This was subsequently applied to the treatment of people with dementia, and contrasted with the predominant approach of the time, which was very much embedded in a medicalised model. The biomedical model focuses on the treatment of the neurological symptoms of dementia in isolation to other factors. While it is recognised that people with dementia have difficulties related to memory, language and orientation in time and place, these do, of course, vary from one person to another and over time. A purely medical model can struggle to account for these variations in experience; given the disease process may not vary greatly across individuals.

Where the biomedical model of dementia focuses on changes to the brain alone, the biopsychosocial model recognises that biological changes interact with psychological and social factors. Biological factors also include health related issues: a person with dementia is no less likely than anyone else in their age group to experience, for example, pain related to arthritis, cardio-vascular disease or problems with sight and hearing. Recognising biological factors is critical for supporting the well-being of people with dementia. For example, people with dementia may need, but not receive, appropriate analgesia if their 'aggression' is viewed as a symptom of dementia when it is caused by an alternative condition.

The psychological component relates to the factors associated with the mind and emotions of the person with dementia, such as personality and sense of self. The social component encompasses aspects of the person's lived experience, which are significantly influenced by the broader social context, including relationships, and external environment, including cultural, historical, economic and political factors. There are overlaps and interconnections between all three dimensions of the biopsychosocial approach, and some of the important aspects of the experience of people with dementia still do not sit easily within any of these categories.

One of the proponents of person-centred care for people with dementia was Tom Kitwood. Kitwood contrasted the person-centred approach with the biomedical model, and argued that psychological and social factors make a significant contribution to the experience and presentation of dementia. Kitwood (1993) explained his theory of dementia using the following 'equation': $D = P + B + H + NI + SP$. In this equation, D – the presentation of dementia in any one person – is influenced by P – Personality; B – Biography, or life history; H – Health (including other physical or mental health problems, sensory deficits, etc); NI – Neurological impairment (the extent of difficulty with memory and other cognitive skills); and SP – Social psychology (the extent to which the social environment meets, or fails to meet, the person's needs).

Person-centred cognitive interventions therefore need to take account of all of these factors, meaning that a thorough assessment of people's needs is therefore required before embarking on an intervention (see the section below). Addressing people's needs in the context of the biopsychosocial framework is consistent with taking a holistic approach that addresses the physical health, psychological and social needs of an individual. Most cognitive interventions will aim to slow down neurological symptoms of changes, impacting on the biological level. In addition, cognitive rehabilitation paradigms may introduce goals aimed at enhancing activity or understanding about its importance, also acting on the biological level. At the psychological level, cognitive interventions might address recent changes in personality and behaviour, anxiety and depression, catastrophic reactions, and coping and defensive mechanisms. Interventions may, to different extents, also have a social component to address issues associated with isolation, lack of social contact or lack of meaningful social engagement.

13.5 Selecting an appropriate cognitive intervention

In this section, we draw together the information about evidence-informed approaches to improving cognitive functioning in dementia with the tenets of person-centred approaches to suggest how to apply knowledge in the human context of living with dementia. As we have seen above, albeit still limited, there is a growing body of evidence about how different aspects of cognition, such as autobiographical memory, prospective memory and metamemory work, are affected by dementia; and there is also evidence that each of the 'big three' approaches to cognitive intervention can have positive benefits for people with dementia. Cognitive training is most likely to have discrete effects on the domains that are the focus of practice, cognitive stimulation has a wider impact across cognition possibly through reducing excess disability and improving confidence, and cognitive rehabilitation is suited to addressing specific difficulties in everyday living through its tailored use of restorative and compensatory strategies based on refined understanding of everyday memory.

Deciding which approach might be helpful for a particular person with dementia involves undertaking a holistic assessment. This needs to include careful assessment of the nature of the difficulties arising from the dementia from the perspective of the person as well as others who are closely involved. We need to consider the context and environment in which the person lives, their cognitive and social resources, their awareness of their problems and their ways of coping with them, i.e., we need to take a biopsychosocial approach. Broad discussion of the needs of the person with dementia, which considers the impact of dementia on life in general, is essential, and much preferable over a narrow assessment of level of dementia or of cognitive functioning per se. A biopsychosocial assessment would normally begin with a semi-structured interview(s) with the person themselves, as well as any close relative(s) who are also affected by the dementia, and would then be supplemented by further behavioural, cognitive or biomedical tests as necessary. Where dementia is advanced and it is hard for the person to communicate their needs verbally, then observation rather than conversation will take a more central place. In this context, an approach such as Dementia Care Mapping can be used (Brooker, 2005). A person-centred, biopsychosocial formulation can then inform the prioritisation of needs and the best approach to employ to address them. Some of the key aspects are briefly outlined below.

13.5.1   Cognitive functioning

The need for cognitive intervention depends on the way cognitive impairment is affecting the person's day-to-day life. This sounds simple but necessitates development of a reflective, informed consideration of the interplay between cognitive functions and everyday activity in the life of the person with dementia. It means that the clinician conducting cognitive assessment should be guided by motivation in relation to intervention rather than intellectual curiosity or a disengaged wish to provide comprehensive information.

Despite these caveats, in-depth cognitive assessment, based on knowledge of information processing, is invaluable in outlining areas of impaired and conserved functioning. This informs areas that could be a focus of intervention and strategies that may be successfully implemented. The assessment needs to go beyond simple cognitive screening to test functioning in a more sophisticated way in each relevant cognitive domain. Exploration of memory, for example, should include assessment of long-term and working memory, retrospective, prospective and meta-memory, consideration of visual and orally presented material, learning across trials in addition to single trial assessment, and free and cued recall as well as recognition. Where possible, standardised tests should be used but need to be chosen with the overall level of dementia in mind. Detailed discussion of selection of tests is beyond the scope of this chapter (see Lezak, Howieson, Bigler, & Tranel, 2012).

Many people with dementia find standardised testing of cognitive functioning uncomfortable, so a clear explanation and justification needs to be presented to the person with dementia and their consent needs to be gained. Attention must be paid to rapport and motivation, with breaks if the person becomes fatigued or discouraged, and time needs to be given to de-briefing and explanation of the outcomes.

13.5.2   Relational considerations and resources

It is widely acknowledged both that dementia affects not only the individual but also the family, and that family members are hugely instrumental in supporting relatives with dementia in the community. In considering cognitive approaches, service providers therefore should consider carers' needs in their own right, and not only think about them as a helpful resource to assist the person with dementia.

Carer stress is quite widespread and multi-determined. It may be associated with changes in the balance of the relationship related to responsibility (e.g., for household finances) or extra work (e.g., extra washing), frustration about the impact of memory problems (e.g., repetitive questions), tiredness (e.g., from interrupted sleep), worry (e.g., the person with dementia being at risk) or loneliness (e.g., change in the relationship). Primary sources of stress are often related to issues with a cognitive dimension that could be a focus of cognitive intervention. Where using a cognitive rehabilitation approach, it will be important to consider the carer's priorities in balance with those of the person with dementia.

Where a core dyad is involved, typically spouses, but also sometimes parent and adult-child, a relational perspective is helpful in prompting exploration of whether there is convergence or divergence between understanding, priorities and goals. Providing care in the context of a wider and longer-term relationship means that long established patterns of interaction and perceptions influence reactions to the changes brought about by dementia. Some couples may work constructively together to face dementia, whereas others may 'work apart' or may come to diverge over time (Keady & Nolan, 2003). Where there are differences, it may be that preliminary steps need to be taken before cognitive interventions can be used, to assist person-centred understanding of dementia and to generate some optimism that the approach is worth trying.

Cognitive rehabilitation is usually carried out in the domestic setting and has to be supported by others in the household to be successful. If compensatory adaptations are to be made – for example, labelling kitchen cupboard doors to assist with finding items – then the carer needs to understand and agree to this approach. If restorative approaches are used, then a carer is often key in prompting the person with dementia to put strategies in place, and might be closely involved in assisting with fading cues, or spaced rehearsal. Cognitive training is more often a solitary activity, so could be carried out without assistance, although where a person with dementia needs a prompt to do training, it is helpful to have understanding and commitment also from the carer. Cognitive stimulation, on the other hand, is usually carried out in a service setting and so could give a stressed carer some time to themselves, while also allowing the person with dementia to combat excess disability. This approach may therefore be possible even when differences in perspective exist between carer and the person with dementia.

People with more advanced dementia may be living in care home settings where the context is of communal living and care is provided by care assistant staff. In these settings and with greater levels of cognitive impairment, interventions will need to be differently applied. Some key considerations would be: adapting cognitive stimulation to the levels of functioning (e.g., appealing to emotional memories triggered through the senses), and focusing on compensatory and environmental strategies.

13.5.3   Awareness and coping

Aside from the profile and relational issues, levels of awareness and usual coping strategies of the person with dementia also need to be taken into account in considering cognitive interventions. Awareness is a complex construct. It is influenced by neuro-degeneration but also by the social milieu and the individual's psychology, and is undoubtedly altered in dementia. Awareness is not global but related to its object, and it occurs at different levels, from the explicit, which can often be voiced, to the implicit, which is shown in behaviour (Agnew & Morris, 1998). Early in dementia, there is varying awareness between individuals in how well they seem to recognise changes in their cognition. It may be that someone does not show a high level of reflective meta-awareness, but is aware of online difficulties in memory: for example, as they carry out a task. Not only are there individual differences in awareness but there may also be differences associated with the type of dementia. Those with behavioural variant fronto-temporal dementia, for example, may be less likely to have rounded awareness (Eslinger et al., 2005), yet those with semantic dementia may be acutely aware of their expressive difficulties (Gorno-Tempini et al., 2011).

Explicit strategies involving behavioural goals for the person with dementia are far easier to implement if a person is aware of their cognitive problems and prepared to tackle them in a problem-focused way, than if they have less full awareness and/or prefer to cope by using emotion-focused strategies. Where awareness is limited, it may still be possible to put cognitive stimulation in place, as its social medium may still be acceptable to the person. Similarly, environmental adaptations or passive compensatory strategies can still be implemented and may provide benefit where explicit and active cognitive rehabilitation cannot be employed.

Awareness is a phenomenon that includes automatic and unconscious processes as well as conscious ones, and it forms the backdrop to coping. Coping, in psychological parlance, usually refers to the efforts, both cognitive and behavioural, a person makes to respond in a situation where there are demands that exceed their usual resources (Lazarus & Folkman, 1984). Like awareness, coping occurs in reference to its object; thus, someone with dementia may be coping with memory problems, or coping with changes in a relationship. An individual can be seen as having a coping repertoire that may be narrow or broad, and rigid or flexible. There is, not surprisingly, some research that indicates that flexibility is important to adaptation. Although individual coping differs from one situation ('object') to another, individuals often have a general coping style, which can be characterised as approach (or problem-solving) or avoidant (or emotion-focused). Approach coping tends to be pro-active and involves the person trying to find ways of stopping the source of the stress, either behaviourally (e.g., finding a way not to get lost, or finding a strategy to re-learn forgotten names) or cognitively (e.g., blaming embarrassment on the dementia rather than the self), whereas an avoidant coping strategy tends to be less direct and does not tackle the source (e.g., ceasing to go out so as not to have the stress of getting lost; or turning to alcohol or relaxation tapes to overcome the embarrassment of forgetting someone's name). Studies of coping with a diagnosis of dementia have found these broad styles are echoed in the way a person responds to the diagnosis (Clare, 2003), with some accommodating the diagnosis into their sense of self (self-adjusting) and others fending it off (self-maintaining), and that both problem-focused and avoidant coping are demonstrated through the actions of people with mild to moderate dementia when they are confronted by their memory problems (Oyebode, Motala, Hardy, & Oliver, 2009).

The three approaches to cognitive intervention would seem to fit differently with different coping styles. Cognitive training might appeal to a person who has a problem-focused approach where they like to feel they have mastery and control over a situation; and similarly, cognitive rehabilitation might also better suit someone who has a problem-focused approach; whereas cognitive stimulation might be amenable to those with approach or avoidant styles.

13.6   Summary

In summary, there are a range of cognitive-based interventions designed to enhance the everyday function of people with different types of dementia. However, in order for the intervention to succeed, it is essential that a person-centred approach is taken to assessing the suitability and implementation of the intervention. Person-centred approaches are known to best support the well-being of people with dementia. The development of person-centred cognitive-based interventions is in line with national and international policy, in a landscape where pharmaceutical interventions for people with dementia are limited.

References

Addis, D. R., & Tippett, L. J. (2004). Memory of myself: Autobiographical memory and identity in Alzheimer's disease. *Memory, 12*, 56–74.

Agnew, S. K., & Morris, R. G. (1998). The heterogeneity of anosognosia for memory impairment in Alzheimer's disease. *Aging and Mental Health, 2*, 7–19.

Baddeley, A. D. (2004). The psychology of memory. In A. D. Baddeley, M.D. Kopelman, & B.A. Wilson (Eds.), *The Essential Handbook of Memory Disorders for Clinicians*. London: John Wiley & Sons, Ltd.

Bahar-Fuchs, A., Clare, L., & Woods, B. (2013). Cognitive training and cognitive rehabilitation for mild to moderate Alzheimer's disease and vascular dementia. *Cochrane Database of Systematic Reviews, 6*, CD003260.

Banaji, M.R., & Crowder, R.G. (1989). The bankruptcy of everyday memory. *American Psychologist, 44*, 1185–1193.

Bernhardt, T., Maurer, K., & Froelich, L. (2002). Influence of a memory training program on attention and memory performance of patients with dementia. *Zeitschrift fuer Gerontologie und Geriatrie, 35*, 32–38.

Bird, M. (2001). Behavioural difficulties and cued recall of adaptive behaviour in dementia: Experimental and clinical evidence. *Neuropsychological Rehabilitation, 11*, 357–375.

Birks, J., & Harvey, R. J. (2006). Donepezil for dementia due to Alzheimer's disease. *Cochrane Database of Systematic Reviews*, CD001190.

Brooker, D. (2005). Dementia Care Mapping: A review of the research literature. *The Gerontologist, 45*, 11–18.

Bruce, D. (1985). The how and why of ecological memory. *Journal of Experimental Psychology-General, 114*, 78–90.

Bunce, D. (2003). Cognitive support at encoding attenuates age differences in recollective experience among adults of lower frontal lobe function. *Neuropsychology, 17*, 353–361.

Cermak, L.S., & O'Connor, M. (1983). The anterograde and retrograde retrieval ability of a patient with amnesia due to encephalitis. *Neuropsychologia, 21*, 213–234.

Clare, L. (2003). Managing threats to self: Awareness in early stage Alzheimer's disease. *Social Science and Medicine, 57*, 1017–1029.

Clare, L. (2004). Assessment and intervention in dementia of Alzheimer type. In A. D. Baddeley, B. A. Wilson, & M. Kopelman (Eds.), *The Essential Handbook of Memory Disorders for Clinicians* (pp. 255–283). London: Wiley.

Clare, L. (2008). *Neuropsychological Rehabilitation and People with Dementia*. Hove: Psychology Press.

Clare, L., Bayer, A., Burns, A., Corbett, A., Jones, R., Knapp, M., . . . Whitaker, R. (2013). Goal-oriented cognitive rehabilitation in early-stage dementia: Study protocol for a multi-centre single-blind randomised controlled trial (GREAT). *Trials, 14*.

Clare, L., Linden D. E. J., Woods, R. T., Whitaker, R., Evans, S. J., Parkinson, C. H., . . . Rugg, M. D. (2010). Goal-oriented cognitive rehabilitation for people with early-stage Alzheimer disease: A single-blind randomized controlled trial of clinical efficacy. *American Journal of Geriatric Psychiatry, 18*, 928–939.

Clare, L., Wilson, B. A., Breen, K., & Hodges, J. R. (1999). Errorless learning of face-name associations in early Alzheimer's disease. *Neurocase, 5*, 37–46.

Conway, M.A., & Pleydell-Pearce, C.W. (2000). The construction of autobiographical memories in the self-memory system. *Psychological Review, 107*, 261–288.

Craik, F.I.M. (1986). A functional account of age differences in memory. In H.H.F. Kilx (Ed.), *Human Memory and Cognitive Capabilities*. North Holland: Elsevier.

Crovitz, H.F., & Daniel, W.F. (1984). Measurements of everyday memory – toward the prevention of forgetting. *Bulletin of the Psychonomic Society, 22*, 413–414.

Davis, R. N., Massman, P. J., & Doody, R. S. (2001). Cognitive intervention in Alzheimer disease: A randomized placebo-controlled study. *Alzheimer Disease and Associated Disorders, 15*, 1–9.

Department of Health. (2009). *Living Well with Dementia: A national dementia strategy*. London: Department of Health.

Dunlosky, J., & Connor, L.T. (1997). Age differences in the allocation of study time account for age differences in memory performance. *Memory and Cognition, 25,* 691–700.

D'Ydewalle, G., Bouckaert, D., & Brunfaut, E. (2001). Age-related differences and complexity of ongoing activities in time- and event-based prospective memory. *American Journal of Psychology, 114,* 411–423.

Einstein, G.O., & McDaniel, M.A. (1990). Normal aging and prospective memory. *Journal of Experimental Psychology-Learning Memory and Cognition, 16,* 717–726.

Einstein, G.O., Richardson, S.L., Guynn, M.J., Cunfer, A.R., & McDaniel, M.A. (1995). Aging and prospective memory – examining the influences of self-initiated retrieval-processes. *Journal of Experimental Psychology-Learning Memory and Cognition, 21,* 996–1007.

Engel, G. L. (1977). The need for a new medical model: A challenge for biomedicine. *Science 196,* 129.

Eslinger, P. J., Dennis., K., Moore, P., Antoni, S. S., Hauck, R., & Grossman, M. (2005). Metacognitive deficits in frontotemporal dementia. *Journal of Neurology, Neurosurgery and Psychiatry, 76,* 1630–1635.

Fernández-Ballesteros, R., Zamarron, M. D., Tarraga, L., Moya, R., & Iniguez, J. (2003). Cognitive plasticity in healthy, mild cognitive impairment (MCI) subjects and Alzheimer's Disease patients: A research project in Spain. *European Psychologist, 8,* 148–159.

Folstein, M., Folstein, S. E., & McHugh, P. R. (1975). "Mini-mental state": A practical method for grading the cognitive state of patients for the clinician. *Journal of Psychiatric Research, 12,* 189–198.

Gatz, M., Fiske, A., Fox, L., Kaskie, B., Kasl-Godley, J., & McCallum, T. (1998). Empirically Validated psychological treatments for older adults. *Journal of Mental Health and Aging, 4,* 9–46.

Gorno-Tempini, M. L., Hillis, A. E., Weintraub, S., Kertesz, A., Mendez, M., Cappa, S. F., . . . Grossman, M. (2011). Classification of primary progressive aphasia and its variants. *Neurology, 76,* 1006–1014.

Graham, K. S., & Hodges, J. R. (1997). Differentiating the roles of the hippocampal complex and the neocortex in long-term memory storage: Evidence from the study of semantic dementia and Alzheimer's disease. *Neuropsychology, 11,* 77–89.

Haxby, J.V., Gobbini, M.I., Furey, M.L., Ishai, A., Schouten, J.L., & Pietrini, P. (2001). Distributed and overlapping representations of faces and objects in ventral temporal cortex. *Science, 293,* 2425–2430.

Henry, J.D., MacLeod, M.S., Phillips, L.H., & Crawford, J.R. (2004). A meta-analytic review of prospective memory and aging. *Psychology and Aging, 19*(1), 27–39.

Hodges, J. R., & Graham, K. S. (2001). Episodic memory: Insights from semantic dementia. *Philosophical Transactions of the Royal Society B: Biological Sciences,* 356, 1423–1434

Holden, U., & Woods, R. T. (1995). *Positive Approaches in Dementia Care* (3rd edition). Edinburgh: Churchill Livingstone.

Hopper, T., Bourgeois, M., Pimental, J., Qualis, C., Hickey, E., Frymark, T., & Schooling, T. (2013). An evidence-based systematic review on cognitive interventions for individuals with dementia. *American Journal of Speech-Language Pathology, 22,* 126–145.

Jones, S., Livner, A., & Bäckman, L. (2006). Patterns of prospective and retrospective memory impairment in preclinical Alzheimer's disease. *Neuropsychology, 20,* 144–152.

Keady, J., & Nolan, M. (2003). The dynamics of dementia: Working together, working separately or working alone? In M. Nolan, U. Lundh, G. Grant, & J. Keady (Eds.), *Partnerships in Family Care: Understanding the caregiving career* (pp. 15–32). Buckingham: Open University Press.

Kitwood, T. (1993). Towards a theory of dementia care: The interpersonal process. *Ageing and Society, 13*(1), 51–56.

Kopelman, M.D., Wilson, B.A., & Baddeley, A. D. (1989). The autobiographical memory interview – a new assessment of autobiographical and personal semantic memory in amnesic patients. *Journal Of Clinical And Experimental Neuropsychology, 11*(5), 724–744.

Koriat, A., Ben-Zur, H., & Sheffer, D. (1988). Telling the same story twice – output monitoring and age. *Journal of Memory And Language, 27*(1), 23–39.

Kvavilashvili, L., & Ellis, J. (1996). Let's forget the everyday/laboratory controversy. *Behavioral and Brain Sciences, 19,* 199–200.

Lazarus, R. S., & Folkman, S. (1984). *Stress, Appraisal and Coping.* New York: Springer.

Lezak, M. D., Howieson, D. B., Bigler, E. D., & Tranel, D. (2012). *Neuropsychological Assessment* (5th edition). USA: OUP.

Loewenstein, D. A., Acevedo, A., Czaja, S. J., & Duara, R. (2004). Cognitive rehabilitation of mildly impaired Alzheimer's disease patients on cholinesterase inhibitors. *American Journal of Geriatric Psychiatry, 12,* 395–402.

Lorant-Royer, S., Munch, C., Mescle, H., & Lieury, A. (2010). Kawashima versus Super Mario! Should a game be serious in order to stimulate cognitive aptitudes? *Revue européenne de psychologie appliquee, 60*(4), 221–232.

McDaniel, M. A., & Einstein, G. O. (2007). *Prospective Memory: An overview and synthesis of an emerging field.* Thousand Oaks, CA: Sage.

National Institute for Health and Clinical Excellence (NICE). (2006). Dementia: Supporting people with dementia and their carers in health and social care. *NICE clinical guideline 42,* November. Retrieved from www.nice.org.uk/guidance/cg42

Nelson, T.O., & Narens, L. (1990). Metamemory: A theoretical framework and new findings. In G. H. Bower (Ed.), *The Psychology of Learning and Motivation: Advances in research and theory* (Vol. 26, pp. 125–174). Chicago/London: Academic Press, Inc.

Orrell, M., Aguirre, E., Spector, A., Hoare, Z., Woods, R. T., Streater, A., . . . Russell, I. (2014). Maintenance cognitive stimulation therapy for dementia: Single-blind, multicentre, pragmatic randomised controlled trial, *British Journal of Psychiatry, 204,* 454–461.

Orrell, M., Spector, A., Thorgrimsen, L., & Woods, B. (2005). A pilot study examining the effectiveness of maintenance Cognitive Stimulation Therapy (MCST) for people with dementia. *International Journal of Geriatric Psychiatry, 20,* 446–451.

Orrell, M., Yates, L. A., Burns, A., Russell, I., Woods, R. T., Hoare, Z., . . . Orgeta, V. (2012). Individual cognitive stimulation therapy for dementia (iCST): Study protocol for a randomized controlled trial. *Trials, 13,* 172. doi:10.1186/1745-6215-13-172

Owen, A. M., Hampshire, A., Grahn, J. A., Stenton, R., Dajani, S., Burns, A. S., . . . Ballard, C. G. (2010). Putting brain training to the test. *Nature, 475*(7299), 775–778.

Oyebode, J. R., Motala, J., Hardy, R., & Oliver, C. (2009). Coping with challenges to memory in people with mild to moderate Alzheimer's disease: Observation of behaviour in response to analogues of everyday situations. *Aging and Mental Health, 13,* 46–53.

Piolino, P., Desgranges, B., Belliard, S., Matuszewski, V., Laleve, C., De La Sayette, V., & Eustache, F. (2003). Autobiographical memory and autonoetic consciousness: Triple dissociation in neurodegenerative diseases. *Brain, 126,* 2203–2219.

Prull, M.W., Gabrieli, J.D.E., & Bunge, S.A. (2000). Age-related changes in memory: A cognitive neuroscience perspective. In F.I.M. Craik & T. A. Salthouse (Eds.), *The Handbook of Aging and Cognition* (2nd edition). Mahwah, NJ: Lawrence Erlbaum Associates.

Quayhagen, M. P., Quayhagen, M., Corbeil, R. R., Hendrix, R. C., Jackson, J. E., Snyder, L., & Bower, D. (2000). Coping with dementia: Evaluation of four nonpharmacologic interventions. *International Psychogeriatrics, 12*(2), 249–265

Robinson, A.E., Hertzog, C., & Dunlosky, J. (2006). Aging, encoding fluency, and metacognitive monitoring. *Aging Neuropsychology and Cognition, 13*(3–4), 458–478.

Salthouse, T. A. (2006). Mental exercise and mental aging: Evaluating the validity of the "use it or lose it" hypothesis. *Perspectives on Psychological Science, 1,* 68–87.

Smith, S. J., Souchay, C., & Conway, M. A. (2010). Over–general autobiographical memory in Parkinson's disease. *Cortex, 46*(6), 787–793.

Smith, S. J., Souchay, C., & Moulin, C. J. A. (2012). Awareness of prospective memory performance in Parkinson's. *Neuropsychology, 25*(6), 734–740.

Snowden, J., Griffiths, H., & Neary, D. (1996). Semantic-episodic memory interactions in semantic dementia: Implications for retrograde memory function. *Cognitive Neuropsychology, 13,* 1101–1137.

Souchay, C., & Isingrini, M. (2004). Age related differences in metacognitive control: Role of executive functioning. *Brain and Cognition, 56*(1), 89–99.

Spector, A., Gardner, C., & Orrell, M. (2011). The impact of Cognitive Stimulation Therapy groups on people with dementia: Views from participants, their carers and group facilitators. *Ageing & Mental Health, 15*(8), 945–949.

Spector, A., Orrell, M., & Woods, B. (2010). Cognitive Stimulation Therapy (CST): Effects on different areas of cognitive function for people with dementia. *International Journal of Geriatric Psychiatry, 25*(12), 1253–1258.

Spector, A., Thorgrimsen, L., Woods, B., Royan, L., Davies, S., Butterworth, M., & Orrell, M. (2003). Efficacy of an evidence-based cognitive stimulation therapy programme for people with dementia: Randomised controlled trial. *British Journal of Psychiatry, 183,* 248–254.

Tulving, E. (1985). Memory and consciousness. *Canadian Psychology-Psychologie Canadienne, 26*(1), 1–12.

Williams, H. L., Conway, M. A., & Cohen, G. (2008). Autobiographical memory. In G. Cohen & M. A. Conway (Eds.), *Memory in The Real World* (pp. 21–81). Hove: Psychology Press.

Wilson, B. A. (1997). Cognitive rehabilitation: How it is and how it might be. *Journal of International Neuropsychological Society, 3,* 487–496.

Woods, B., Aguirre, E., Spector, A. E., & Orrell, M. (2012). Cognitive stimulation to improve cognitive functioning in people with dementia. *Cochrane Database of Systematic Reviews,* CD005562.

Woods, B., Spector, A. E., Jones, C. A., Orrell, M., & Davies, S. P. (2005). Reminiscence therapy for dementia. *Cochrane Database of Systematic Reviews,* CD001120.

14

AUGMENTING FAMILIAR APPLIANCES TO ASSIST PEOPLE LIVING WITH DEMENTIA

Damien Renner, David Reid, Mark Barrett-Baxendale, Davide Bruno and Hissam Tawfik

14.1 Introduction

Individuals living with dementia require substantial care and are often forced to move from their home environment into facilities providing appropriate care services (O'Neill et al., 2014). Extensive care (such as medical care) impacts significantly on the economy, with projected disastrous effects on publicly funded health care services over the next quarter of a century (Helal, Chen, Kim, Bose, & Lee, 2012). Additionally, the ongoing global increase in age expectancy is leading to significant shifts in the demography of the general population, which is becoming progressively elderly. This conundrum emphasises the need for economically viable technologies that can be used to support independent living, and could substantially reduce the caring burden.

Dementia is an umbrella term for a number of progressive, irreversible and organic brain diseases currently affecting approximately 35.6 million people across the world (Aloulou et al., 2013). Depending on the type of dementia (e.g., Alzheimer's disease), different symptoms will be more prominent and emerge earlier. For instance, in the case of vascular dementia, which is the second most common type of dementia and is due to extensive vascular damage to the brain, executive dysfunction is pre-eminent (e.g., Jefferson, Gentile, & Kahlon, 2011; Rainville et al., 2002). Executive dysfunction is characterised by a disruption of high order cognitive abilities, such as attention and problem solving, and typically results in difficulties with sequencing of tasks and in performing tasks simultaneously (Orpwood, Gibbs, Adlam, Faulkner, & Meegahawatte, 2005). With many seemingly simple tasks requiring the completion of a series of subtasks in a specific order (e.g., making a cup of tea), many daily activities necessitate the ability to perform a series of higher order cognitive functions effectively. For example, *attention* is required to keep track of where one is within the sequence of tasks, *memory* is needed to remember the sequence, *problem solving* would be required if any change to the normal procedure becomes necessary, and so on. This ability is progressively impaired in people with dementia (e.g., Calderon et al., 2001), potentially leading to avoidance of activities that may become too difficult, thus spurring a vicious cycle of inactivity, fear of failure and embarrassment, loss of self-esteem and depressive feelings (Orpwood et al., 2010).

To overcome the deficits that accompany dementia, in recent years, there has been an effort to provide assistive technology to support and improve the quality of life experienced by people living with dementia. However, this effort is met with many important challenges. For instance, people with dementia have been noted to prefer familiar objects, with displays of extreme anxiety often following the introduction of novel technologies into one's home (Orpwood et al., 2005). With this in mind, the purpose of this chapter is to describe the design and prototype of a new assistive device that attempts to minimize both complexity and unfamiliarity, while providing support to the end user. This device is designed to replicate the support naturally provided by a carer via the monitoring of progress made within a specified task, and by delivering audio-based instructions where necessary. The system also attempts to be as simple as possible, removing the need to learn a new task or system.

The proposed device falls into the general category of *reminding technologies*. Reminding technology can be regarded as one of the most unobtrusive technologies for individuals with dementia. Through providing reminders at appropriate times, it offers a solution enabling users to perform daily activities independently, as they are no longer required to memorise the information and recall it at the right time (Koldrack, Luplow, Kirste, & Teipel, 2013; O'Neill et al., 2014). Additionally, research has highlighted the importance of providing cues to help an individual complete a task, thus supporting the work carried out within this chapter (Aloulou et al., 2013; Smith, 2013; Van Den Heuvel, Jowitt, & McIntyre, 2012).

14.2   Related work

Innovative technologies are rapidly emerging that offer caregivers the support and means to assist older adults with cognitive impairments, and facilitate continued living in a home environment (Mahoney et al., 2007). There are three main types of technologies currently available on the market: monitoring technology, detection technology and assistive technology. With *monitoring technology*, data about the user's status is sent to an authorised person, such as a carer, for the purposes of monitoring their current condition. The user has little to no interaction with the system. In *dementia detection systems*, the user will interact with the system (e.g., completing a questionnaire) and the results will be forwarded to the relevant professional body (e.g., a general practitioner). The professional body will analyse the results and contact the user to inform them of the findings. This type of system can be used to diagnose dementia and to track the progression of dementia (e.g., collecting monthly results and producing a correlation to show the level of deterioration). Finally, with *assistive technology*, the focus is to help the user perform daily activities. Here, a person with dementia may autonomously interact with the system via a programme of step-by-step assistance. This chapter focuses on designing an assistive technology.

A wide range of companies in recent years have developed reminder-based software that operates by prompting users to facilitate task completion. These programmes use task reminders and display the correct order of the subtasks. *MemoJog*, for example, is a mobile-based programme that allows carers to set up and deliver text-based reminders to a person they care for, and to monitor their activity. A carer records prompts that are stored on a remote server. Later, these prompts are transmitted to the mobile device, and the carer is alerted if the end user does not acknowledge a reminder. For example, a carer may set a reminder to alert the user at 6 pm to eat their meal; if the user does not acknowledge this reminder, an alert is then sent to the carer. Morrison, Szymkowiak and Gregor (2004) tested *MemoJog* for a period of 12 weeks, asking 12 participants to carry out ten specified tasks and recording their performance. The study participants were elderly individuals experiencing memory problems. The results showed that users were able to carry out more complex tasks with the aid of this system than without, showing that reminders technologies can play an important role in augmenting quality of life. However, problems were noted regarding the reliability of network coverage, battery life, sensitivity of buttons, and text size. These limitations highlight the importance of having a robust system to use with individuals with dementia (e.g., not relying on network coverage or battery powered devices), and suggests that text-based cues may not be effective due to potential age related impaired vision.

Donnelly et al. (2008) developed a mobile phone-based video streaming system that utilises everyday technology. The system targets individuals with mild dementia, and provides users with video-based reminders and prompts. This is achieved by the user's carer recording personalised messages, and then setting scheduled dates and times of delivery (e.g., a carer may record a message telling the user to eat their lunch to be displayed at 13:00). This system was piloted with 27 pairs of users/carers and has gone through several iterations and improvements. Interestingly, the handsets used by the user were modified in later versions of the product to allow for a single button being used for interaction. O'Neill, Mason and Parente (2011) conducted a study where nine participants were monitored without the system, then later with the system, and then again without the system, and observed that the system helped users organise their routine effectively; four participants stated that it was as successful as their current reminding methods/system (Mason, Craig, O'Neill, Donnelly, & Nugent, 2012). Although based on a limited sample, this study highlights that usage of multimedia-based reminders delivered via technological systems can be an effective tool to increase independence in users with mild forms of dementia.

14.3   Understanding the user to help the user

During the initial to middle stages of dementia, cognitive deficits are mainly apparent in episodic memory (memory for specific events; see also Chapter 1) and executive function (e.g., planning, sequencing and attention). Executive function processes are essential for goal-driven actions, thus impairment in this domain can have a detrimental effect on one's ability to perform everyday tasks (Wherton & Monk, 2006). Therefore, the aim of this chapter is to describe the design, development and evaluation of a proof-of-concept prototype that demonstrates the role technology can play in supporting those with impaired executive functioning. The work focuses on supporting the user with the task of making a cup of tea. This task is appropriate because at any point in the task, the individual is engaged in a subtask, while needing to maintain a sense of its position within the whole series of activities. Additionally, the task of making a cup of tea has been considered by previous research and established as a non-trivial task to use for this type of research (Mayer & Zach, 2013). Finally, the fundamental concept of task ordering demonstrated in making a cup of tea can be applied to a wide range of scenarios.

Before a prototype can be designed, it is vital to understand and make valid appraisal of all of the symptoms and resulting problems associated with dementia. After conducting an extensive literature review, we propose the following as the most important assumptions (Table 14.1).

TABLE 14.1 User assumptions

Assumption Number	Assumption	Implication
1	User has difficulties performing sequential and simultaneous tasks due to impaired working memory (Orpwood et al., 2005)	The system should provide support for the ordering of tasks being carried out
2	The user will be more competent in a familiar environment (Wherton & Monk, 2008)	The system must be flexible. For example, it must be applicable to both traditional stove kettles, and electric kettles
3	Providing cues to the user will increase their performance (Brennan, Giovannetti, Libon, Bettcher, & Duey, 2009; Vézina, Robichaud, Voyer, & Pelletier, 2011)	The system must provide cues in a timely and appropriate manner
4	The graphical user interface (GUI) is a major cause of distress when individuals with dementia attempt to use technology (Mosa, Yoo, & Sheets, 2012)	It is paramount that the system proposes an alternative to the GUI – computer vision could monitor the activities
5	People with dementia are unable to learn new tasks and may become anxious interacting with new technology (Orpwood et al., 2005)	The user must not be required to interact with the system directly (e.g., using sensors to monitor the progress instead); thus, the system will become invisible to the user

Following these directions, we describe below a system we have developed by augmenting a familiar and common home appliance, a kettle, which provides reminders to a user. The process of developing a system such as this is especially useful in that it highlights the potential issues with the development of assistive technologies for people with dementia, and suggests a number of conceptual as well as practical questions. Moreover, by modifying an existing and familiar appliance, we show that assistive technologies do not require a radical reimagining of a person's living environment, but can be implemented within habitual surroundings by operating a number of relatively small modifications. The smooth and painless insertion of a new technology within an existing environment with minimal alterations should also help overcome the general resistance to using and adopting new technological systems.

14.4   Proposed system to support independent living

This project adopted an iterative user-centred design process due to the fact that there is a well-specified end user. This required the understanding of the users' needs, of the tasks to be carried out, and of context, which contributes to a conceptual understanding of what the system should do for users and how it should be designed (Petrie & Bevan, 2009).

In principle, assistance for individuals with dementia usually follows one of two forms. First, the user could be relieved completely from a task that they regularly experience problems with if, for example, the carer completes the task for them. The second option involves providing support that accommodates for the user's impaired functions by suitable means, as, for example, providing cues where needed (see Table 14.2 for a list of processes and related cognitive functions). The second option has been regarded as more suitable due to the fact that it motivates the usage of the remaining mental resources, possibly delaying the process of deterioration (Koldrack, Luplow, Kirste, & Teipel, 2013). Therefore, assistive technologies are aimed at providing appropriate information and/or cues to the user in a timely manner. To achieve this, we must have a thorough understanding of the environment surrounding the individual, thus creating a context aware system

TABLE 14.2 Processes and functions

Action	Function
Plan making a cup of tea	Executive function and decision making
Remember the location of all the elements	Memory
Ensure that they notice the kettle has finished boiling	Attention
Add milk and sugar to the cup, at the correct point in the process	Planning

TABLE 14.3 System processes

Event	Result
A user presses a button located near the kettle	The entire process is started. An audio file will be played telling them to add water to the kettle and turn it on. This supports with the planning of making a cup of tea
Start the kettle	The sensor will monitor the temperature and play an audio file once it has boiled. The audio file will say, "now pour the water into your mug"
Pour the kettle	The sensor will monitor the accelerometer to tell when it has been poured. Once it has been poured, it will play an audio file telling the user to add milk and/or sugar, thus completing the entire process. If required, the audio instruction may outline the location of the milk and sugar
Add milk and sugar	The behaviour is not monitored by the system

(Skillen, Chen, Nugent, Donnelly, & Solheim, 2012). It was decided that for this project, the system would replicate the support naturally provided by a carer. The user is monitored during the process of making a cup of tea, while audio instructions are provided at key steps. The system utilises several sensors to monitor the user's progression, enabling the system to calculate when the user is engaged in a subtask so that instructions can be provided at the appropriate time in anticipation of the next subtask. For example, once the temperature sensor detects values greater than 98°C (boiling water), an audio file instructs the user to pour the water into a mug.

Table 14.3 shows the processes that occur within the system, highlighting the 'event' and the 'result'. If the user 'forgets' to press the button, the system will continue to provide audio instructions, while skipping the first audio file. Figure 14.1 shows all of the processes in a storyboard fashion.

Koldrack et al. (2013) argues that a system that adapts to the users' abilities may be more easily accepted rather than specialised devices, which may have to be regularly updated each stage of decline. With this in mind, the designed system is intended to be flexible in regards to the capabilities of the user. This is achieved by having the system respond to key points within the process of making a cup of tea (e.g., when the kettle has boiled is detected by the system directly). Therefore, the carer can easily adapt the audio files that are played to the user over the progression of the disease, ensuring that they are suitable for the user, without the system requiring modifications. For example, a person with a mild form of dementia may hear "now add milk and sugar into the mug", whereas a person at a more advanced stage may hear "take the milk out of the fridge and the sugar from the cupboard above the kettle; now add a small amount of milk and two teaspoons of sugar into your mug".

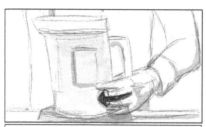

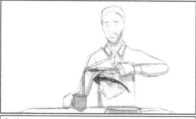

Action:	**Action:**
The user presses a button located on or near the kettle	The water inside the kettle is boiling (tracked via the temperature sensor inside the kettle)
Response:	**Response:**
The first audio file is played (e.g. 'David, make sure there is water inside the kettle before you turn it on')	The second audio file is played (e.g. 'David, pour the water into your mug')

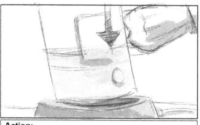

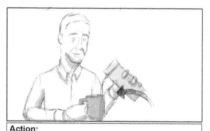

Action:	**Action:**
The kettle is returned to the dock (detected via the accelerometer)	David adds milk and sugar to his cup of tea
Response:	**Response:**
The third audio file is played (e.g. 'David, now add some milk and sugar to your mug. Enjoy your cup of tea')	This action is not monitored, thus no response is provided

FIGURE 14.1 Storyboard.

14.5 Prototype implementation and evaluation

The system developed consists of sensors, an embedded device, an audio shield and a kettle. The following parts were selected: an Arduino Uno embedded device (to perform all of the operations), an Adafruit Wave Shield (to play the audio files), a DS18B20 temperature sensor (to monitor the temperature within the kettle), an ADXL335 3 axis accelerometer (to detect when the kettle has been poured), an SD card (to store the audio files) and a speaker. The temperature sensor was placed inside the kettle, whereas the accelerometer was attached to the outside of the kettle. Figure 14.2 shows a visual diagram of the system. A video of the prototype being demonstrated can be accessed at http://youtu.be/YAUFyVJyUWo.

A carer would normally support the person living with dementia by monitoring their progress through a specific task and by providing spoken cues when needed. The system proposed here attempts to imitate monitoring by utilising sensors to track the progression made in the task and by giving audible feedback at appropriate times. It is proposed this operation should be as *natural* as possible by not

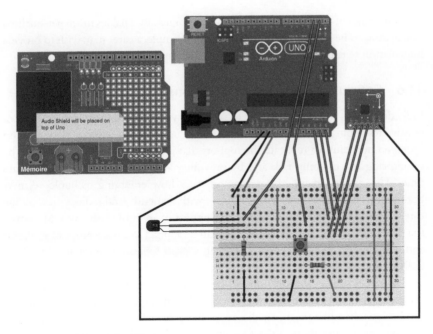

FIGURE 14.2   Schematic (this image was created with Fritzing).

explicitly requiring the user to learn how to use this new piece of equipment. As the system uses direct sensors, it is less likely that they would be affected by external environmental factors such as ambient heat or humidity. The accuracy of the timings of the audio cues is critical, as misleading information may cause confusion and distress to the user.

Research conducted by Orpwood et al. (2010) highlighted the confusion latency can cause by creating an audio player that had a small, but appreciable, delay in playing music after the 'play' button was pressed. Even small delays led to the participants pressing the button multiple times. In light of this, the system created is not only very responsive, but also filters out multiple button presses.

Specific modality is also engineered into the system. For example, when the user is tilting the kettle to fill it with water, the system will behave differently to when the kettle is tilted to pour out the water. The accelerometer only becomes active once the kettle is boiled, which increases the fault tolerance of the system and reduces the chances that misleading information is inadvertently given to the user.

The system has preloaded default audio instructions, which can be modified by the carer by replacing the files stored on the SD card. This flexibility is allowed given that whether a familiar or unfamiliar voice should be used within the system is an open question. On the one hand, if the system speaks with the carer's voice, the user may become confused since the carer is not physically present; on the other hand, using the carer's voice might be preferable due to its familiarity. It is also possible that different solutions may be preferable for different people, or at different stages of the disease. The system's flexibility also enables more personalised instructions to be stored on the system, as, for example, a carer may wish to provide information regarding the location of a specific item.

14.6   Conclusions and future directions

Individuals with dementia struggle to utilise new devices. Therefore, the design of assistive technology needs to consider carefully user interface aspects. The solution proposed here aims to replicate the support that is naturally provided by a carer by monitoring the ongoing task and by providing audio instructions at appropriate times. The system described here demonstrates how emerging technologies may both promote independent living for those with dementia, and reduce stress on the carer by providing additional and natural support in an unobtrusive way. Moreover, the fundamental concepts in this chapter can be applied to a wide range of scenarios and tasks, which could potentially result in a *smart home* environment, suitable for individuals with dementia.

The rather bulky (and off-putting) electronics currently used in the prototype can easily be incorporated onto a single chip design (e.g., Tinyduino and Femtoduino devices). In addition, the small sizes of these devices open up the possibility of including them directly into the 13-amp plug itself. Furthermore, existing electric kettle manufacturers can implement this system into their kettles with very little changes to the design due to the fact that a kettle already has the necessary sensors to detect when water is boiling, and when it has been returned to the dock.

There is very little research conducted into systems for supporting an individual with dementia that do not require users to interact directly with the technology, and most systems use graphical user interfaces (GUI), which may be too unfamiliar for people with emerging memory problems and dementia. With this in mind, we propose that future assistive technology designers should look into autonomous and ubiquitous systems, and the roles these systems can play in supporting individuals with cognitive impairments. Current research has highlighted the level of stress caused to users with dementia by having difficulties in attempting to control a system, either by manipulating a physical device or using a GUI. Using systems that do not require learning how to interact with the technology, as in our example, could overcome this problem. However, it should also be noted that if care is not taken, it is possible to design automatic, autonomous, ubiquitous systems that relinquish control from the user and frustrate and confuse them.

References

Aloulou, H., Mokhtari, M., Tiberghien, T., Biswas, J., Phua, C., Kenneth Lin, J.H., & Yap, P. (2013). Deployment of assistive living technology in a nursing home environment: Methods and lessons learned. *BMC Medical Informatics and Decision Making, 13*, 42–42.

Brennan, L., Giovannetti, T., Libon, D.J., Bettcher, B.M., & Duey, K. (2009). The impact of goal cues on everyday action performance in dementia. *Neuropsychological Rehabilitation, 19*, 562–582.

Calderon, J., Perry, R.J., Erzinclioglu, S.W., Berrios, G.E., Dening, T.R., & Hodges, J.R. (2001). Perception, attention, and working memory are disproportionately impaired in dementia with lewy bodies compared with Alzheimer's disease. *Journal of Neurology, Neurosurgery, and Psychiatry, 70,* 157–164.

Donnelly, M.P., Donnelly, M.P., Nugent, C.D., Nugent, C.D., Craig, D., Craig, D., & Mulvenna, M. (2008). Development of a cell phone-based video streaming system for persons with early stage Alzheimer's disease. Paper presented at the *30th Annual International Conference of the IEEE Engineering in Medicine and Biology Society,* 5330–5333.

Fasola, J., & Mataric, M.J. (2009). Robot motivator: Improving user performance on a physical/mental task. Paper presented at the 4th ACM/IEEE International Conference on Human-Robot Interaction (HRI), 295–296.

Helal, S., Chen, C., Kim, E., Bose, R., & Lee, C. (2012). Toward an ecosystem for developing and programming assistive environments. *Proceedings of the IEEE, 100,* 2489–2504.

Jefferson, A.L., Gentile, A. M., & Kahlon, R. (2011). Vascular Dementia. In A. E. Budson & N. W. Kowall (Eds.), *The Handbook of Alzheimer's Disease and Other Dementias.* Oxford, UK: Wiley-Blackwell. doi:10.1002/9781444344110.ch2

Knapp, M., Prince, M., Albanese, E., Banerjee, S., Dhanasiri, S., & Fernandez-Plotza, J.-L. (2007). Dementia UK – the full report. *Alzheimer's Society,* IX–X.

Koldrack, P., Luplow, M., Kirste, T., & Teipel, S. (2013). Cognitive assistance to support social integration in Alzheimer's disease. *Geriatric Mental Health Care, 1,* 39–45.

Mahoney, D., Purtilo, R., Webbe, F., Alwan, M., Bharucha, A., Adlam, T., . . . Becker, S. (2007). In-home monitoring of persons with dementia: Ethical guidelines for technology research and development. *Alzheimer's & Dementia, 3,* 217–226.

Mason, S., Craig, D., O'Neill, S., Donnelly, M., & Nugent, C. (2012). Electronic reminding technology for cognitive impairment. *British Journal of Nursing, 21,* 855–861.

Mayer, J., & Zach, J. (2013). Lessons learned from participatory design with and for people with dementia. Proceedings of the *15th international conference on Human-computer interaction with mobile devices and services,* 540–545. doi:10.1145/2493190.2494436

Morrison, K., Szymkowiak, A., & Gregor, P. (2004). Memojog – An Interactive Memory Aid Incorporating Mobile Based Technologies. *Mobile Human-Computer Interaction – Mobile-HCI 2004,* 481–485.

Mosa, A.S.M., Yoo, I., & Sheets, L. (2012). A systematic review of healthcare applications for smartphones. *BMC Medical Informatics and Decision Making, 12,* 67.

O'Neill, S.A., Mason, S., & Parente, G. (2011). Video Reminders as Cognitive Prosthetics for People with Dementia. *Ageing International, 36,* 267–282.

O'Neill, S.A., McClean, S.I., Donnelly, M.D., Nugent, C.D., Galway, L., Cleland, I., . . . Craig, D. (2014). Development of a technology adoption and usage prediction tool for assistive technology for people with dementia. *Interacting with Computers, 26,* 169–176.

Orpwood, R., Chadd, J., Howcroft, D., Sixsmith, A., Torrington, J., Gibson, G., & Chalfont, G. (2010). Designing technolgy to improve quality of life for people with dementia: User-led approaches. *Universal Access in the Information Society, 9,* 249–259.

Orpwood, R., Gibbs, C., Adlam, T., Faulkner, R., & Meegahawatte, D. (2005). The design of smart homes for people with dementia – user-interface aspects. *Universal Access in the Information Society, 4,* 156–164.

Petrie, H., & Bevan, N. (2009). The evaluation of accessibility, usability and user experience. In C. Stephanidis (Ed.), *The Universal Access Handbook.* London: Taylor & Francis.

Rainville, C., Amieva, H., Lafont, S., Dartigues, J., Orgogozo, J., & Fabrigoule, C. (2002). Executive function deficits in patients with dementia of the Alzheimer's type: A study with a Tower of London task. *Archives of Clinical Neuropsychology: The Official Journal of the National Academy of Neuropsychologists, 17,* 513–530.

Skillen, K., Chen, L., Nugent, C.D., Donnelly, M.P., & Solheim, I. (2012). A user profile ontology based approach for assisting people with dementia in mobile environments. Proceedings of the *2012 Annual International Conference of the IEEE*, 6390–6393.

Slegers, K., Wilkinson, A., & Hendriks, N. (2013). Active collaboration in healthcare design: Participatory design to develop a dementia care app. *CHI '13 Extended Abstracts on Human Factors in Computing Systems*, 475–480.

Smith, G.E. (2013). Everyday technologies across the continuum of dementia care. Proceedings of the *Annual International Conference of the IEEE*, 7040–7043.

Van Den Heuvel, E., Jowitt, F., & McIntyre, A. (2012). Awareness, requirements and barriers to use of assistive technology designed to enable independence of people suffering from dementia (ATD). *Technology and Disability, 24*(2), 139–148.

Vézina, A., Robichaud, L., Voyer, P., & Pelletier, D. (2011). Identity cues and dementia in nursing home intervention. *Work, 40,* 5–14.

Wherton, J. P., & Monk, A. F. (2006). Designing cognitive supports for dementia. *ACM SIGACCESS Accessibility and Computing*, 28–31.

Wherton, J.P., & Monk, A.F. (2008). Technological opportunities for supporting people with dementia who are living at home. *International Journal of Human–Computer Studies, 66,* 571–586.

INDEX

Information in tables and figures is indicated by page numbers in *italics*.